AF782328

EMERGENCY PSYCHIATRY

EMERGENCY PSYCHIATRY

DOUGLAS A. RUND, M.D., F.A.C.E.P.
Associate Professor and Director,
Division of Emergency Medicine,
Department of Preventive Medicine,
The Ohio State University,
Columbus, Ohio

JEFFERY C. HUTZLER, M.D.
Assistant Professor and Chief, Consultation-
Liaison Service, Department of Psychiatry,
The Ohio State University,
Columbus, Ohio

with 37 *illustrations*

The C. V. Mosby Company

ST. LOUIS TORONTO 1983

MOSBY

A TRADITION OF PUBLISHING EXCELLENCE

Editor: Julia Allen Jacobs
Assistant editor: Catherine H. Converse
Manuscript editor: Selena V. Bussen
Design: Jeanne Bush
Production: Jeanne A. Gulledge, Barbara Merritt

Copyright © 1983 by The C.V. Mosby Company

All rights reserved. No part of this publication may be reproduced, stored in a retrieval system, or transmitted, in any form or by any means, electronic, mechanical, photocopying, recording, or otherwise, without prior written permission from the publisher.

Printed in the United States of America

The C.V. Mosby Company
11830 Westline Industrial Drive, St. Louis, Missouri 63146

Library of Congress Cataloging in Publication Data

Rund, Douglas A.
Emergency psychiatry.

Bibliography: p.
Includes index.
1. Psychiatric emergencies. I. Hutzler, Jeffery C.
II. Title.
RC480.6.R86 1984 616.89'025 82-25885
ISBN 0-8016-4216-7

C/VH/VH 9 8 7 6 5 4 3 2 1 02/B/214

To my parents

Carl and Caroline

D.A.R.

In loving memory of

Nadine W. Hutzler

1910-1983

J.C.H.

PREFACE

The purpose of this book is to enable the emergency physician to understand and deal effectively with patients who have psychiatric disorders. It is our firm conviction that recognition and management of psychiatric disorders in the emergency patient need not be inordinately difficult. The diagnosis of psychiatric disorders has been made far more straightforward with the American Psychiatric Association's adoption of clear clinical criteria for psychiatric illness in the 1980 version of the *Diagnostic and Statistical Manual of Mental Disorders* (third edition), the DSM-III. Relatively simple treatment regimens can be remarkably effective when applied in the proper circumstance.

The initial emphasis of the text is that of determining which mental and behavorial disorders are organic and which are not. The differentiation between these two categories of disorders is of major importance in determining the direction of further assessment and treatment and can usually be accomplished rather easily in the emergency department.

The next emphasis is to clarify psychoses, affective disorders, and personality disorders. These classifications of disease are often avoided by physicians who have in the past been confused, if not bewildered, by conflicting terminology, various "schools" of psychiatric thought, and imprecise diagnostic criteria for these clinical conditions.

The text also deals with several common problems in the emergency department from a psychiatric perspective: patient-defined emergencies; the violent or combative patient; psychiatric emergencies associated with death, suicide, anxiety syndromes, panic attacks, or somatoform disorders; and the patient who signs out or refuses treatment. The text concerns itself with therapeutic techniques, including both interpersonal and pharmaceutical therapy for psychiatric illness.

Our objective is to make emergency physicians as comfortable and adept with psychiatric disorders as they are with medical or surgical disorders and to ultimately improve the care of the psychiatrically impaired patient in the emergency department.

We are indebted to those who helped to make this book possible. Christine Dailey, Jacqueline Parris, Pamela McDougall, and Pam Furney created superior manuscript from our handwritten versions. Cathy Converse of The C.V. Mosby Company kept us amply supplied with professional advice and continuing encouragement. Catherine Khoury, Gerald Chever, Jim O'Harra, Debra Slusher, and William Lanier provided invaluable assistance in preparing our illustrations, and special thanks go to an incomparable Gary Smith for his facile display of mood and movement. Martin D. Keller,

Lee Jansen, and the American Red Cross furnished additional photographic material from their collections; Steve Moon rendered line drawings with his characteristic style; Ed Whitehead provided invaluable assistance in our library searches; Dr. Charles Whitfield helped us greatly in our thinking and in our presentation of alcohol syndromes; and Steven R. Schneir created a fine preliminary draft of Chapter 21.

Finally, we are indebted to our families who tolerated our preoccupation with this text during the long months of its preparation.

Douglas A. Rund
Jeffery C. Hutzler

CONTENTS

EMERGENCY PSYCHIATRY

1 EMERGENCY PSYCHIATRY
the medical model

Psychiatric illness is remarkably common in patients who seek care in emergency departments. Psychiatric problems constitute the primary reason for 10% of the patients visiting one urban hospital.[1] The prevalence of active psychiatric illness in emergency patients seeking care for *any* reason was as high as 38% in a fairly recent study using standardized research criteria for psychiatric diagnoses.[2] This represents an enormous group of patients to be evaluated by emergency physicians.

The psychiatric disorder may not be apparent from the patient's chief complaint, and the immediate clinical problem may seem unrelated to an underlying psychiatric disorder. By contrast, the psychiatric condition may be so florid that it outshines all others, disrupting normal functioning of the department and the composure of the staff. Such conditions demand attention, and the emergency physician must act immediately to bring both the patient and the situation under control.

Some conditions are far more common than others. Substance abuse, depression, anxiety, and acute situational reactions are huge social and medical problems that appear regularly and predictably in emergency practice.

The emergency physician and psychiatrist are now able to collaborate on both the clinical management and investigation of these disorders far more easily than in the past because their respective disciplines are progressing. Emergency medicine is moving to identify and explore its clinical content; psychiatry is moving toward the medical model.

Both the science of psychiatry and the discipline of emergency medicine are on pathways that allow the development of a skillful and compassionate approach to the problem of the "psychiatric patient" in the emergency department (Fig. 1-1). To fully appreciate the developments that make this approach possible, we can briefly review the evolution of each specialty.

PSYCHIATRY: HIPPOCRATES TO DSM-III
Origins

The science of psychiatry is rooted in ancient observations of disordered behavior and thought. Hippocrates wrote of madness, delirium, and "fears and terrors (which) assail us, some by night and some by day. . . All these things we endure from the brain when it is not healthy."[3] This early viewpoint was a precursor of the "medical

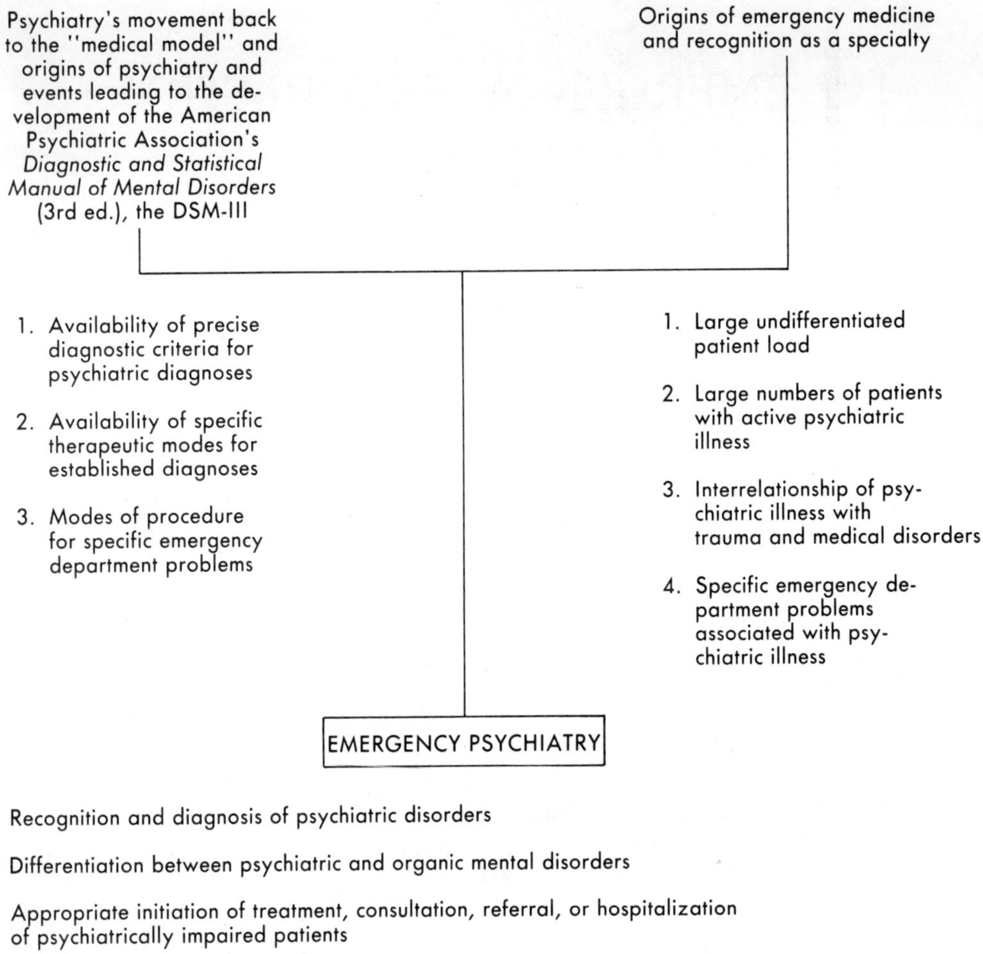

Fig. 1-1. Development of emergency psychiatry made possible by application of major advances in both psychiatry and emergency medicine.

model'' concepts of psychiatry, which are most prevalent today; that psychiatric illness is similar to other types of medical illness. Psychiatric conditions can be evaluated rationally, can be defined according to their clinical characteristics, and can be treated with therapies that are indicated for a given diagnosis.

Dichotomy of mind and body

Plato is given historical credit for establishing the notion that mind and body, *psyche* and *soma,* were separate entities. The dichotomy of mind and body continued as the dominant concept through the middle ages and was fostered by religious scholars who viewed the human soul as separate and distinct from the human body.

After many centuries we once again view the individual as a whole. Biochemical processes that affect the body affect the mind, and disorders of thinking, behavior, and emotions certainly affect the body. This holistic concept builds bridges of understanding between the medical practitioner and the psychiatrist, and it forms a foundation that allows the emergency physician to understand current concepts of psychiatric illness.

The medical model presented emphasizes medical (organic) causes of abnormal thought and behavior. We recognize that biochemical and perhaps structural abnormalities of brain tissue produce syndromes of abnormal thought and behavior. In some syndromes (like schizophrenia) underlying pathology is not fully understood; antipsychotic drug therapy of the disease controls the symptoms (hallucinations, delusions) just as drug therapy for certain medical conditions controls the symptoms of pain or fever.

Clinical psychiatry

The clinical discipline of psychiatry emerged gradually in the eighteenth and nineteenth centuries and was intermittently influenced in one direction or another by individual theories, terminologies, and therapeutic methods. The impact of Freud, for instance, profoundly influenced psychiatry in the late nineteenth and early twentieth centuries.

Various Freudian theories that explained abnormal thought and behavior on the basis of "delayed oral gratification stage" or "inadequate development of superego" were barely comprehensible for practicing physicians. For many, these theories created mystery instead of understanding and resembled more an art form or a philosophical system than science or useful medical knowledge.

Psychiatry was finally recognized as a specialty in the United States in 1934 with the establishment of the American Board of Psychiatry and Neurology.[4] Since that time, psychiatry has moved deliberately into the medical realm. Becoming firmly established as a "medical" discipline, psychiatry has sharpened and refined its clinical science.

DSM-III

The American Psychiatric Association first adopted standardized nomenclature for psychiatric diagnoses in 1952. The publication of this nomenclature in the *Diagnostic and Statistical Manual of Mental Disorders,* (1st ed.)[4] provided the practicing psychiatrist and medical community with a set of established diagnoses. Ideally, patients given a specific diagnosis had certain clinical characteristics specific for that diagnosis. Communication could flow among all physicians about diagnosis, effects of therapy, and patient prognosis.

In 1968 a second edition, the DSM-II,[5] was published with a set of revised terminology. The need for even more precise diagnostic criteria and terminology for psychiatric illness remained, however. Feighner and his colleagues took constructive steps to formulate explicit criteria for psychiatric diagnoses that allowed reproducible psychiatric research and meaningful clinical communication especially between the psychiatrist and nonpsychiatrist.[6] They identified 14 psychiatric diagnoses with precise diagnostic criteria; most of the data needed for the diagnosis could be obtained at the bedside. The illnesses identified in this early work were the following: primary affective disorders (depression and mania), secondary affective disorders, schizophrenia, anxiety neuroses, obsessive compulsive neurosis, phobic neuroses, hysteria, antisocial personality, alcoholism, drug dependence, mental retardation, organic brain syndrome, homosexuality, and transsexualism. The potential advantage of the emergency physician having precise terminology and clear-cut criteria for psychiatric illness was enormous. Physicians could now make clinical psychiatric diagnoses based on specific clinical criteria. Psychiatrists had developed the roots of a diagnostic nomenclature, which was as specific, or even more specific, than many other medical specialties.

The work of Feighner emphasized standardized terminology and clear criteria for psychiatric diagnoses. The collection of one cluster of symptoms and signs comprised one diagnosis, whereas a different cluster defined a different diagnosis. With increasing experience the psychiatric community further crystallized its diagnostic thought. The result was the latest edition of the *Diagnostic and Statistical Manual of Mental Disorders,*[7] published in 1980. Commonly abbreviated as the DSM-III, the *Diagnostic and Statistical Manual* is available from the American Psychiatric Association, Washington, D.C., both as a full-sized textbook and as a pocket-sized reference with the essential diagnostic criteria for terminology and code numbers for psychiatric illnesses. It also has easy-to-understand flowcharts (or decision trees) to enhance rapid, bedside diagnosis.

EMERGENCY MEDICINE

Origins

The science of emergency medicine, in one respect, has its historical roots in the most primitive attempts to deal with acute injury, illness, and life-threatening events. The development of emergency medicine as a formal discipline, however, has a far more recent beginning. The enormous growth of emergency medicine in the last 20 years has been largely the result of changing societal behavior, changing social demands, and technological improvements in the immediate management of life-threatening conditions.

The economic basis for the increase in the number of hospital-based emergency physicians is the tremendous increase in the volume of patients seeking care in the emergency department. In 1958 the nation's hospitals reported 18 million emergency patient visits. In 1968 the number reported was 44 million,[8] and by 1977 the number had risen to 76 million[9] annual patient visits. The reason for the increase included a general societal drift away from stable relationships with providers of essential services, decreasing relative numbers and availability of general practioners and primary care physicians, and third-party payment policies that reimburse the fees incurred for hospital emergency services but not for office-based medical care.

The lack of availability of primary physicians has been most acute in inner-city communities and rural areas, and although the coming increase in physician supply may improve many problems of physician availability, the importance of emergency medicine is not likely to diminish. The medical community and the public fully expect competent emergency physicians to be available at all times to provide initial management of acute medical, surgical, and psychiatric conditions in the hospital emergency department.

The proportion of patients with life-threatening illnesses in most emergency departments is no more than 5% to 10%, compared to 15% to 20% for those with illnesses and injuries that make hospitalization necessary. The most salient characteristic of emergency patients is that they often arrive in large numbers and have illnesses that run the gamut from the most minor to the most serious.

The early leaders in academic emergency medicine were originally from the discipline of surgery.[10] Therefore it was reasonable that an emphasis on the immediate management of trauma was felt early in the development of emergency medicine. Since the first automobile accident in 1899, the incidence of trauma had grown to become the leading cause of death in persons under 30 years of age, which also made the emphasis on early trauma management a reasonable expectation.

As the overall content of emergency practice is fully elaborated, however, conditions like psychiatric illness and substance abuse continue to surface as major problems. Many of the current leaders in emergency medicine are nonsurgeons or graduates of a residency program in emergency medicine. As they try to understand the problems that arise in their clinical practice, psychiatric conditions stand out as major dilemmas.

Specialty status

The American Board of Emergency Medicine was approved in 1979, and the scientific underpinnings of the discipline continue to emerge. In creating a new body of knowledge and a unique mode of clinical practice specific for emergency medicine, it has been necessary initially to draw heavily from established disciplines and create mutual approaches to shared clinical problems. Psychological disorders are specifically identified as an integral part of the Emergency Medicine Core Content.[11] Continued collaborative analysis of psychiatric problems in the emergency setting will undoubtedly be fruitful, and the general movement of psychiatry toward the medical fold facilitates such cooperation. It is with this collaborative approach in mind that we have written this text.

EMERGENCY PSYCHIATRY

The management of patients with abnormal behavior or thought processes in the emergency department is bound to be influenced by the setting. The pace is fast. The patient problem may be complex and often extremely serious. The pressure to make rapid decisions with minimal data is ever present and insistent, yet the physician must be able to evaluate each patient quickly and succinctly without significant loss of accuracy. Similarly, treatment and disposition must be accomplished in a concise fashion with reasonable certainty that the treatment will be effective and almost absolute certainty that the treatment will do no harm. Our presentation of emergency psychiatry must then be relevant and applicable in the emergency setting. Some therapies involve medication, and some involve active listening and crisis intervention. These latter therapies are techniques that can be accomplished by a physician or a nonphysician.

The treatment of these patients is similarly influenced by the attitudes of the entire emergency staff. It is not secret that physicians, nurses, and clerical staff seem to dislike the confrontation with psychiatric patients. The disturbing behavior of such patients bothers us, and we often blame them as if they purposefully try to disrupt our emergency schedule. Some of the distaste for dealing with psychiatric patients can, in our opinion, be decreased with increasing knowledge by providing the emergency physician and team with effective diagnostic tools, straightforward management approaches to psychiatric illness, and perhaps most importantly of all, an understanding of the patient and his disease.

Our thesis is perhaps controversial. We feel that the emergency physician should be just as capable of initiating proper early therapy in psychiatric disorders as in those of the cardiovascular system. Similarly, just as the treatment of some cardiovascular disorders require consultation with a cardiologist and hospitalization, certain psychiatric illnesses are complex and time consuming; the physician should be able to recognize these disorders and seek the appropriate psychiatric consultation, psychiatric referral, or hospitalization for the patient.

Throughout this text certain fundamental principles of emergency psychiatric care are emphasized. The following are three of the principles of emergency psychiatric care.

1. Immediate stabilization of the patient and the situation is usually the physician's first management priority.
2. Recognition of medical conditions that cause the abnormal thought or behavior should be an early responsibility of the emergency physician.
3. Psychiatric consultation and/or mandatory hospitalization may be the only logical conclusion of the emergency physician's encounters with these patients.

Stabilization

Certain emergency situations require immediate stabilization. The violent patient must be brought under control immediately for the protection of everyone involved. Early restraint of such patients requires adequate manpower and proper techniques. The concept of stabilization applies to other psychiatric emergencies as well. Such emergencies may include a suicide attempt, a substance abuser, or a psychotic patient. The concept of stabilization is critically important in the practice of emergency medicine, since this is an environment where things happen quickly and unexpectedly. Throughout this text, the concept of early stabilization is applied to specific patients, situations, and problems that seem to involve psychiatric disorders.

Medical conditions

Certain abnormalities of thought and behavior are caused by medical conditions, obvious physical alterations in brain tissue, or abnormalities in brain function as a result of exogenous or endogenous substances. When abnormal thought or behavior is caused by such conditions, the disorder is labeled *organic*. Such abnormalities of thought or behavior are called *organic mental disorders*. The specific mental disorder created by a "medical" condition is labeled according to its presumed cause. Examples of organic mental disorders include *hypertensive* encephalopathy, *hepatic* encephalopathy, *drug* intoxication, *alcohol* intoxication, and *alcohol* withdrawal.

Medical conditions that commonly cause abnormalities of thought and behavior are often missed by the medical doctor because of the rush to get the psychiatric patient *out* of the emergency department and *into* the hands of a psychiatrist. It is estimated that up to 30% of patients referred to psychiatrists have medical disorders that cause "psychiatric" symptoms. Paradoxically it is the psychiatrist who then must evaluate the patient to discover the responsible "medical" pathology.

For the emergency physician, the consideration of organic mental disorder must be paramount in the approach to the psychiatric patient. Some of these medical disorders may be life-threatening, and the only early clue to their presence may be bizarre behavior, hallucinations, or "crazy" speech. Some of the life-threatening conditions include meningitis, encephalitis, poisoning, hypoxia, or hypoglycemia.

In this text two broad categories of illness are considered. The terms *organic* and *functional* are used. Organic, as mentioned previously, refers to disorders that have underlying medical or structural pathology. Functional disorders are those for which the medical, structural, or chemical cause is unknown and for which the ultimate treatment is often within the province of the psychiatrist. These "functional" disorders include schizophrenia, generalized anxiety disorders, and personality disorders. When there is no underlying medical cause, the affective disorders (depression and mania) are also considered to be in the functional category. Some functional disorders respond to psychotherapy and/or psychoactive medications. Both of these broad classes of therapy constitute some of the special skills of the psychiatrist. The principles and limited application of these therapies can be learned by the emergency physician.

Consultation and hospitalization

Questions that frequently arise in the emergency care of the psychiatric patient (and one that invariably arises at 3 o'clock AM) are where to obtain immediate psychiatric consultation and where to hospitalize the patient, even against his will.

The general answer is that consultation is called for if there is doubt and that hospitalization is necessary if there is a danger of harm coming to the patient or others if he is not hospitalized. More specific recommendations with guidelines for consultation and hospitalization are presented as particular disorders are considered.

SUMMARY

Throughout this text we deliberately use the terminology and diagnostic criteria of the DSM-III. It is our firm belief that this allows the emergency physician to begin the study of emergency psychiatry at "square one." The terminology is current and new, explicit and concise, and, in our opinion, it enables the emergency physician to be an accurate psychiatric diagnostician.

Though we recognize that the DSM-III is not accepted by everyone and will undoubtedly be revised again in the future, it does provide a starting point for collobora-tion. It offers a common vocabulary and a common conceptual framework for understanding psychiatric illness. In our opinion, it forms an excellent basis for the presentation of emergency psychiatry.

REFERENCES

1. Krome, RL, Wilson, RF, and Walt, AJ. The organization of the modern emergency department. In Walt, AJ, and Wilson, RF, *Management of trauma: pitfalls and practice*. Philadelphia: Lea & Febiger, 1975.
2. Summers, WK, Rund, DA, and Levin, ML. Psychiatric illness in a general urban emergency room: daytime versus nighttime population. *Journal of Clinical Psychiatry,* 1979, *40*(8), 340-343.
3. Mora, G. Hippocrates, the sacred disease in historical and theoretical trends in psychiatry. In Freedman, AM, Kaplan, HI, and Sadock, BJ, *Comprehensive textbook of psychiatry* (3rd ed.). Baltimore: The Williams & Wilkins, Co., 1980.
4. American Psychiatric Association. *Diagnostic and statistical manual of mental disorders* (1st ed.). Washington, D.C.: The Association, 1952.
5. American Psychiatric Association. *Diagnostic and statistical manual of mental disorders* (2nd ed.). Washington, D.C.: The Association, 1968.
6. Feighner, JP, et al. Diagnostic criteria for use in psychiatric research. *Archives of General Psychiatry,* Jan. 1972, *26,* 57-63.
7. American Psychiatric Association. *Diagnostic and statistical manual of mental disorders* (3rd ed.). Washington, D.C.: The Association, 1980.
8. George, JE. Emergency re-entry to health care. *Hospital Topics,* Oct. 1969, *47,* 69-74.
9. American Hospital Association. *Hospital statistics* (1977 ed.) Chicago: The Association, 1977.
10. Mattox, KL. Reflections on "turf" and "young turks." *Annals of Emergency Medicine,* Jan. 1980, *9*(1), 69-70.
11. American College of Emergency Physicians. Emergency medicine core content. *Journal of American College of Emergency Physicians,* Jan. 1979, *8*(1), 39.

2 APPROACH TO THE PATIENT

The patient with grossly abnormal behavior or thought is easily recognized by virtually everyone involved in his care. The patient's first words to the emergency staff may sound the alarm: "The underground psyches keep coming out and biting me," or "The radios are telling me to kill myself."

Alternatively, the circumstances of the patient's police arrest or the summoning of an ambulance may provide the obvious clues: "He was standing on the corner with his pants down shouting at everyone," or "She was found unconscious with several empty pill bottles and a suicide note near her bedside."

When the abnormal behavior is not so obviously deviant and the disorder of thinking is subtle, the patient may enter the emergency department with a variety of midleading, obscure, or nonspecific complaints, including the notorious "sick all over" complaint frequently associated with an affective disorder (like major depression). A history of trauma or a complaint primarily related to injury is frequently related to alcoholism, substance abuse, or antisocial personality disorder.

The stages in the management of psychiatric patients in the emergency department are as follows:

- Recognition of abnormal behavior or thought
- Stabilization of the patient and the setting
- Alertness for medical emergencies
- Interview
- Physical examination
  - Vital signs
  - Head and neck
  - Further examination as needed and/or tolerated by the patient
- Testing
- Consultation if needed
- Admission or discharge

It cannot be emphasized too strongly that patient stabilization and the search for an organic mental disorder are fundamental skills for the emergency physician.

STABILIZATION

As in the management of any medical disorder, the first priority in the emergency management of psychiatric disorders is the stabilization of the patient and the situation.

Stabilization requires that steps are taken immediately to protect the patient and the staff from further harm. It also prevents anticipated problems by gathering the necessary treatment resources ahead of time.

For instance, in the case of the truly violent patient, hospital security, police, or strong hospital orderlies provide a show of force and should be summoned immediately to restrain the patient quickly and effectively. Attempts by a single physician or nurse to "talk the patient down" or to gently restrain him are fraught with great hazard and generally threaten the psychotic patient who is, in fact, afraid of his uncontrollable impulses. On the other hand, stabilization of the suicidal patient requires both medical treatment for the overdose or injury and constant observation by the staff to assure that the attempt is not repeated in the emergency department.

ALERTNESS FOR MEDICAL EMERGENCIES

Certain medical emergencies cause psychosis. Hypoglycemia, meningitis, hypertensive encephalopathy, or drug overdose may actually be the emergency that requires immediate medical treatment. The clinician must remain alert to the possibility of organic causes of psychosis or mental disturbance throughout the patient's management. This important topic is discussed in greater detail in the following chapter.

INTERVIEW

The interview is really the heart of the psychiatric assessment. Since the disorders are those of thought content, thought process, and behavior, there can be no substitute for listening carefully to what the patient says. The techniques of conducting a successful interview are as much a craft and skill as are the techniques used in suturing lacerations or in reducing dislocations, and they take no longer. The skill of interviewing requires paying attention to certain fundamental principles and allowing a given period of time. The realities of emergency practice are often less than ideal for the interview. Unscheduled interruptions, time limitations, and the justifiable priority given to life-threatening conditions are routine in emergency practice (Fig. 2-1). The discussion of the interview is presented in the context of realities of everyday practice.

Purpose of the interview

The psychiatric interview has the following three goals: (1) to establish a positive physician-patient relationship, (2) to elicit information about the patient's condition, and (3) to permit observation of the patient's behavior.[1,2]

Establishment of a positive relationship is of great importance during both the evaluation and the treatment phases of the patient's management. The physician should try to create a rapport or communication that ideally allows cooperative and harmonious interaction between the patient and physician. The gathering of information about the patient involves two very essential components: listening to him and asking carefully thought out questions that should yield responses leading to an accurate diagnosis.

The final purpose of the interview is extremely important for psychiatric diagnosis. The observation of the patient's behavior may be among the most important clues to the

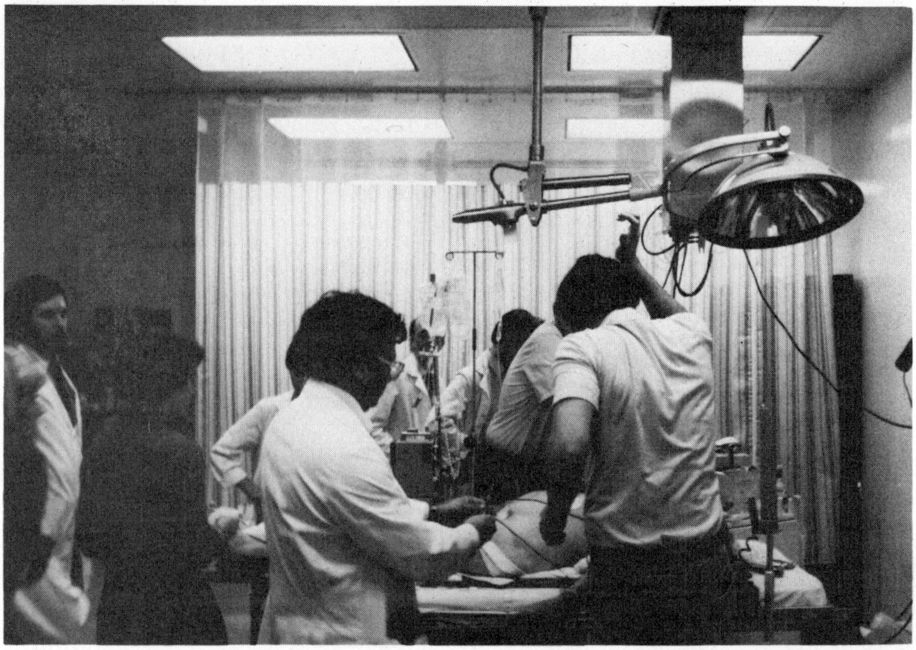

FIG. 2-1. The realities of emergency medicine often are not ideal for a calm psychiatric assessment. It may be difficult for the inexperienced physician to complete a cardiac resuscitation and move immediately to a comfortably seated interview with a psychiatric patient. With purpose and practice, however, such skills can be mastered.

diagnosis. The patient may move and talk very slowly (suggesting substance abuse or major depression), stop speaking in midsentence, listen to auditory hallunications, or fidget and move about continuously (suggesting mania). Accurate observation of this behavior usually requires that the physician be in the "listening mode" rather than the "talking mode."

Requirements for a successful interview

Time. The interview cannot take an inordinate amount of time in the emergency department. Very few emergency practices allow over 15 minutes for an interview. Most do allow, however, 3 to 10 minutes of uninterrupted interview time. Although this is possibly the most important concept in interviewing, it is probably the most difficult for the emergency physician to practice. The successful interview requires that the physician take at least some period of time, predetermined perhaps before the interview, and listen to the patient. This time spent initially is far more valuable than an interview obtained while the physician dashes in and out of the patient's cubicle, asks a few questions, darts away again, and returns, appearing hurried, harassed, or angry. Though these emotions may reflect the day-to-day reality of emergency practice, a successful interview requires that they be replaced by an appearance of calm and sympathetic understanding. The calm attitude also sets the tone for the rest of the emergency department staff and saves time later.

Privacy. The setting of the interview should be one that allows the patient to feel a sense of privacy. The emergency department is hardly secluded and quiet. A great deal can be accomplished, however, by drawing the curtains around the patient's cubicle to provide as much "psychological privacy" as possible. If an individual room is available, however, this affords even more privacy.

Whenever possible emergency department personnel should not interrupt the interview for the first 3 to 5 minutes. All the people involved in discussing the patient's chief complaint (nurses, medical students, social workers, or psychologists) should be present during the first few minutes of the interview. They should remain throughout the interview or wait until the conclusion for an introduction.

Anyone attending the interview, including the physician, should not be distracted with other duties, such as leafing through charts, answering telephones, or shifting around in the examining area. Ideally, all the personnel involved in the interview should be seated comfortably. This imparts a sense of calm, receptive listening. Attempts to provide an atmosphere compatible with the establishment of good rapport inevitably save time later in the patient's managment. With a more effective communication style, the patient gives better information initially, and this prevents unnecessary tests or repeat evaluations subsequently.

Phases of the interview

It is helpful to think of the interview as having the following three phases:

Phase I

A. Introductions

B. Chief complaint and present problem

   1. Open-ended, undirected, unhurried explanation by the patient of his major problem; physician response should be understanding, calm, and nonjudgmental
   2. Observation of patient behavior and general appearance

Phase II

A. Probing, specific questions leading to diagnosis if needed (e.g., responses for diagnosis of major depression according to the DSM-III diagnostic criteria)

B. Mental status examination

Phase III

A. Brief summary statement by physician

B. Concise statement of tests to be performed and reason for testing

Each phase has a distinct purpose and specific techniques that are effective. In the beginning the interview is calm and open ended; the ideal response mode is the "understanding" response. In the middle phase the interviewer requires specific information; the response mode may be the "probing" response. In the final stage a summary is made to the patient about the interview, and the plans for further evaluation are

FIVE TYPES OF RESPONSES THAT CAN BE GIVEN BY A HEALTH CARE PROFESSIONAL IN AN INTERVIEW

Understanding response

Emphasis on the patient's feelings or point of view indicates that the professional cares about how the patient feels rather than the factual content of his concerns.

EXAMPLE Patient: I'm worried that I will lose my job if I have to stay in the hospital.
Interviewer: You seem to feel anxious about staying in the hospital.

Hostile response

A hostile response antagonizes or humiliates the patient. It reflects the professional's anger and implies or states that the patient's feelings are inappropriate.

EXAMPLE Patient: I'm worried that I will lose my job if I if I have to stay in the hospital.
Interviewer: I wouldn't recommend hospitalization unless you needed it. Stay or go, it's your choice!

Probing response

A questioning response that implies that the patient must give more information so that the interviewer can provide an answer or solution to the problem.

EXAMPLE Patient: I'm worried that I will lose my job if I have to stay in the hospital.
Interviewer: What kind of work do you do?

Evaluative response

A judgment is made about the patient's feelings, and the professional implies or openly states how the patient *should* feel and what he *should* do.

EXAMPLE Patient: I'm worried that I will lose my job if I have to stay in the hospital.
Interviewer: You can probably get another job fairly easily with your education and work experience.

Reassuring response

A reassuring response, in effect, denies that the patient has a problem and reassures him that he need not feel as if he does.

EXAMPLE Patient: I'm worried that I will lose my job if I have to stay in the hospital.
Interviewer: Don't worry about that at all; you probably have some sick leave coming. We'll take care of everything with your employer.

Adapted from Bernstein, L, and Bernstein, RS. *Interviewing—a guide for health professionals*. New York: Appleton-Century-Crofts, 1980.

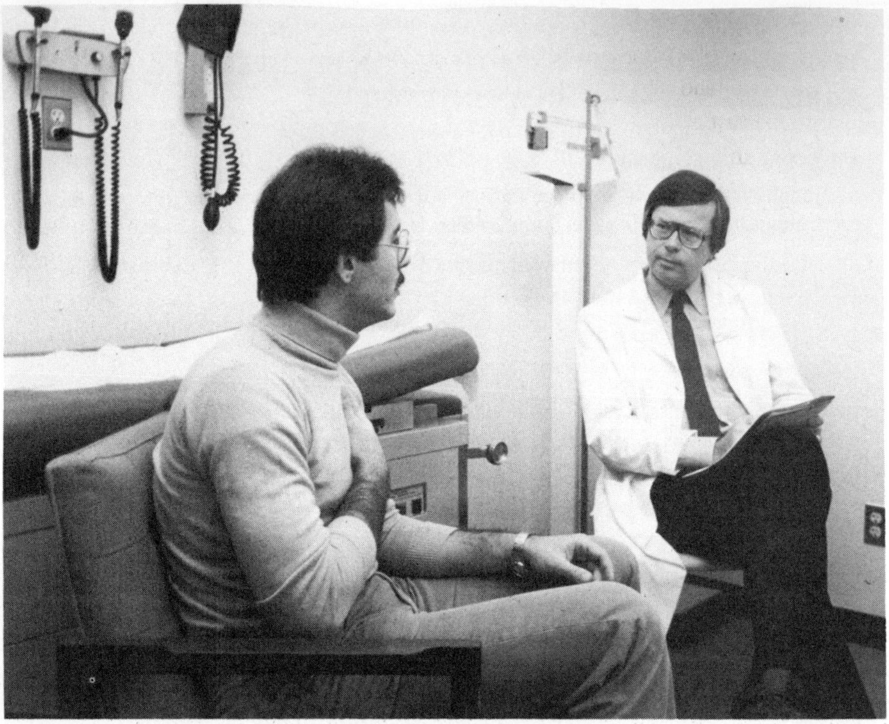

FIG. 2-2. In the ideal interview situation both physician and patient are seated comfortably, and interruptions are minimized.

outlined; the responses may be "evaluative" or "understanding." These response modes are outlined in the box on p. 13 and discussed later in this chapter.

Beginning the interview—phase I. The physician should enter the emergency department in a brisk but unhurried manner, be seated, and come to rest before beginning the interview. The physician who searches for a pen, paper, chart, or begins to examine the patient before establishing some rapport gives the signs of hurriedness and distraction. This may cause the patient to feel increasingly anxious or panicked; he may feel that he is not being listened to carefully. Chatting briefly with the patient as an opening to the interview is helpful, but should be quite brief. The patient generally expects the physician to "get down to business" with meaningful questions. If the patient is seated, the doctor should also be seated (Fig. 2-2). If the patient is lying on a cart, it may be helpful for the physician to sit beside the cart so that his head is at the same level or slightly above the level of the patient's head. This avoids the rather overwhelming situation of having someone tower over the patient. The towering posture does not lend itself to open and trusting conversation.

An organized interview requires that time be taken to elicit the patient's chief complaint and the history of the present problem. Usually the physician can allow a certain time limit to get this very important initial information and to establish a sense of calm communication with the patient. Three to 5 minutes is adequate in most cases.

The initial interview primarily involves the physician listening and the patient talking. An attentive and open technique is helpful. The technique of nodding and maintaining eye contact with the patient can be easily learned. Since the physician is often actually tired, angry, or stressed, it is helpful to consciously practice these techniques until they are habitual, just as are certain styles of auscultation.

Body language. The patient's movement and posture generally reveal important information about physical and psychological health. The hostile patient with arms akimbo, legs set wide apart, and eyes staring boldly, ready for a confrontation or the depressed patient with slow movement, slow speech, "sighing respiration," and head bowed forward illustrate highly informative portraits.

The interviewer has the opportunity to enhance communication with body language. Ideally the interviewer should be seated leaning slightly forward in a receptive "open" position. Nodding and maintaining a body posture similar to that of the patient suggests sympathy and a willingness to listen. If the patient leans forward, the interviewer leans forward; if the patient reaches out, the physician can respond by holding the patient's hand. Too much physical contact or "laying on of hands," however, may be damaging and threatening early in the interview.

The "talkative" patient. A garrulous or overly verbose patient can prolong an interview unnecessarily. The interviewer should interrupt such a patient at a relatively appropriate point and tell him that he appears quite anxious and is giving the physician more information than he can use at the moment. This avoids a hostile response and helps to structure the rest of the interview and to provide time to ask questions and receive short replies. The interviewer who conveys a sense of irritation, or constantly interrupts in a hostile or provoked way, makes the patient more anxious and may actually increase his verbosity. Most people who are talking "too much" are anxious; the less anxiety they feel, the less they will "babble."

Searching for a diagnosis—phase II. The middle part of the interview is a period of information gathering that should lead toward a specific diagnosis. The questioning may progress from general to more specific queries. If time permits, it is helpful to ask a question and allow the patient to develop his own story at his own pace with gentle guidance by the interviewer. If too many questions are asked in rapid sequence without providing an interval for an answer, the patient can easily become confused. During this middle phase of the interview, the physician may want to ask questions that satisfy the precise criteria for a specific diagnosis.

If depression is suspected, the interviewer asks about appetite, sleep habits, guilt, and other specific questions for the diagnosis of major depression. If the suspected condition is schizophrenia, the interviewer inquires about the patient's early days, school experience, previous psychiatric treatments and hospitalization, and any specific delusions or hallucinations the patient volunteers.

Summary and plans—phase III. The end of the interview should include a brief summary statement from the physician and a clear and consise statement about the investigations that are needed for the patient's further evaluation. The explanation of tests and their purpose reduces the patient's anxiety. Any procedures that are going to be ordered should be explained briefly and carefully in straightforward, easily understandable terms. The patient can be asked if he has any questions about the procedures.

Interviewer responses

Verbal responses. The type of response by the interviewer to the feelings expressed by the patient determine the ease with which information can be elicited throughout the interview. Five types of verbal response have been identified by Bernstein and Bernstein[2] and are presented in the boxed material listed earlier. The responses fall into five categories: understanding, hostile, probing, evaluative, and reassuring.

Understanding response. The understanding response permits the patient to clarify his feelings. The response indicates that the professional is interested in the patient's feelings, or point of view, and communicates this interest to the patient. The emphasis of the professional must be on how the patient *feels* rather than the factual content of his concerns.

The understanding response is nearly always appropriate in the early, open-ended part of the interview. This response reinforces the patient's feeling of trust, establishes a satisfactory physician-patient relationship, creates rapport, and increases the patient's participation in the interview. Once the interviewer identifies the patient's feelings, not the content of what is said, the interviewer can reflect these feelings back to the patient.

If the patient, for instance, complains about the long wait in the emergency department, the callous nurses, and the questionable competence of the physicians, the interviewer should identify the feeling as one of anger, or perhaps frustration. The proper understanding response *then reflects this feeling, not the specific content of the thought.* The interviewer correctly answers, for example, "I gather that you're feeling pretty angry right now." This allows the patient to elaborate, to vent emotion, and perhaps to explain his feelings.

Hostile response. A hostile response antagonizes or humiliates the patient. It reflects the professional's anger and implies or states that the patient's feelings are inappropriate. When the patient complains about the long wait, for instance, the hostile response may be, "Well, why don't you just go to another hospital if this is so bad!" Although the hostile response is a rather natural reaction to such anger, it is counterproductive and should be avoided by the interviewer who wants to obtain more information.

Probing response. The probing response implies that the patient must give more information so that the interviewer can provide an answer or solution to the problem. It may simply involve asking a question for more specific information. Probing responses to the patient who feels depressed and "bad all over," for instance, would be, "How are you sleeping," and "How is your appetite?"

The probing response is often required in phase II of the interview. The examiner has a general idea of the nature of the patient's disorder, but needs responses to specific questions to fulfill the criteria required to make a particular diagnosis. Specific questions about sleep patterns, appetite, guilt, and ability to concentrate complete the DSM-III screening for suspected depression.

Evaluative response. An evaluative response is one in which the interviewer makes a judgment about the patient's feelings; the professional implies or openly states how the patient *should* feel and what he should do.

The patient who has guilty feelings about something, for instance, may be told by the interviewer that "guilt is a natural reaction and you should have some guilt or you wouldn't be normal." Or the advice may be the opposite: "Guilt isn't healthy for you, wipe it out of you mind and try to never feel guilty about these things again."

The evaluative response has some usefulness in day-to-day conversation and certain types of physician-patient communication, but it is of limited help in gaining information during the interview. It provides a summary value judgment and does not probe for the patient's feelings.

Reassuring response. A reassuring response, in effect, denies that the patient has a problem. It reassures the patient that he does not have a problem or that he need not feel as bad as he does. The patient who complains about the long wait could be reassured by statements like the following: "Don't worry; waits like this are common. This is our normal routine. We take the sickest patients first . . . so cheer up and be glad you're not that sick. We'll take you as soon as we can." The reassuring response, intended to soothe and comfort the patient, essentially denies the problem and thus cuts off the continued flow of information from the patient about his feelings.

Nonverbal responses. Nonverbal responses can certainly convey a great deal of information to the patient during the interview. If the interviewer appears bored, angry, or excessively hurried, the patient will be reluctant to lay out his deepest concerns. With some practice, the interviewer should be able to adopt an open, receptive posture and a facial expression reflecting concern and interest. Practice is important in developing these nonverbal skills because they may be needed at a time when the emergency physician actually feels overwhelmed by fatigue or by concerns about the urgent problems of other patients. As with the verbal responses, adoption of nonverbal techniques and mannerisms that communicate understanding and receptiveness ultimately results in the most effective evaluation of patients with psychiatric disorders.

SUMMARY

An effective approach to the psychiatric patient in the emergency department can be as easily learned as any other patient care skill. It requires attention to certain basic principles of patient management, like stabilization; a constant vigilance for underlying medical conditions causing the behavioral or thought abnormality; a skillful interview; and a concern for the patient that leads to immediate treatment, consultation, hospitalization, or discharge with appropriate follow-up arrangements.

REFERENCES

1. Sheppe, WM, Jr., and Stevenson, I. Techniques of interviewing. In Leif, HI, Leif, FU, and Leif, NR (Eds.), *The psychological basis of medical practice*. New York: Praeger Publishers, Inc., 1980.
2. Bernstein, L, and Bernstein, RS. *Interviewing: a guide for health professionals (3rd ed.)*. New York: Appleton-Century-Crofts, 1980.

3 ORGANIC MENTAL DISORDERS

Organic mental disorders are mental conditions characteristically resulting from diffuse impairment of brain tissue function from any cause.[1] Organic disorders are perhaps most easily thought of as mental disorders caused by various medical conditions, gross or histological pathological changes of the central nervous system, poisoning, illness, injuries, and infections. They are thus distinguished in clinical practice from functional (or idiopathic) disorders. Functional disorders are considered to be primarily psychiatric in nature and not the result of diffuse dysfunction of brain tissue. The distinction between the two may someday blur as more is learned about cellular and biochemical abnormalities in psychiatric disease. For now, however, the distinction is clinically useful. The distinction affects the choice of treatment, the estimation of prognosis, and the need for medical and psychiatric treatment. As is later discussed, organic disorders have definite clinical components that allow the physician to distinguish them from functional disorders. These clinical components usually include the history of the problem, physical findings, and laboratory data that can be obtained in the emergency department.

When evaluating a psychiatric patient in the emergency department, one of the most important questions regarding the patient's illness is, "Could this behavior be the result of an organic cause?" The ability to distinguish organic from functional disorders is a critically important skill for emergency physicians. Organic mental disorders, particularly those associated with drugs and alcohol, are important causes of behavioral and thought disturbances in emergency patients; some organic disorders initially showing signs and symptoms of psychosis such as poisoning, meningitis, and hypoxia may be life-threatening. Causes of organic mental disorders that may be found in emergency patients are listed with an indication of the frequency of occurrence.

1. Alcohol
   a. Intoxication
   b. Withdrawal
2. Drug associated
   a. Intoxication
   b. Side effects
3. Poisoning

4. Seizure or postictal confusion
5. Endocrine disorders (primary hypoglycemia)
6. Circulatory failure
7. Hypoxia
8. Infection
    a. Meningitis
    b. Encephalitis
    c. Sepsis
9. Head trauma
10. Cerebral hemorrhage
11. Tumor
12. Disturbance of growth
13. Disturbance of nutrition
14. Chronic dementia of unknown cause
15. Hepatic failure
16. Renal failure
17. Hypertensive encephalopathy

Other organic disorders may be overlooked entirely as the emergency physician focuses on the more highly visible abnormal thought or behavior. It has been reported that there is a major organic component in a large percentage of patients referred from emergency departments to psychiatrists. Many of the patients referred to psychiatrists by other physicians or hospitalized on a psychiatry ward have undiagnosed physical disorders.[4] For many of these patients, the physical disorder contributed significantly to the severity of the psychiatric symptoms.[3,4]

The discussion presented here focuses on clinical recognition of the more common organic mental disorders seen in emergency practice and on a limited consideration of their treatment.

CLINICAL FEATURES

When an emergency physician sees a patient demonstrating odd behavior or telling an odd story, a high level of suspicion that these behavioral abnormalities are the result of an organic cause must be maintained. Among the clinical features of organic mental disorders that generally distinguish them from psychiatric (functional or idiopathic) disorders are the following characteristics:

History

1. Recent or abrupt onset of the disorder with no previous history of psychiatric illness, treatment, or personality problems
2. Psychosis in patients over 40 years of age with no previous psychiatric illness
3. Incontinence of stool or urine
4. Recent hospitalization
5. Medications (name, dose, duration, reason for prescription)
6. Alcohol abuse
7. Drug use

Physical examination

1. Abnormal vital signs
2. Diaphoresis
3. Nystagmus
4. Abnormal mental status

Physicians have a well-recognized reluctance to examine psychiatric patients. Emergency physicians generally like to transfer these patients to the care of a psychiatrist as rapidly as possible, and psychiatrists may be reluctant to extensively examine their patients because of emotional attitudes that may be generated in patient and therapist (transference and countertransference) or because they feel their patients have few relevant physical findings.[5]

We suggest in this chapter that the emergency physician at least examine the patient's general appearance, measure vital signs, and perform a head and neck examination. In general, of course, the more comprehensive the examination, the more likely it is that a physical ailment will be found.

A part of the examination sometimes omitted, but of critical importance in distinguishing organic mental disorder from functional disorder, is the mental status examination.

Mental status

The mental status examination includes assessment of the following areas:

1. Orientation
2. Memory
3. Intellectual functioning
4. Judgment
5. Affect

Orientation. Orientation refers to the patient's awareness of his surroundings (place), time (day, month, year), and situation (circumstances surrounding present problem).

Memory. Memory refers to the patient's recall of facts, events, impressions, or sensations. The patient may exhibit impairment of memory for recent events (last few minutes or hours) or for past events (last few months or years).

Intellectual functioning. The patient with organic brain syndrome usually has decreased intellectual functioning severe enough to interfere with social or occupational activity. The patient has difficulty with simple mathematical calculations and with abstract thinking.

Judgment. Judgment refers to the mental process involved in forming an opinion based on evaluating and comparing different types of information. Patients with impaired judgment also frequently exhibit poor impulse control. Typical questions to elicit information about a patient's judgment involve the construction of a hypothetical situation and the patient is asked to respond as if he were in that situation and were required to make some judgments.

Emotional lability and impared affect. Affect refers to the patient's observable emotions—what the patient appears to feel. Does the patient laugh or cry, and do the feelings seem appropriate for the situation? Affect is usually described as normal (full), depressed (sad), flat (no emotion), or inappropriate (not corresponding to the situation).

TYPES OF ORGANIC MENTAL DISORDERS

Organic mental disorders are classified according to their specific cause. In the past, however, several organic syndromes have been identified according to the patient's behavior and clinical course. Because these clinical patterns are widely recognized, the terms that label such patterns are presented here with their currently accepted definitions.

Acute versus chronic

In the past a significant distinction was made between acute and chronic organic disorders. Acute brain syndrome implied that the disorder had a sudden onset, resulted in delirium or coma, and was reversible, or ended in a resolution of the acute symptoms. Chronic, on the other hand, implied in addition to the slow onset of dementia, that the condition was irreversible or permanent. Although these distinctions are perhaps helpful in nosology, they cannot be precisely determined without long-term observation and are thus of limited value in the emergency department. These distinctions are not used in the DSM-III.

Delirium

Delirium is a well-recognized clinical entity that describes organic brain syndromes with particular characteristics. Delirium results from a diffuse impairment of brain tissue function. The patient typically has clouding of consciousness with decreased clarity of awareness of the environment. Sensory perception and recognition are altered. The disorder is typically transient with periods of intervening improvement in thought.

Though the patient's consciousness is clouded in delirium, he is able to respond to verbal stimuli. The familiar clinical portrait of the delirious patient is that of a restless, bedridden person thrashing about, "talking out of his head," and perhaps experiencing hallucinations. There is usually severe impairment of orientation and memory in delirium. Delirium is typically resolved within a week and rarely lasts longer than 1 month. If the symptoms persist indefinitely, the patient is reclassified to the categories of dementia or amnestic syndrome.

A summary of the current criteria for the diagnosis of delirium is the following:

1. Clouding of consciousness.
2. At least two of the following:
   a. Perceptual disturbance or hallucinations
   b. Incoherent speech
   c. Sleep disturbance
   d. Increased or decreased psychomotor activity

DIAGNOSTIC CRITERIA FOR DELIRIUM

A. Clouding of consciousness (reduced clarity of awareness of the environment), with reduced capacity to shift, focus, and sustain attention to environmental stimuli.
B. At least two of the following:
   1. Perceptual disturbance: misinterpretations, illusions, or hallucinations
   2. Speech that is at times incoherent
   3. Disturbance of sleep-wakefulness cycle, with insomnia or daytime drowsiness
   4. Increased or decreased psychomotor activity
C. Disorientation and memory impairment (if testable).
D. Clinical features that develop over a short period of time (usually hours to days) and tend to fluctuate over the course of a day.
E. Evidence, from the history, physical examination, or laboratory tests, of a specific organic factor judged to be etiologically related to the disturbance.

From American Psychiatric Association. *Diagnostic and statistical manual of mental disorders* (3rd ed.). Washington D.C.: The Association, 1980, p. 107.

3. Disorientation and memory impairment.
4. Transient, fluctuating course.
5. Clinical or laboratory evidence of a specific organic cause.

Dementia

Dementia is characterized by impairment of intellectual abilities severe enough to interfere with social or occupational functioning and implies a more chronic disorder than delirium. Although memory impairment is common to both syndromes, it is the predominant symptom of dementia. Impairment of memory may be so severe that the patient forgets how to perform common daily activities like getting dressed, setting the table, preparing a meal, or driving a car.

Patients with severe dementia can rarely function independently. The diagnosis may not be immediately apparent, however, because these patients often retain their superficial social and conversational skills despite gross memory impairment. The patient's behavioral changes are usually first reported by the family or other persons who share living quarters with the patient. The family may relate, for instance, that the patient's personality and personal hygiene have changed. The patient may have become withdrawn and unkempt over several months or years, or may have become immodest or reckless.

The mental status examination provides quick clinical confirmation if dementia is suspected. Memory, judgment, and intellectual functioning show the greatest impairment. The cause of the dementia may be treatable. Such causes include normal pressure hydrocephalus, chronic subdural hematoma, hypothyroidism, brain tumor, hepatic in-

DIAGNOSTIC CRITERIA FOR DEMENTIA

A. A loss of intellectual abilities of sufficient severity to interfere with social or occupational functioning.
B. Memory impairment.
C. At least one of the following:
   1. Impairment of abstract thinking, as manifested by concrete interpretation of proverbs, inability to find similarities and differences between related words, difficulty in defining words and concepts, and other similar tasks
   2. Impaired judgment
   3. Other disturbances of higher cortical function, such as aphasia (disorder of language due to brain dysfunction), apraxia (inability to carry out motor activities despite intact comprehension and motor function), agnosia (failure to recognize or identify objects despite intact sensory function), "constructional difficulty" (e.g., inability to copy three-dimensional figures, assemble blocks, or arrange sticks in specific designs)
   4. Personality change, i.e., alteration or accentuation of premorbid traits
D. State of consciousness not clouded (i.e., does not meet the criteria for Delirium or Intoxication, although these may be superimposed).
E. Either (1) or (2):
   1. Evidence from the history, physical examination, or laboratory tests, of a specific organic factor that is judged to be etiologically related to the disturbance
   2. In the absence of such evidence, an organic factor necessary for the development of the syndrome can be presumed if conditions other than Organic Mental Disorders have been reasonably excluded and if the behavioral change represents cognitive impairment in a variety of areas

From American Psychiatric Association. *Diagnostic and statistical manual of mental disorders* (3rd ed.). Washington D.C.: The Association, 1980, pp. 111-112.

sufficiency, vitamin deficiencies, chronic heavy metal poisoning, neurosyphilis, or recurrent seizures.

A summary of the current critieria for the diagnosis of dementia is the following:

1. Loss of intellectual abilities of sufficient severity to interfere with social or occupational function.
2. Memory impairment.
3. One or more of the following:
   a. Abstract thinking impairment
   b. Judgment impairment
   c. Aphasia or apraxia
   d. Personality change
4. Delirium not present.
5. Clinical or laboratory evidence of organic etiology, or the disorder does not fit the criteria for other organic mental disorders.

Amnestic syndrome

The amnestic syndrome is a specific form of mental disorder that has as its central feature impairment of short- and long-term memory in a patient who shows no clouding of consciousness. The patient typically cannot learn new material (remembering three items for 5 minutes) or remember previously learned material like his birthplace, early employment, or the names of previous presidents. The disorder may be caused by bilateral destruction or damage to certain diencephalic and medial temporal structures like the mamillary bodies and hippocampus. Head injury, hypoxia, or infarction of the brain in the distribution of both posterior cerebral arteries may cause the syndrome.

Organic hallucinosis

Recurring hallucinations may be the result of a specific organic cause, like phencyclidine (PCP) ingestion or alcohol withdrawal. When a specific organic cause is known and the patient has no clouding of consciousness or delirium, organic hallucinosis may be diagnosed and labeled with its specific etiology (e.g., phencyclidine hallucinosis or alcohol withdrawal hallucinosis).

Organic affective syndrome

Certain organic factors can cause depression or mania. Reserpine or hypothyroidism, for instance, may cause symptoms of depression, whereas amphetamine or hyperthyroidism can cause symptoms of mania.

Substance-induced organic mental disorders

The most common cause of organic mental disorders is related to drug or alcohol intoxication, drug or alcohol withdrawal, and medication effects. In many cases the cause of the patient's mental dysfunction is so obvious that it is not thought of as an organic mental disorder; alcohol intoxication is an example. In other cases the history of substance abuse is either not available or not immediately obvious on clinical grounds. Toxicological screening helps greatly.

DIAGNOSIS OF ORGANIC MENTAL DISORDERS

Family interview

The emergency physician may save a great amount of time and effort if included in the early assessment of the puzzling psychiatric patient is a conversation with the patient's relatives or friends about their perceptions of any changes in behavior or thinking. Close relatives are often able to detect subtle changes in personality before major changes in the patient's orientation, memory, or thinking develop. It also allows the physician to find out *how suddenly* the changes have occurred. Additionally, the patient's relatives or friends should be questioned about past or present:

1. Medical illness
2. Psychiatric disorders

3. Medications
4. Drug abuse

Specific questions may include the following:

1. Has any change occurred in behavior?
2. What kind of change has occurred?
3. How fast has this change occurred?
4. Have there been any other unusual behavioral changes in the past few weeks or days?
5. Have these changes occurred before?
6. Are these changes truly unusual or bizarre for the patient, or are they variants of his customary behavior?

Certain symptoms should always alert the clinician to the possibility of organic mental disorder. Incontinence of the stool or urine is an example. This symptom should be taken seriously and a diligent search for an organic cause is justified. A history of regular use of *any* medication is important. Over-the-counter preparations like Nervine contain bromide; Sominex contains atropine-like compounds. Both could cause abnormal behavior and thinking. Similarly, nonpsychotropic drugs like cardiovascular medication or antibiotics can cause adverse mental reactions and should be noted by the physician.

Finally, a clear history of psychiatric disorders with the same symptoms and treatment may save an enormous amount of time. The patient may have discontinued the medication on his own, for instance, and a call to his psychiatrist and reinstitution of the medication may solve the problem simply.

Patient interview

In the patient interview it is important to remember that patients conform to the structure of the setting in which they find themselves; that is, in a highly structured interview situation, emergency department roles are clearly defined. The physician is a knowledgeable authority figure, and the patient is requesting help. In this light, some patients who have organic illnesses tend to display minimal behavioral or thinking abnormalities. Patients with organic mental disorders frequently try to minimize their deficits, but they become disorganized and the diagnosis is apparent under certain conditions, which can be created during the interview. With this in mind, the approaches discussed in Chapter 2 are helpful.

First the clinician should ask the patient an open-ended question such as, "Why are you here," or "What problems are you having," and then should listen for 3 minutes (time these with a clock). If 3 minutes is not feasible (e.g., the ambulance service has called ahead that they are bringing in a patient with cardiac arrest), at least some period of silence is helpful. This part of the evaluation is undoubtedly the most difficult to master for the action-oriented emergency physician. Even if the patient does not initially appear to be talkative, the pressure of his anxiety during silence encourages him to talk.

During this time the interviewer should sit calmly to help allay the anxiety of the patient. The patient should be observed for slurred speech, eye-blinking (patients who hallucinate often look at the source of voices or blink frequently), a staggering gait, or other obvious gross neurological problems. Stereotyped or repetitive phrases or thoughts suggest psychosis. Patients who have organic illness often try to maintain social conversations and superficial discussions to present themselves as normal; they are often fearful of their deficit and try to "cover it up." This is an example of denial and is a relatively frequent phenomenon in patients with an organic mental disorder.

If the patient appears disorganized, has slurred speech, and is having trouble "making sense," it is important to go on with the interview and screen for organic dysfunction. Similarly, if the patient falls asleep during this nonstimulating period, an organic disturbance should be suspected. Following the open-ended questions period, a brief mental status examination is useful and easy to perform.

If the patient does not appear confused or disorganized during the 3-minute, open-ended session, formal mental status questioning usually demonstrates a deficit in patients with an organic mental disorder. Patients with functional disorders, by contrast, do not demonstrate the same degree of difficulty with mental status examination and typically are able to correctly answer questions that test orientation, memory, and intellect.

Mental status examination

Mental status questions can be introduced gently with such phrases as, "I am going to ask you a few questions to see how well you are concentrating." Oftentimes patients with organic mental disorders laugh and joke about the questions to avoid answering. They should, nevertheless, be gently pressed to answer each question.

Previously published mental status examinations are simple to perform and yield data that evaluate the five clinical features of organic mental disorder: orientation, memory, cognitive functioning, affect, and knowledge of general information. The questions suggested by Fauman and Fauman[6] include the following:

1. What is the name of this place, or where are you now?
2. Where is this place located (address)?
3. What is today's date?
4. What is the month now?
5. What year is it?
6. How old are you?
7. When were you born (month)?
8. When were you born (year)?
9. Who is the president of the United States?
10. Who was the president before him?

The first five questions are to test orientation and the latter five cognition. The first five questions assess whether the patient knows where he is and the current date. The last five require that the patient have at least some memory of past and recent events. If defects are noted in answering these questions, more accurate tests of cognition functioning, like simple mathematical calculations, can be performed.

Spatial orientation

Patients who have an organic mental disorder (ie, suffer from either delirium or dementia) can be tested quickly and sensitively with the following device: A circle is drawn on a blank piece of paper, and the patient is asked to pretend that it is the face of a clock and put in the numbers as though it were a clock. The patient should be able to space the numbers appropriately around the circle and place the hands correctly (Fig. 3-1, *A*). The small hand is usually midway between the 2 and 3, and the long hand points to the 6. Watching the patient do this may help to determine how well organized he is, how quickly he can place the numbers on the clockface, and whether he needs to place the 12, 3, 6, and 9 to organize himself better.

Patients who have difficulty with this first task probably have an organic mental disorder like delirium. Patients who have a mild organic disorder may have difficulty spacing the numbers on the clockface. They may not realize their difficulty until they are putting in the last few numbers and then they have to squeeze them in the upper left hand quadrant. Patients with a mild to a moderate delirium may recognize their error when they are finished, but may be unable to repeat the process correctly (Fig. 3-1, *B*).

One of the most common errors made in a delirious or demented patient is seen in Fig. 3-1, *C*. The patient shows perseveration, and although he may be able to write several numbers in sequence, the numbers move off the clockface and continue down the sheet of paper. Usually the patient does not recognize the error, even if it is specifically mentioned.

In Fig. 3-1, *D*, the patient with mild delirium or dementia may correctly place the numbers on the clockface, but then write in 2:30 rather than, as he is directed, place the hands in a position indicating 2:30. These patients can often correct their mistake, although with difficulty, if it is called to their attention.

The clockface exercise tests for several organic deficits: spatial orientation, ability to follow directions, immediate memory, and concentration. A patient with even a mild organic deficit has trouble completing this task, which makes it a simple screening device. If space on the record permits, the clockface can be recorded on the chart. The physician following the patient can monitor the patient's recovery or progress by comparison of the initial clockface to subsequent ones drawn by the patient. When this kind of severe deficit is noted in the emergency department, the physician should suspect a disruption in the functioning of the central nervous system and should search for an acute underlying medical problem.

Another test of spatial orientation is that used in the National Institute of Mental Health (NIMH) Diagnostic Interview Schedule (DIS). The patient is given a card or

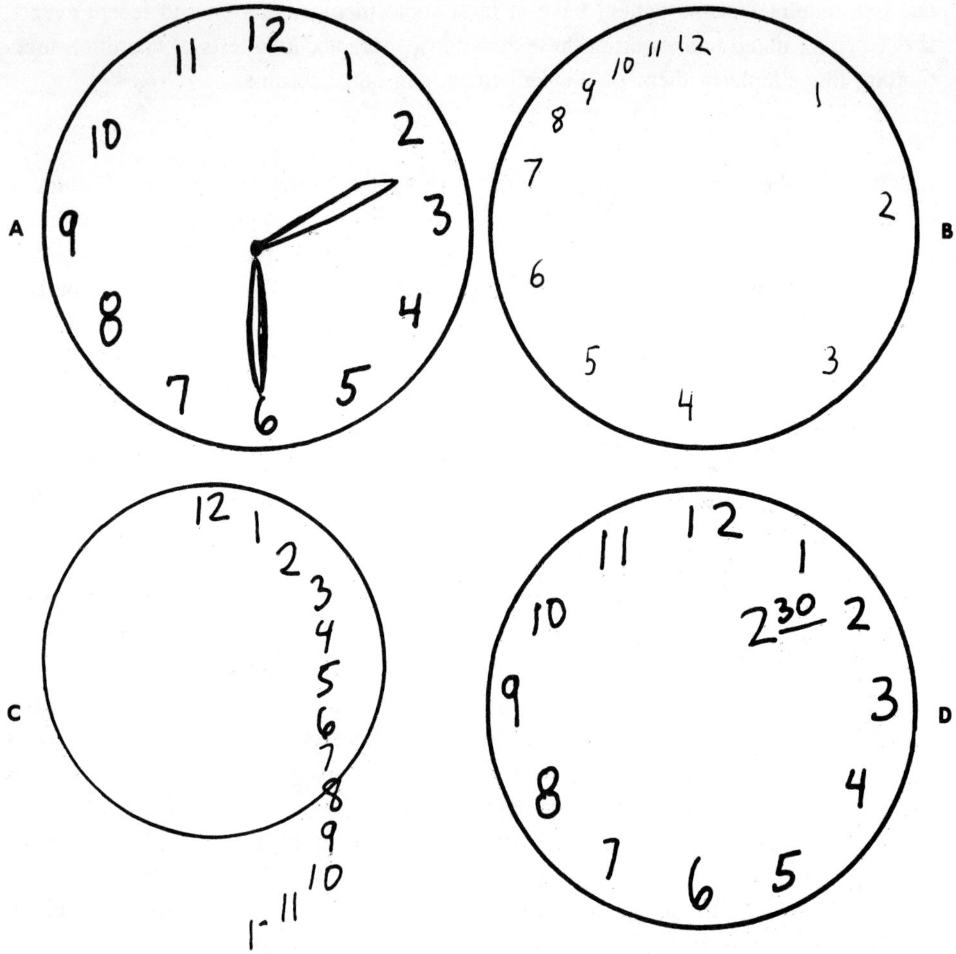

FIG. 3-1. A, Correct reproduction of clockface, including numbers and positions of hands to indicate the time of 2:30. Note small hand midway between *2* and *3*. Clock numbers are well spaced. **B,** Occasionally this drawing occurs in moderate delirium or dementia. The patient is somewhat disorganized, lacks perspective, is unable to "plan ahead." **C,** Common clockface in moderate to severe delirium or dementia. Patient is perseverating, disorganized. **D,** Occasionally seen in mild delirium or dementia. The hands are left out, and *2:30* is written in.

page showing the drawing portrayed in Fig. 3-2. He is then given a blank page and asked to reproduce the figure. A satisfactory or "correct" response is a drawing of two five-sided figures and one intersection.

As a continuation of the testing, the examiner can ask the patient to turn the paper over, write any sentence on the back, and hand it back. The three actions are graded separately: (1) turn the paper over, (2) write a sentence, (3) hand the paper back.[7]

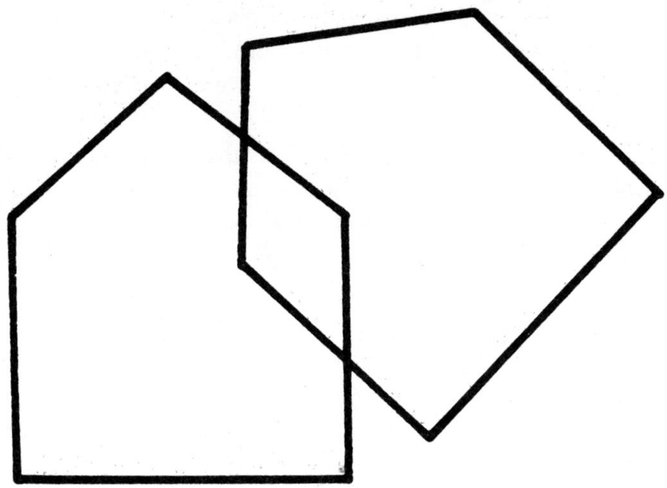

FIG. 3-2. Intersecting pentagon used in NIMH Diagnostic Interviews Schedule (DIS).

Testing specific mental functions

It is often helpful to separately test the five components of organic mental disorder. Frequently patients with an organic disorder fluctuate in their abilities so that a waxing and waning of the level of consciousness or attention should be noted. The following methods rather specifically evaluate each component.

Orientation. The patient should be asked the day, date, and year. He should be asked where he is and why he is there. These questions test orientation in terms of time, place, and situation, respectively.

Intellectual function. The patient should be asked to repeat between five and seven numbers forward and be able to repeat approximately five numbers backwards. It is helpful for the examiner to use part of his or her social security number so that this can be done easily and without mistakes. Calculation ability is also tested by asking the patient to count backwards from 100 by sevens (serial sevens). The patient may be asked to spell a five-letter word like *world* backwards (d-l-r-o-w).

Memory

Immediate. The patient should be given a sequence of items to remember such as the name of a city, a color, and a type of flower. Five minutes later, after other questioning is completed, the patient is asked to recall the items. Specific items, for instance, could be New Orleans (city), blue (color), and carnation (flower).

Recent. Recent memory can be tested by asking about something that happened several hours ago, such as what food the patient ate during his last meal. The answer should be substantiated by a relative or friend.

Remote. Remote memory involves distant events. The following are common questions for remote memory: Where were you born? How far did you go in school? Who was the president before this one? "Where were you employed on your first job?

Judgment. A question for evaluating judgment involves giving the patient a situation and asking him what he would do. The examiner may ask, for instance, "If you were in a crowded theater and you detected smoke or fire, what would you do?" The correct answer, obviously, is that the patient would call the smoke or fire to the attention of the manager or usher, or that he would help other patrons out of the theater quietly and in an orderly fashion.

Affect. The patient's emotional tone should be noted while the examination is taking place. The patient's mood should seem appropriate for what he is discussing and should remain relatively stable if he is in a normal emotional state. It is particularly important to note inappropriate giggling, laughter, sadness, or complete indifference (la belle indifference).

Hallucinations. Hallucinations are apparent perceptions of external objects or noises that the patient experiences when no such objects or noises actually exist. Questioning the patient about hallucinations or delusions may be very informative. The sensory modality involved, the content of the hallucation, and the way in which the patient reacts are important in separating an organic versus a functional (psychotic) cause. Occasionally the hallucinations are so striking that they form the dominant part of the initial impression and are the major clue to the physician that the patient's behavior and thinking are abnormal and that an organic hallucinosis is present.

Senses involved

Visual. If the patient experiences visual hallucinations, the cause is more likely to be the result of an organic disorder, perhaps of an electrolyte disorder like hypocalcemia; of ingestion of substances like lysergic acid diethylamide (LSD) or mescaline, which are known to cause visual hallucinations; or of the alcohol withdrawal syndrome with delirium (delirium tremens).

Tactile. Tactile (haptic) hallucinations are also most suggestive of an organic disorder. The feeling of "bugs" crawling on or under the skin is known as formication. Alcohol withdrawal delirium (delirium tremens) or cocaine intoxication may cause this syndrome.

Olfactory. Sensations of strong or pungent smells may be associated with the aura of temporal lobe epilepsy (uncinate fits).

Auditory. Isolated auditory hallucinations suggest that a functional disorder is present. The schizophrenic, for instance, may report that he is hearing voices or whispers or someone shouting at him. Auditory hallucinations are also associated with alcohol withdrawal hallucinosis, however, and may take the form of voices or unformed sounds like buzzing or hissing.

Perception and reaction. When initiating the discussion about hallucinations, the interviewer may want to begin by couching the questions with phrases such as "Sometimes people under a lot of stress hear voices or see things when no one is around. Has this ever happened to you?'' Often patients with an organic disorder report hallucinations or delusions as ''ego alien''; that is, they know that they are hearing voices or having visual hallucinations and they are frightened by them and feel that these happenings are ''strange.'' They report them in a frightened manner and particularly stress that they know that the hallucinations are ''unreal.'' Patients with a functional disorder, such as schizophrenia, often are not aware that the hallucinations or delusions are inappropriate; they incorporate the hallucinations into their perception of reality and typically report them as though they were real.

Physical examination

The importance of the physical examination should not be forgotten in the initial evaluation of the patient with bizarre behavior. Most of the essential components of the examination can be performed without asking the patient to disrobe. The physician can assess the general appearance, behavior, vital signs, signs of head injury (contusion, ecchymoses, hemotympanum, cerebrospinal fluid (CSF) drainage from nose or ear), eye movements, pupils, fundus, and mental status without having the patient undress. Though such a limited examination is simple, it must be done. It is not sufficient to label the patient as purely psychiatric without at least a screening examination for serious medical conditions that may cause or be associated with the behavioral or thought abnormalities. In most cases the patient eventually permits disrobing for a more complete examination.

Vital signs. Vital signs are among the first pieces of patient data available to the physician in the emergency department and are most important in evaluating the patient with abnormal behavior in whom an organic disorder is suspected. As a general rule, if the vital signs deviate greatly from the norm, a medical illness should be suspected; as the vital signs become more and more abnormal, the estimated seriousness and urgency of the condition should increase as well.

Examples of abnormal vital signs in organic brain disorders are myriad but include, for instance, hypertension in amphetamine intoxication and tachycardia in thyrotoxicosis. Examples of abnormal vital signs in medical conditions that can cause organic mental disorders are shown in relation to expected deviation in Table 3-1.

TABLE 3-1. Examples of abnormal vital signs in disorders that may produce an organic mental disorder

Vital sign	*High*	*Low*
Blood pressure	Amphetamines	Hypoadrenalism
Pulse	Thyrotoxicosis	Hypothyroidism
Respiratory rate	Ketoacidosis	Opiates
Temperature	Meningitis	Hypothermia

Head. The main physical findings sought in an examination of the head are those of past or recent trauma. Hematoma, ecchymosis, lacerations, or palpable bony defect suggest that trauma may be responsible for some or all of the mental symptoms.

Eyes. Paralysis of extraocular gaze and nystagmus are present in Wernicke's encephalopathy, and more specific gaze paresis can result from intracranial neoplasm (sixth nerve disruption) or infratentorial lesions. Pupillary abnormalities may be noted, as in symmetrical pinpoint pupils associated with opiate intoxication or dilated pupils in atropine poisoning. Asymmetrical pupils suggest a structural lesion. Papilledema on funduscopic examination suggests an intracranial mass or lesion, such as a neoplasm.

Ears. Hemotympanum suggests a basilar skull fracture and may be present in a very agitated patient. Basilar skull fracture often causes restless, combative behavior in the acute phase.

Neck. Rigidity of the neck is a characteristic finding in meningitis and subarachnoid hemorrhage, but may be part of the generalized muscular rigidity of extrapyramidal syndromes associated with parkinsonism or phenothiazine toxicity.

Chest and heart. The general physical examination must include an examination of the chest and heart. Since hypoxia or cerebral hypoperfusion can cause mental and behavioral abnormalities, pulmonary and cardiac examinations are helpful. The barrel-chested, dyspneic patient may pace about at night because his hypoxia prevents him from sleeping and causes restless, confused behavior.

The clinician may detect the midsystolic click and systolic murmur of mitral valve prolapse in a patient with recurrent panic attack or may find an S_3 gallop, cardiomegaly, and rales that suggest heart failure in the confused patient.

Abdomen. Evidence of hepatic disease such as hepatomegaly or ascites should be noted. Hepatic encephalopathy is an important cause of organic mental disorder.

Rectum. The presence of blood in the gastrointestinal tract is noted by a rectal examination and stool guaiac determination for occult blood. Hepatic encephalopathy in the patient with chronic liver dysfunction is often triggered by gastrointestinal hemorrhage, presumably because the breakdown of blood in the intestine is associated with elevated blood ammonia levels.

Extremities. The extremities may show clubbing in disorders that cause chronic hypoxia or hairless, shiny skin in lower extremities affected by arteriosclerotic vascular disease.

Skin. Examination of the skin may reveal needle tracks or other evidence of intravenous drug use. A dermal rash may suggest an infectious process, drug reaction, or evidence of an autoimmune disorder with vasculitis.

Neurological

Mental status. The mental status portion of the neurological examination has already been described. The level of consciousness can be determined by noting the patient's responses to tactile and verbal stimuli. To avoid confusion with different coma scales and nomenclature (lethargy, stupor, somnolence, and obtundation, for instance), the examiner may merely describe the response to various stimuli. These descriptions could be the following: "Responds to sternal pressure by decerebrate posturing," "Opens eyes with verbal stimuli, but falls asleep without continuing stimulation."

Neurological deficit. A focal neurological deficit, such as weakness of a particular muscle group, localized sensory loss, or isolated or unilateral cranial nerve deficit, suggests that a specific portion of the brain is damaged or impaired. The impairment may be the result of infarction, hemorrhage, tumor, abscess, or injury.

Ataxia. Disturbances in gait may be characteristic in certain organic disorders. The ataxic, broad-based gait, for instance, so commonly associated with alcohol intoxication or certain drug intoxications can reflect thiamine deficiency and Wernicke encephalopathy. Ataxia usually indicates organic disease. Other disturbances of gait may be a shuffling gait caused by extrapyramidal dysfunction in Parkinson's disease or the ataxic gait of Wilson's disease, a reversible cause of organic mental disorder.

Dysarthria. Dysarthria may be the result of some form of intoxication like phenytoin. Dysarthria and dysphagia occurring together suggest a pseudobulbar palsy caused by small, multiple cerebrovascular lesions.

Nystagmus. Nystagmus may be present in organic disorders that are otherwise difficult to differentiate from psychiatric disorders; vertical and horizontal nystagmus may be present in phencyclidine intoxication, horizontal nystagmus in phenytoin intoxication, and a peculiar rotatory nystagmus in amphetamine intoxication.

Tremors. Tremors are an important clue to the presence of an organic mental disorder. Fine tremor is characteristically associated with hyperthyroidism. A rather coarse intention tremor may be present in patients suffering from alcohol withdrawal; a resting tremor, "pillrolling," may be a feature of extrapyramidal syndrome; and *asterixis,* a "flapping" tremor associated with hepatic encephalopathy, is most easily noticed when the wrists are dorsiflexed and the hands jerk or "flap" forward intermittently.

Seizures. Seizures always imply an organic disturbance and may be seen in epilepsy, alcohol withdrawal, barbiturate withdrawal, anoxia, and tricyclic antidepressant poisoning.

Pathological reflexes. The presence of so-called pathological reflexes is highly suggestive of an organic mental disorder. These reflexes include the plantar, snout, suck, and glabellar. The plantar response is elicited by stroking the bottom of the foot with a firm object like the handle of a reflex hammer. An extension of the great toe usually indicates a physical disease or impairment of the more developed portions of the central nervous system, like the cerebral cortex. The snout reflex (puckering of the mouth when the upper lip is tapped) and the suck reflex (movement of the mouth toward the stimulus when the cheek is stroked) indicate similar impairment of higher central nervous system areas. The glabellar reflex is elicited by tapping the forehead just above the bridge of the nose (the glabella). The normal response is to blink in response to each glabellar tap only. A patient with extrapyramidal disease, like Parkinson's disease, continues to blink indefinitely each time he is tapped.

Laboratory studies

Certain laboratory studies are obtained routinely when an organic mental disorder is suspected. These studies include a complete blood count, urinalysis, electrolytes, blood urea nitrogen, glucose, calcium, serological test for venereal disease (VDRL), and x-ray films of the chest. Skull films may be appropriate for patients with a history or physical evidence of severe head injury. Arterial blood gases are invaluable when the problem may be related to hypoxia or hypercapnia. More specialized blood studies that may be indicated include thyroid function, liver function, and serum magnesium tests.

Studies that involve more patient risk, are expensive, or involve repeated measurements over a few days generally require hospital admission. Examples include lumbar puncture, computerized axial tomography of the brain, and electroencephalogram.

Toxicology. Toxic substances may appear in the blood of patients with bizarre behavior or thought. When the diagnosis of an apparent mental disorder is in doubt, a blood sample should be tested for some of these toxic substances. Toxicological screening panels can include tests for barbiturates, salicylates, amphetamines, narcotics, alcohol, phenytoin, hallucinogens, and heavy metals. If intoxication is suspected, a qualitative screen identifies the toxin and a quantitative measurement determines the serum level of the intoxicant.

CAUSES OF ORGANIC MENTAL DISORDERS

Organic disorders may be the result of such a myriad of causes that the entire listing would include disorders of virtually every body system. Some of these causes are listed early in this chapter. In the emergency department, however, certain causes are far more prevalent than others, and some causes are lethal. Anderson lists seven causes of psychosis that "may cause serious complications or death in a short time" if not recognized.[8] These causes are as follows:

1. Infection—meningitis or encephalitis
2. Hypoglycemia
3. Hypertensive encephalopathy
4. Wernicke encephalopathy
5. Hypoxia—diminished cerebral oxygen transfer
6. Intracranial hemorrhage
7. Poisoning

Other rather common causes include the following:

8. Drug intoxication and withdrawal
9. Organ failure
10. Head injury
11. Seizure disorder and the postictal state

Infection

The patient with headache, high fever, and nuchal rigidity is fairly easily diagnosed as having bacterial meningitis. The patient with bacterial meningitis who has agitation, disorientation, and hallucinations may not be so easily recognized. Since bacterial meningitis is highly lethal when untreated, yet so responsive to antibacterial therapy, it is one of the causes of disordered thought or behavior that must be considered early in the assessment of psychiatric patients. Other infections like viral meningitis, encephalitis, or generalized sepsis should be included in the differential diagnosis. Fever, nuchal rigidity, and leukocytosis facilitate the diagnosis of infection, but in questionable cases a lumbar puncture may be necessary.

Hypoglycemia

As the blood glucose level decreases, the patient becomes hungry, confused, stuporous, and eventually comatose. Seizures may occur in association with these lowered glucose levels. Some patients may, however, react to lowered glucose levels with bizarre behavior and inability to think clearly. Some become violent and combative. Early clinical clues to the presence of hypoglycemia may be a profuse diaphoresis and pupillary dilatation associated with adrenergic stimulation. The emergency medical service (EMS) team or the patient's family may provide the valuable information that the patient is diabetic; they may know the insulin dosage, the most recent pattern of use, and the dietary intake on the day of admission. Hypoglycemia can be fatal if not detected rapidly and yet is easily corrected with glucose. The condition should always be included in the quick mental checklist of organic conditions that should not be overlooked when evaluating the patient with abnormal behavior or thought.

Hypertensive encephalopathy

Severe hypertension, especially when associated with a rather abrupt rise in blood pressure, may cause encephalopathy. The affected patient typically complains of a severe headache, then becomes progressively more confused. The patient may be restless, delirious, or even combative. The measurement of an elevated blood pressure (diastolic above 140 mm Hg) strongly suggests the diagnosis in an acutely confused patient. Rapid lowering of the blood pressure with nitroprusside should eventually reverse the mental symptoms.

Wernicke's encephalopathy

The Wernicke encephalopathy syndrome, consisting of ataxia, ophthalmoplegia, and mental change is caused by thiamine deficiency and is most commonly seen in alcoholics. It is discussed in greater detail in Chapter 8.

Hypoxia

Since glucose and oxygen are essential substrates for cerebral metabolism, it is not surprising that a deficiency of either substance causes impairment in thinking and behavior. Hypoxia may be associated with various acute cardiopulmonary disorders like pneumonia, pulmonary embolism, or congestive heart failure or with traumatic disorders like flail chest tension pneumothorax or hemothorax. The diagnosis of hypoxia in such cases is usually fairly easy to make from the clinical history and the measurement of a low arterial blood oxygen level. Hypoxia may be caused by various chronic conditions as well. A patient with chronic lung disease may function well at a certain level of hypoxia that develops over years. When such a patient develops confusion, memory loss, restlessness, and insomnia, he may be developing a pneumonia that lowers his already low oxygen level even further. The new level of hypoxia cannot be so easily tolerated, and new mental symptoms become apparent.

Since hypoxia may develop rapidly in acute cardiovascular events or trauma, respirator-ventilated patients who develop agitation must undergo arterial blood gas evaluation immediately. The following case example illustrates the point.

CASE EXAMPLE 1

A 19-year-old man was involved in an automobile accident and was transferred to a university hospital after 24 hours in the intensive care unit of the first hospital. The patient was intubated, and a left-sided chest tube was in place. Shortly after arrival he became acutely agitated and tried to pull out the endotracheal tube. The initial diagnosis by the house staff was "intensive care unit (ICU) psychosis." An arterial blood gas measurement demonstrated a Po_2 of 36 mm Hg. A chest x-ray film revealed diffuse pulmonary haziness characteristic of adult respiratory distress syndrome. The percentage of delivered oxygen was increased, and the patient's agitation subsided completely.

The clinician must avoid the pitfall of making a diagnosis like ICU psychosis in the emergency department. The patient should be carefully evaluated and all possible causes of agitation or confusion should be considered because hypoxia and shock, for example, are more likely to arise in the victim of severe multiple injuries.

Intracranial hemorrhage

Intracranial hemorrhage can produce acute behavioral alterations before other changes are detected. A patient with sudden subarachnoid hemorrhage may cry out with pain and appear acutely agitated. The patient with intracerebral bleeding may develop clouding of consciousness and focal neurological impairment that is not apparent until specific neurological testing is conducted.

Chronic subdural hemorrhage may cause personality disturbance and an organic mental disorder. Alcoholics with liver and blood coagulation impairments are particularly prone to repeated head injury and development of a chronic subdural hematoma. Since it is sometimes difficult to distinguish changes caused by a subdural abnormality from those caused by psychiatric or alcohol-related mental disorders, a computerized tomography (CT) scan may be indicated in certain cases.

CASE EXAMPLE 2

A 62-year-old man was brought to the emergency department by his family who reported that he was not "acting right" and was sleepy all the time. There was no history of known psychiatric disorders or psychiatric hospitalization, though the family reported that the patient drank alcohol fairly heavily (1 to 2 pints per day) on the weekends. Physical examination revealed a mute, somnolent male with "waxy flexibility" of the arms. The patient would allow his arms to be raised or formed to any shape, and he held them in that position. He had a wide-based ataxic gait but there were no lateralizing neurological signs. A diagnosis of "catatonic schizophrenia" was made by the early examiners, and psychiatric consultation was obtained. Because of the acute onset of the disorder, somnolence, and ataxia, a toxicology screen and CT scan were obtained. The CT scan revealed a large left parietal subdural hematoma. Craniotomy and evacuation of the subdural hematoma resulted in the patient's nearly complete recovery.

Poisoning

Poisoning includes toxicity from prescribed or other legitimate medication, drugs of abuse, and toxicants from a variety of other substances that may be ingested. Poisoning that causes psychosis early in its use may result from ingestion of poisonous mushrooms like *Amanita muscaria,* which contain high levels of an atropine-like alkaloid. Other toxic substances that may cause psychosis include lead, camphorated oils, bromides, and polycyclic chlorinated insecticides.

Occasionally psychosis precedes death when there is rapid absorption of massive amounts of drugs. Persons who swallow condoms full of cocaine to smuggle them into this country may experience this syndrome when the condoms rupture in the stomach or intestine. The "body packer" syndrome is characterized initially by delirium and confusion. The treatment includes supportive care and rapid laparotomy to surgically remove any remaining drug or drug packet.[9]

Drug intoxication and withdrawal

Recreational drug use is so widespread that any emergency physician suspects drug intoxication when a young person has an altered sensorium. Amphetamines can produce a syndrome identical to paranoid schizophrenia. Lysergic acid diethylamide (LSD), phencyclidine (PCP), and others are hallucinogens that create hallucinations and other symptoms of psychosis.

Drug withdrawal may also precipitate psychotic symptoms. Narcotics and barbiturates produce some of the most serious drug withdrawal syndromes. Barbiturate withdrawal is particularly lethal.

Selected drug intoxication syndromes and their treatment are presented in Chapter 6. Substances that can cause intoxication, withdrawal, and other psychiatric symptoms are listed in Table 3-2. When there is doubt about the cause of an organic mental syndrome, a toxicology screening battery is justified and recommended. Furthermore, from a medical-legal viewpoint, a toxicology screen may be very important. An emergency department physician or other attending physician may be later asked in court to testify about a patient's behavior. Being able to testify either positively or negatively, regarding a toxicology screen, is extremely important under these conditions and is always asked about in a court of law. If a patient refuses such a blood test, it should be noted clearly in the chart.[10]

TABLE 3-2. Substances that can create an organic mental disorder as a result of intoxication or withdrawal from the substance

Substance	*Intoxication*	*Withdrawal*	*Other*
Alcohol	X	X	Hallucinosis
Barbiturate	X	X	
Opioid	X	X	
Cocaine	X		
Amphetamine	X	X	Delirium
Phencyclidine	X		Delirium
Tobacco		X	
Caffeine	X		
Cannabis	X		Delusional disorder
Hallucinogen*			Hallucinosis; delusional disorder, affective disorder

Adapted from American Psychiatric Association. *Diagnostic and statistical manual of mental disorders* (3rd ed.). Washington, D.C.: The Association, 1980.
*The hallucinogens can cause delusional disorders and affective disorders, as well as hallucinations.

CASE EXAMPLE 3

A 19-year-old man was brought to the emergency department by his mother who reported that he had been "acting strange" since the previous evening. There was no history of psychiatric illness, and he had seemed "normal" to his family previously. The patient looked somewhat blankly around the room, commenting on the "beautiful pictures" on the bare walls of the examining cubicle.

The patient's urine was tested and found positive for PCP. Although he steadfastly refused to confess to its use, the visual hallucinations, abrupt onset of psychosis, and blank stare were characteristic of a drug-induced psychosis and provided the clinical clues in this case.

Medication. Prescription medication like methaqualone (Quaalude, Sopor) and ethchlorvynol (Placidyl) may be taken in relatively large quantities, especially by younger patients, to "get high" or in a suicide attempt. Many prescriptions or over-the-counter medications, however, can cause symptoms and signs of a mental disorder, even when taken as prescribed.

Antidepressants, tranquilizers, anticonvulsants, and antihistamines can produce organic mental effects. A cardiovascular medication like propranolol hydrochloride may produce visual hallucinations, depression, and even catatonia. Other antiarrhythmics and antihypertensive medications have similar effects; the depression associated with reserpine or methyldopa is a well-known example.

Over-the-counter preparations commonly contain multiple medications in one tablet. Certain ingredients are more likely to produce delirium or psychosis than others. The scopolamine hydrobromide in sleeping pills (Sominex, Compoz) has been associated with toxic delirium, especially in the elderly.

A thorough and meticulous medication history from the family is invaluable in the evaluation of patients with mental or behavioral abnormalities. A toxicological screening battery is strongly advised for patients with previously unrecognized dementia, delirium, or psychosis.

Alcohol syndrome. Alcohol intoxication and withdrawal are such common causes of organic mental disorders in the emergency department that they are considered separately in Chapter 8. The major challenge for the emergency physician is to be able to distinguish the atypical alcohol syndrome and to diagnose an alcohol syndrome when it complicates the medical or psychiatric disorder.

Organ failure

Renal failure. The organic mental disorder associated with renal failure usually includes memory loss, disorientation, and lethargy. The elevated blood urea nitrogen and creatinine levels may be the first clues to acute renal failure. Chronic renal failure, however, is generally recognized by the patient's characteristic sallow appearance, and, in many cases, by the surgical arteriovenous anastomosis or Gortex graft for hemodialysis.

CASE EXAMPLE 4

A 48-year-old man with a history of psychiatric hospitalization was brought in by his elderly parents "to see the psychiatrist." They reported that he was mad because they left him alone for a week while they were on vacation and that he had refused to eat or drink anything while they were gone. Now that they had returned, the patient did not know the day of the week, the month, or the year. He was unable to subtract 7 from 100 and could not remember three items for 30 seconds.

The fact that the family "wanted to see the psychiatrist" could have led to an inappropriate psychiatric referral by the triageur. Because the patient was disoriented and had impaired intellectual functioning and memory, a blood profile including hemoglobin, electrolytes, blood urea nitrogen (BUN), and glucose was obtained. The results showed a BUN of 146 mg/dl, creatinine level of 22.5 mg/dl, and potassium level of 8.5 m Eq/liter. A rectal examination showed a markedly enlarged prostate. The patient was admitted with a diagnosis of renal failure secondary to prostatic urethral obstruction.

Hepatic failure. The full-blown portrait of hepatic failure should be easy to recognize. The patient may have some or all of the following classical findings: ascites, ecchymoses, telangiectasia, palmar erythema, gynecomastia, and jaundice. The associated organic mental disorder involves memory loss, poor intellectual functioning, and nonspecific personality change. Asterixis, the flapping tremor of the outstretched hands, is an associated sign that can be helpful in making the diagnosis.

Subtle mental changes caused by early hepatic failure may be noted only by close friends or family. They may report that the patient is increasingly forgetful and absent-minded or shows other signs of confusion. A brief mental status examination of such a patient can establish a memory defect or subtle change in intellect, even when the patient performs well in preliminary light conversation and demonstrates appropriate, though superficial, social skills.

Head injury

The altered state of consciousness caused by head injury ranges from coma to mild confusion. Cerebral concussion occurs when there is loss of consciousness, amnesia for the event, or a transient neurological dysfunction following the injury. Though consciousness is regained, the patient may remain confused for several hours. In an attempt to reorient themselves, such patients frequently and repeatedly ask, "What happened?" or "How did I get here?" despite explanations of the events.

CASE EXAMPLE 5

A 24-year-old man was brought to the emergency department by two men who pushed him out of the car and drove away. He was brought into the department by hospital security guards who found him lying in the parking lot yelling and shouting. Although he was restrained by the two guards, he struggled continuously and tried to break free. He was obviously combative and hostile and refused to let anyone touch him. He continued to spew verbal abuse and curse the hospital staff. The patient was placed in leather restraints and examined. A right-sided parietal hematoma and abrasions were noted on inspection of the head, and examination of the ear revealed a right hemotympanum. The patient was hospitalized; 24 hours later his sensorium cleared, and he remembered having a motorcycle accident (no helmet) and losing consciousness.

The head-injured patient may initially display agitation or violent behavior. This seems to be particularly common in the patient (like the one presented) who has a basilar skull fracture. The case just described emphasizes the need for a basic physical examination of the head, neck, eyes, ears, and nose of the patient with abnormal behavior or thought.

The head injury may be more severe than a straightforward concussion. The injury may include subdural hemorrhage, epidural hemorrhage, or intracerebral hemorrhage. Basilar skull fractures seem particularly likely to cause combative, restless behavior.

Even though the head-injured patient may be restless, hostile, or combative, he requires a period of observation to rule out serious intracranial processes. This may entail physical restraint to complete the patient's examination. When possible, sedation is avoided until the full extent of the injury is known, and the patient is observed for 24 hours for neurological deterioration.

Seizure disorder and the postictal state

The diagnosis of postictal confusion is usually easy; someone witnesses a seizure, activates the EMS system, and the patient is brought to the emergency department. As the patient awakens, confusion is accepted as an expected phase of the recovery process. If the seizure is not witnessed by anyone, however, the emergency physician may confront a confused, disoriented patient who denies recent drug or alcohol use. Once again, it is helpful to talk to a relative or friend who can relate a history of prior seizure disorder. Since the natural course of postictal confusion is one of steady improvement over several hours, it is usually sufficient to merely observe the patient in the emergency department until the sensorium clears and a clear history can be obtained.

Other causes

Neoplasm. Cerebral neoplasms are a comparatively rare cause of organic mental disorder in the typical emergency population, but they may cause mental behavioral abnormalities. Like cerebral hemorrhage, their detection is usually relatively easy with a CT scan. The combination of headache and increasingly bizarre behavior and confusion over a period of months or weeks should at least suggest neoplasm as one of the possible diagnoses.

Cerebrovascular disease. Cerebrovascular disease is so common in elderly patients that for years senile dementia was blamed on "hardening of the arteries," implying a defect in cerebral perfusion. These elderly patients may, in fact, have a reversible condition like medication reaction, chronic subdural hematoma, or vitamin deficiency. They deserve at least a basic evaluation before the more irreversible diagnoses of cerebrovascular accident or lacunar syndrome are made.

SUMMARY

Disorders of thought and behavior are extremely common in emergency department patients. The broadly educated emergency physician must be aware of the characteristics of organic mental disorders and be suspicious that each patient with bizarre behavior or disordered thinking has an organic mental disorder, perhaps the result of a reversible cause. A satisfactory history from relatives or friends, a relevant physical examination, and in certain cases, metabolic, toxicological, and radiographic studies are indicated in the assessment of such patients.

REFERENCES

1. American Psychiatric Association. *Diagnostic and statistical manual of mental disorders* (3rd ed.). Washington, D.C.: The Association, 1980.
2. Muecke, LN, and Krueger, DW. Physical findings in a psychiatric outpatient clinic. *American Journal of Psychiatry,* Sept. 1981, *138*(9), 1241-1245.
3. Koranyi, E. Morbidity and rate of undiagnosed physical illness in a psychiatric clinic population. *Archives of General Psychiatry,* 1979, *36*,414-419.
4. Hall, RCW, et al. Unrecognized physical illness prompting psychiatric admissions: a prospective study. *American Journal of Psychiatry,* 1981, *138*(5), 629-635.
5. Weissberg, MP. Emergency room medical clearance: an educational problem. *American Journal of Psychiatry,* 1979, *136*(6), 787-790.
6. Fauman, MA, and Fauman, BJ. The differential diagnosis of organic based psychiatric disturbance in the emergency department. *Journal of American College of Emergency Physicians,* July 1977, *6*(7), 315-323.
7. Robins, L, et al. *National Institute of Mental Health diagnostic interview schedule.* Rockville, Md.: National Institute of Mental Health, 1979.
8. Anderson, WH. The emergency department. In Hackett, TP, and Cassem, NH (Eds.), *Massachusetts General Hospital handbook of general hospital psychiatry,* St. Louis: The C.V. Mosby Co., 1978.
9. Fishbain, DA, and Wetli, CV. Cocaine intoxication, delirium and death in a body packer. *Annals of Emergency Medicine,* 1981, *10*(10), 531-532.
10. Di Sclafani, A, Hall, RCW, and Gardner, GR. Drug induced psychosis: emergency diagnosis and management. *Psychosomatics,* 1981, *22,* 845-855.

4 PSYCHOSES

The central feature in the diagnosis of psychosis involves the patient's perception of reality. The psychotic patient incorrectly interprets external and internal stimuli; acts and speaks "crazy"; and may experience delusions and hallucinations. According to the DSM-III, psychosis is a condition "indicating gross impairment in reality testing (. . .) the individual incorrectly evaluates the accuracy of his or her perceptions and thoughts and makes incorrect inferences about external reality even in the face of contrary evidence."[1]

Recognition of the floridly psychotic patient is usually quite easy. The patient's behavior or thought is clearly abnormal.

The symptoms of psychosis include one or more of the following:

1. "Craziness"
2. Bizarre delusions
3. Hallucinations
4. Grossly disorganized behavior
5. Disorganized thought processes
   a. Incoherence
   b. Illogical thought processes
   c. Loose associations
   d. Poverty of content of speech

RECOGNITION

The craziness may be so obvious that anyone can recognize it. The police officers, bystanders, receptionists, and nursing staff realize that the patient appears crazy, and the physician is warned before the patient is seen. The patient's grossly disorganized behavior may be one of the most obvious clues in this regard. Many such patients have been found wandering in public places with no apparent destination or acting in a bizarre or deviant manner.

The first clue that the patient is psychotic may be that the examiner can make no sense out of the story. It is difficult to follow the patient's account of his reason for being in the department, and one statement does not logically follow the next. The patient may say, for instance, "I came here to see you and my clothes are all dirty." The patient may look at the physician and say, "I have air in my toes. . . .The underground psyches are coming up and biting me." The former complaint represents loose, illogical association, and the latter represents bizarre delusions. By contrast the initial presentation may be more subtle; in these cases the defects in thinking are not evident until the patient has responded to several questions.

Auditory hallucinations may be the first clue to psychosis. The patient stops talking and appears to be listening to something the physician cannot hear, or he may appear to be answering voices. The auditory hallucinations may have a threatening quality. The patient explains that his dead mother and father are whispering bad things about him, for instance. Auditory hallucinations may consist of voices that keep a running commentary on the patient's behavior or thoughts. The schizophrenic patient typically has delusions or hallucinations but no insight into their pathological nature.

Poverty of content of speech means that the speech is adequate in amount but communicates little information. The patient may seem to ramble with words and phrases that are relatively meaningless in themselves and do not bear any clear relation to other words, phrases, and sentences.

STAFF REACTION

Psychotic patients are often frightening to the emergency staff. Because they are irrational and erratic, they represent the unknown and threaten our sense of order and predictability. Because they do not respond to logic and may be violent, they threaten our physical safety. The staff's frightened and apprehensive reaction to even the nonviolent psychotic patient leads to the understandable consequence that these patients are often isolated, confronted by the police, or restrained. These reactions to the nonviolent psychotic patient worsen the situation. The patient typically becomes increasingly fearful, belligerent, and assaultive. The cycle may escalate. As the patient is treated with tighter physical restraints and becomes more physically violent, more restraint is applied. This cycle can usually be avoided.

DIFFERENTIAL DIAGNOSIS

Major categories of illness

The emergency physician should be able to recognize the psychotic patient, evaluate the patient for an organic mental disorder, and obtain psychiatric consultation. Although it is not a requirement that the emergency physician ferret out the precise psychiatric diagnosis, it is helpful to recognize some of the more common psychiatric conditions. The major categories are as follows:

A. Organic mental disorders
B. Schizophrenic disorders
C. Affective disorders
D. Other disorders
   1. Schizophreniform disorder
   2. Brief reactive psychosis
   3. Paranoid disorder

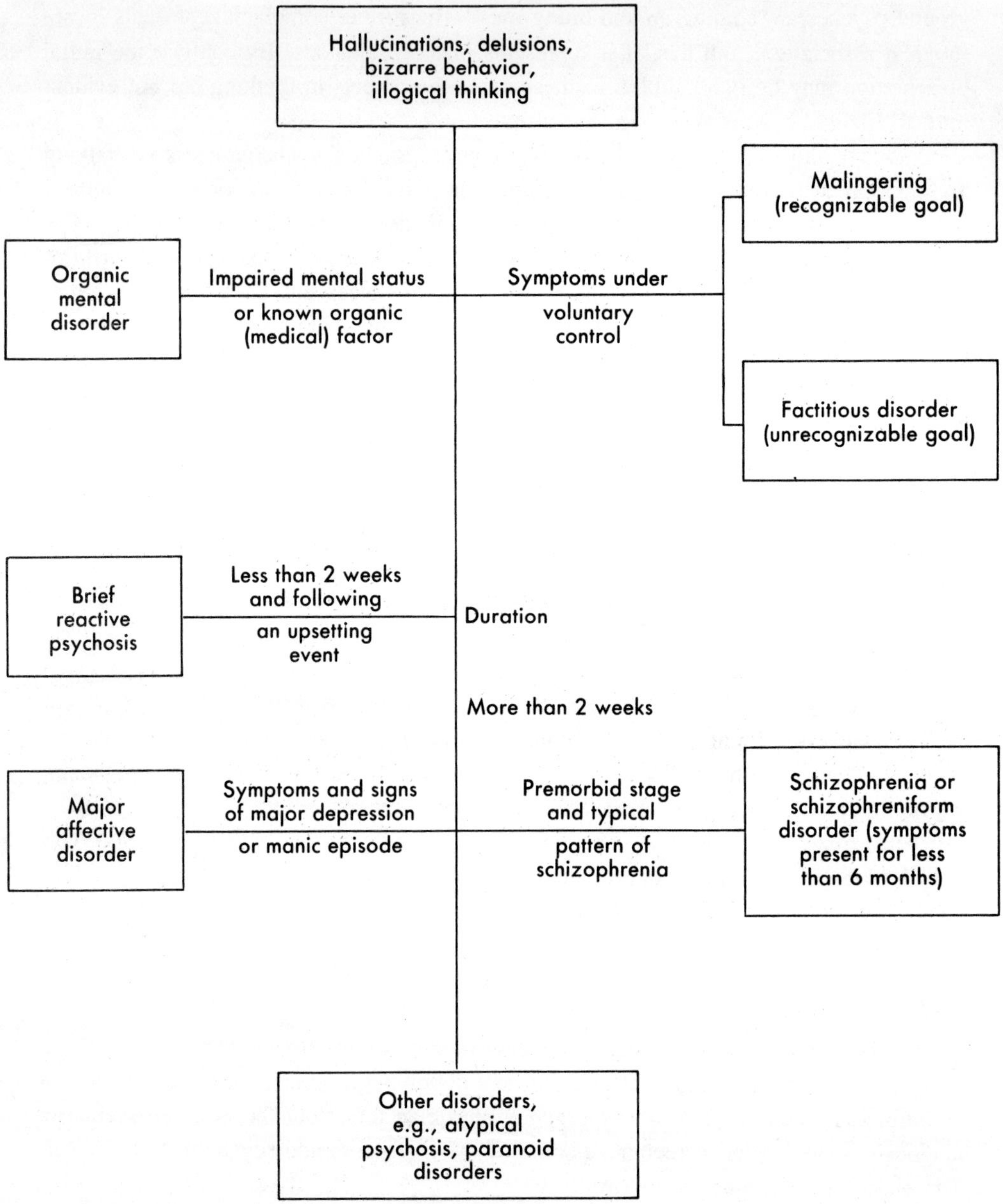

FIG. 4-1. Decision strategies for evaluation of patient with psychotic behavior and thought.

4. Factitious disorders
   a. Malingering
   b. Ganzer syndrome

A decision tree for the differential diagnosis of psychotic features is presented in Fig. 4-1.

TABLE 4-1. Specific schizophrenic disorder diagnoses according to duration of symptoms

Disorder	*Time symptoms must be present to make a diagnosis*
Schizophrenic disorder	6 months
Schizophreniform disorder	2 weeks to 6 months
Brief reactive psychosis	Few hours to 2 weeks

Organic mental disorders. As discussed in Chapter 3, the organic causes of psychosis, especially the life-threatening causes like hypoglycemia, poisoning, and meningitis, must always be suspected when the psychotic patient is evaluated in the emergency department. When organic disorders are ruled out or considered unlikely after a history and physical examination, the schizophrenic and affective disorders should be considered. Other disorders, like paranoid disorder, can cause psychiatric symptoms but are much less common than the three major categories: organic mental disorders, schizophrenia, and affective disorders.

Schizophrenic disorders. Schizophrenia, schizophreniform disorder, and brief reactive psychosis have the same signs and symptoms. Only the duration of the symptoms differentiates them. The schizophrenic disorders require continuous signs of the illness for at least 6 months. Schizophreniform disorders are so designated because the patient appears to have signs and symptoms of schizophreia but these have occurred for less than 6 months but for more than 2 weeks. Brief reactive psychosis has similar signs and symptoms to schizophrenia, but the psychotic disorder has occurred for at least a few hours but no more than 2 weeks' duration (Table 4-1). It is important to differentiate these three disorders, since they have different prognoses.

The schizophrenic patient. Schizophrenic patients who attract the earliest attention of the emergency staff usually are in the midst of some kind of crisis; they may be actively hallucinating, delusional, or talking "out of their heads." When the patient's bizarre behavior attracts the attention of friends, family, police, or a social worker, these people are likely to send or bring the patient to the emergency department, especially when no other source of acute psychiatric care is available.

The major disturbance in a schizophrenic disorder is the patient's content and expression of thought. These disorders of content and expression are commonly characterized as delusions, loosening of associations, and hallucinations.

Delusions. Delusions are ideas or beliefs that have no basis in fact. The DSM-III defines a delusion as "a false personal belief based on incorrect inference about external reality and firmly sustained in spite of what almost everyone else believes and in spite of what constitutes incontrovertible and obvious proof or evidence to the contrary."[1] Frequently patients say that they are being spied on or that others are planning to harm them. These are *persecutory delusions*. Delusions of being controlled are also common. Schizophrenics may complain that people or machines control their minds or thoughts or that they are controlled by "outside forces."

Bizarre delusions are those that are patently false and seem strange to nearly anyone who hears them. The patient may believe, for instance, that the dentist implanted a radio receiver in a tooth when a cavity was filled or that license plates send special messages to him. *Religious delusions* are beliefs that seem incredible yet are not accepted as an article of faith by other members of the religious group. The patient may, for instance, believe that he is Moses or Christ. *Somatic delusions* are those that pertain to the body and its functioning. The delusion that the body is "rotting away inside" is a typical somatic delusion. *Delusions of reference* are beliefs that external events have particular meaning for the patient. The belief that the television actors give messages directed only to the patient or that the traffic lights turn colors only when they know that the patient is approaching are examples of ideas of reference. Another common example is the exaggerated belief that others are talking about or laughing at the patient.

Loosening of associations. The conversation of a schizophrenic typically shows loosening of associations. The patient's ideas shift from one to another without any apparent association. If the loosening of associations is severe, the speech may be incomprehensible or incoherent. The patient may say, for instance, "I have thoughts in my head but can't get the red color out of my pants."

Hallucinations. The schizophrenic patient also has disturbances in perception that usually take the form of hallucinations. The hallucinations are typically auditory. If the patient has visual or tactile hallucinations, an organic mental disorder should be suspected, although these may in some cases be associated with schizophrenia. Usually the hallucinations are in the form of voices speaking to the patient and generally come from outside his head; the patient often looks toward the direction from which the voices seem to be coming. These hallucinations are typically well organized. For instance, the voices may keep a running commentary on the patient's activities, no matter how trivial. The voices are often insulting and may make sexual statements about the patient. Males often report auditory hallucinations accusing them of being homosexuals. Women often report being accused of having sexual relations with many men.

The hallucinations of schizophrenia may be related to a delusion. The patient may hear voices of those who are trying to persecute him, for instance. The auditory hallucinations of an organic mental disorder, by contrast, are poorly organized, like clicks, buzzing, or music, and are unrelated to any delusional system.

Affect. Affect, or apparent emotion, may be impaired in schizophrenia, organic mental disorders, or affective disorders. The affect may be inappropriate. The schizophrenic may discuss a recent death in the family and giggle inappropriately. Alternatively the affect may be blunted or flat. The patient thus displays a flat, apathetic, uncaring emotional tone associated with what would perhaps appear to be a frightening symptom to anyone else.

Other signs of schizophrenia

Disheveled or bizarre appearance. Since the schizophrenic is typically poorly organized, the initial appearance of the schizophrenic without a functioning support system may be that of a disheveled, unkempt, poorly groomed, unclean individual. Alternatively the patient may dress in an outlandish, garish, or bizarre costume, perhaps consistent with his delusions.

Words used in speech. Other symptoms associated with schizophrenia include the formation of neologisms, perseveration, and clang associations. Neologisms are nonsense words that the patient invents. Examples are *cowlow, filmfilm,* and *soball.* Perseveration is the repeating of words or phrases in the speech. The patient may say, for instance, "The traffic lights are out there to see me, see me, see me, see me, see me . . . ." Clang associations are those in which the patient relates to the sound of the word rather than its meaning. The patient may say, for instance, "I hear ringing sounds. I am wringing my hands. Do you hear me ringing?"

Course

Age at onset. The onset is usually during adolescence or early adulthood. This is important in distinguishing the thought disorder of schizophrenia from that of organic mental disorder. The onset of schizophrenia may begin in high school, when the patient withdraws from social situations and begins to perform poorly in school.

The occurrence of thought disorder in late middle age or in the elderly, without a history of psychiatric disorder, must prompt a search for organic mental disorder. The general rule is that schizophrenia rarely appears as a new entity after 40 to 45 years of age.

Premorbid phase. To make the diagnosis of schizophrenia, the signs of illness should be present continuously for at least 6 months. Usually in taking the history from relatives or even the patient, it is possible to define a phase of the illness that is considered prodromal or premorbid. This phase is usually a deterioration from a previous level of adequate social, intellectual, and personal functioning. The patient typically becomes withdrawn, begins to neglect his appearance, may demonstrate some eccentric or unusual behavior, and is noted to have some obvious changes in personality.

Generally speaking, the schizophrenic patient gives a history of having been eccentric, "odd," or "different." The patient may have spent some time in his childhood or adolescence having fewer interpersonal relationships, having been a "loner," and having been somewhat more withdrawn than the usual adolescent. If these symptoms have occurred over the previous several years, the prognosis is poor.

Active phase. The active phase is the period in which the patient usually comes to the emergency department. This is the phase in which the patient exhibits the most obvious impairment of thought, including delusions, loose associations, and hallucinations. The active phase may be associated with some stress that has precipitated the present psychotic picture. A careful history may identify the associated stressful event.

Residual phase. A residual phase usually follows the active phase of schizophrenia. The residual phase is less spectacular than the active phase and is usually characterized by a blunted or flat emotional tone and impairment of social and interpersonal functioning. The patient in the residual phase may also show markedly peculiar behavior, poor personal hygiene, poor grooming, social isolation, bizarre ideation, or vague delusions.

Impairment in schizophrenia. Schizophrenia severely impairs the patient in most areas of functioning. The patient may require someone to supervise him so that he eats appropriately; he typically shows poor judgment, cannot think clearly, and is often hallucinating. Between these episodes, wide individual variations in impairment exist. There may be very little disability in some patients, yet in others the disability may be so severe that institutionalization is required.

Complications. Schizophrenics have a high suicide rate; about 10% of schizophrenics eventually commit suicide. "Command" hallucinations ("the voices") may be telling the patient to jump out of a window or to stab himself. Other types of hallucinations and delusions may cause the patient to act without warning. The patient may experience the delusion that he can fly and suddenly jump from a height or that he can perform similar unrealistic feats that seriously endanger his life. Such patients behave in a totally unpredictable way and respond to stimuli unseen or unheard by others. Since these patients are at such great risk, they must be treated with suicide precautions, psychiatric consultation, and hospitalization.

Predisposing factors. The diagnosis of schizophrenia seems to be more prevalent in patients with poorer economic status. This has several possible explanations. One of the most common theories is that there is a downward social and economic drift in both premorbid and acutely schizophrenic patients because they have impaired social and intellectual skills.

Prevalence. Studies have shown a lifetime prevalence rate of 0.2% to 1%.[3] The incidence of schizophrenia among emergency patients is roughly similar to that of the general population.[4]

Sex ratio. There is no difference in the appearance of this disorder between males and females.

Familial pattern. Family studies of schizophrenics have shown a higher prevalence of schizophrenia among family members. A monozygotic twin of a schizophrenic is more likely to have the disease than a dizygotic twin. Both genetic and social factors, however, seem to be involved in the genesis of schizophrenia.

Affective disorders. The third major category of psychiatric illness in which psychotic symptoms may predominate includes the affective disorders. The affective disorders can be considered disorders of mood. The two extremes of the mood disorders are depression and mania.

Depression. Severely depressed patients may show signs of psychosis. They may experience hallucinations or delusions congruent with their mood. A mood congruent delusion in a depressed patient would be that the "world is coming to an end," that there is an "emptiness within them," or that their "heart has stopped beating."

The vegetative symptoms of major depression are invariably present along with the signs of psychosis. The patient or family can report a decreased (or increased) appetite, severe sleep disturbance, and other symptoms of a major depressive episode. Visual hallucinations in such patients occur most frequently at night.

The interview with the depressed patient in the emergency department may be painfully slow, since these patients frequently show psychomotor retardation and are slow to answer questions. Nevertheless, the interviewer must give the patient time to answer the questions and must ask about suicidal ideation. Since the major risk of depression is suicide, the depressed patient who shows signs of psychosis *must* be hospitalized.

Mania. The manic patient typically has a mood that is expansive and euphoric. Mania causes an intense pressure to speak. A manic patient may therefore speak constantly throughout the first 3-minute period of the interview in the emergency department. Such patients resist attempts to interrupt them. Other early clues to the diagnosis of mania are ideas of grandeur, intense energy, hyperactivity, and diminished judgment.

Psychotic features of mania include hallucinations and delusions. Visual and auditory hallucinations occur in about 25% of manic patients. The hallucinations support their delusions of grandeur. If the patient believes he is a god or a corporate president, for instance, the hallucinations are congruent with the grandiose delusion. Imagined subordinates may speak to him in a deferential or reverent way, and the patient believes he has unlimited money and/or power.

The differentiation of mania from schizophrenia may be impossible in the emergency department, since the initial signs and symptoms of both disorders can be remarkably similar. In general the manic patient is more organized in his thinking than the schizophrenic. The patient with a schizophrenic disorder generally gives answers that are irrational, bizarre, and senseless. The patient with affective disorder (mood disorder) generally responds to questions with answers that are either depressed or euphoric and grandiose. The manic patient, displaying an elevated mood, makes sense in a grandiose way, such as believing that he alone can go to Washington, D.C. to "straighten things out." The manic characteristically has a somewhat warmer relationship to the emergency staff and seems somewhat less bizarre than the schizophrenic.

Even though there are clinical differences, it still may not be possible to distinguish mania from schizophrenia in the abbreviated emergency interview. The manic patient may have intensely grandiose delusions, whereas the schizophrenic may be only mildly delusional and converse fairly rationally.

Despite the lack of precise diagnosis, however, the immediate treatment tactics for the schizophrenic, manic or depressed psychotic patient are basically the same.

Other disorders

Paranoid disorders. Paranoid disorder is a rare illness and is easily differentiated from schizophrenia and affective disorders. Patients with a paranoid disorder have delusions of persecution but a clear sensorium. Though they may feel conspired against, cheated, spied on, or poisoned, they are able to function rather normally in their intellectual and occupational functions. They may have delusional jealousy (conjugal paranoia); the individual is convinced without due cause that his or her mate is unfaithful. Individuals with paranoid disorders are often grandiose, socially isolated, seclusive, or eccentric. They often come to the emergency department complaining about some perceived injustice, although they rarely seek treatment. Typically a relative, associate, or governmental agency brings the patient to the emergency department. The individual's angry or litigious activities may prompt this solution. The duration of paranoid disorder is at least 1 week.

Malingering. The essential feature of malingering is the voluntary production of false psychological (or physical) symptoms in pursuit of some goal that is easily recognized because of the patient's circumstances. The patient who wishes to avoid going to jail directly from the emergency department may feign psychotic symptoms and request psychiatric hospitalization.

Ganser's syndrome. Ganser's syndrome is a rare disorder that is particularly noted among prisoners. The patient with Ganser's syndrome appears awake and alert but typically gives an obviously wrong answer to a simple question. He may give approximate answers to questions (such as $2 + 2 = 5$) rather than totally inappropriate or meaningless responses. While this patient may not be malingering, neither is he psychotic.

Since this rare diagnosis is difficult to make, especially in the compressed atmosphere of the emergency department, psychiatric consultation and a screening for organic mental disorder is most appropriate.

APPROACHING THE PSYCHOTIC PATIENT

The floridly psychotic patient usually acts "crazy." The craziness may take one of three forms.

Type	Symptoms
1	Agitated, hyperactive, pressured speech, hallucinations, delusions
2	Withdrawn but hypervigilant
3	Somatic delusions

In the first form the patient may be hyperactive, agitated, singing, talking, or behaving in an irrational way. Appearing to respond to voices or situations that others do not hear or see, the patient may look to various points around the room, reacting abruptly to hallucinations.

The second type of patient is extremely withdrawn, does not respond to stimuli, yet appears alert, awake, and vigilant. The patient may simply peer anxiously around the room, rock back and forth (standing or sitting), or sit quietly, not focusing on the environment at all. These first two types of patients are usually brought in by another person.

The third type of person has clearly bizarre or delusional complaints such as, "I have snakes in my abdomen," or "I have bad odors coming from my body." The latter are described as foul smelling or feculent. The described odor is not evident to others.

As described in the previous chapter, an organic cause for this apparent irrational behavior should be sought immediately with a history obtained from a friend or relative of the patient and a physical examination including vital signs and laboratory tests. Mental retardation may be suggested by a history of failing and repeating early grades in school, leaving school at an early age, or previous institutionalization.

If the patient is agitated, singing, talking loudly, or generally appears to be "up tight,'' the need for adequate physical force to restrain him should be anticipated. Four or five aides, police officers, security officers, or squadmen should be assembled, yet kept out of sight, unless the patient becomes violent or remains uncooperative.

The ideal early evaluation of the psychotic patient includes an interview with the emergency physician or psychiatrist. If the patient appears calm and assistants with restraints are nearby, the patient can be conducted to a moderately lighted room and seated comfortably. The physician may want to separate himself from the patient by a table or desk, but should not block the patient's direct path to the door. The blockage of a potential escape route may be so threatening that the paranoid patient could become violent. A room with more than one door is preferred for the interview; both patient and physician then have an available escape route.

The initial conversation should be steady and superficial—one spoken with a calm, reasonable tone of voice. The physician indicates that it is understood that the patient is upset, but a few questions need to be asked. This quiet nonthreatening approach avoids comments about the patient's irrational behavior and thinking, that are, in fact, frightening to the patient. It gives a sense of normality and calm to the patient, which helps him control his own irrational thinking and feeling. This in itself has a tranquilizing effect. At no time should the patient be the subject of jokes or laughter within his hearing. This heightens the patient's level of fear and agitation. Joking directly with the patient is never a good idea. The patient usually misinterprets these jokes in a paranoid way.

Physical contact

Unless restraint is required, physical contact should never be made with the psychotic patient because this contact may be interpreted as threatening. For the same reason, the examiners should keep their hands at the side, never shake hands, touch the patient's shoulder, make sudden movements with the hands, or point a finger at the patient (Fig 4-2).

Restraint

When restraint is required, it must be quick, sure, and effective. One attendant or assistant should be available to grab each arm and leg. Leather restraints are then applied to both arms and legs, and perhaps a restraint is applied around the body. This rapid and sure method of restraint prevents harm for everyone concerned and may even decrease the psychotic patient's anxiety and uncertainty that accompany uncontrollable impulses.

During the interview with the restrained or unrestrained patient, the physician may begin with an open-ended question such as, ''When did you start feeling upset like this?'' At this point the patient should ideally be given 1 to 3 minutes by the watch to answer this first question. This is an excellent period to listen to what the patient says, to try to pick up bizarre content, and to assess the tone of voice and apparent emotions associated with the statements. The early clinical impression is usually psychosis if the

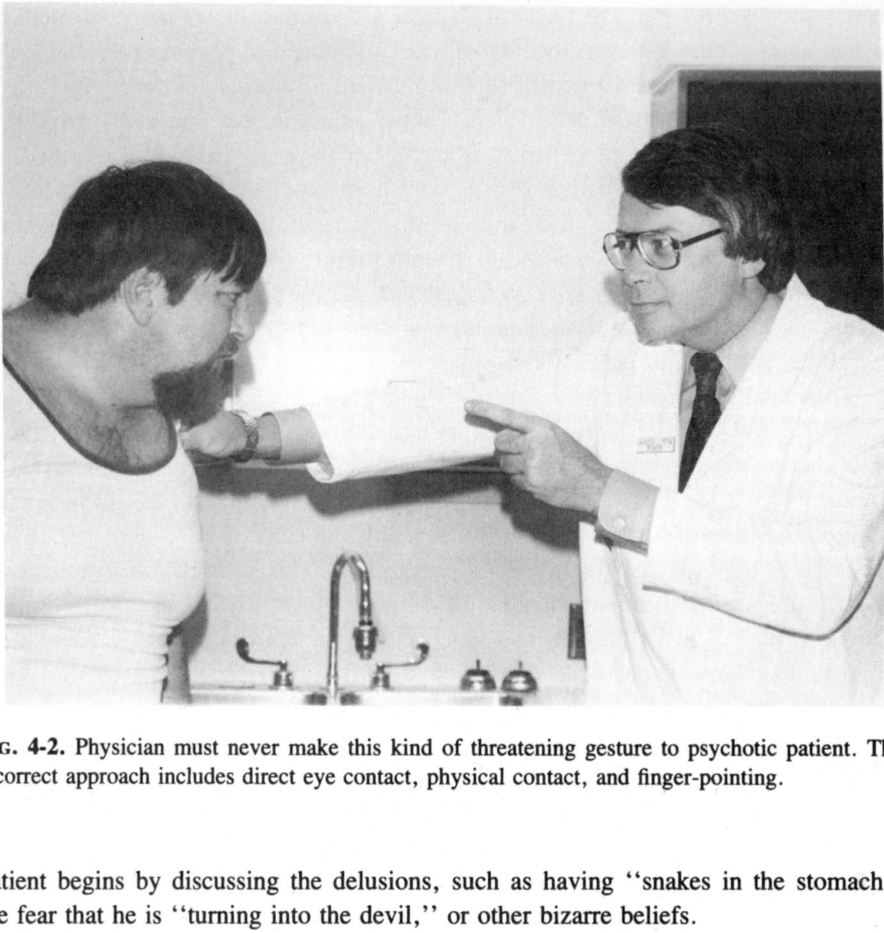

FIG. 4-2. Physician must never make this kind of threatening gesture to psychotic patient. This incorrect approach includes direct eye contact, physical contact, and finger-pointing.

patient begins by discussing the delusions, such as having "snakes in the stomach," the fear that he is "turning into the devil," or other bizarre beliefs.

This initial open-ended approach can be used whether the patient is agitated, withdrawn, or describes strange symptoms. Even the patient who appears entirely unresponsive should be approached in this way. The extremely unresponsive (catatonic) patient may actually be agitated, hypervigilant, and ready to explode. The appearance of a calm and patient examiner is helpful in defusing such patients. Even though it may *seem* impossible for the busy emergency physician to sit quietly and listen to a patient who may not even speak for a full 3 minutes, this early approach may ultimately save time in making an accurate diagnosis and determining disposition.

The second phase of the psychotic patient interview should include questions that enable the physician to determine the general cause of the psychosis from three alternatives: organic mental disorder, schizophrenic disorder, or affective disorder. Table 4-2 lists general areas of questioning and symptoms helpful in distinguishing these three areas of mental disorders. As discussed in Chapter 3, organic mental disorders are likely to cause an abnormal mental status examination, poorly formed tactile or visual hallucinations, and less bizarre delusions than those found in schizophrenic disorders. In

TABLE 4-2. Differentiating features of three major causes of psychosis: organic mental disorders, schizophrenic disorders, and affective disorders

Examination or question	*Organic mental disorder*	*Schizophrenic disorder*	*Affective disorder (mania)*
Orientation	Disoriented (may not know place, day, or time)	Oriented (usually knows place, day, and time)	Oriented
Memory	Short-term memory loss	No memory loss	No memory loss
Intellect	Impaired	Intact	Intact
Hallucinations	Visual or tactile, poorly organized	Auditory, complex, well-organized	Usually absent
Delusions	May be somewhat related to real events in daily life	Bizarre, not usually related to real events in daily life	Grandiose

psychosis caused by an organic disorder, the onset is more likely to be abrupt, and vital signs may be abnormal.

The approach outlined here may seem totally unfeasible to the emergency staff. The emergency physician, for instance, who adeptly resuscitates a cardiac arrest victim one minute may not easily switch attention to a wild-eyed psychotic patient complaining that his insides are "rotting away." The emergency nurse, similarly, may react negatively to the schizophrenic "repeater" who uses up valuable resources needed for patients with acute medical or surgical problems. This is one justification for having either a separate 24-hour emergency psychiatric facility as part of the emergency department or the on-call availability of psychiatrists, psychiatric nurses, or psychiatric social workers. Even if such resources are not available, however, current techniques for medical management of psychosis make early care of the psychotic patient a skill within the province of the emergency physician.

Management

The differentiation between the various psychiatric and medical illness causing psychosis is extremely important for long-term evaluation and treatment. In the emergency department, however, it is quite sufficient for the emergency physician to have the ability to do the following:

1. Recognize psychotic behavior and thought
2. Stabilize the patient and the situation
3. Be able to conduct a basic interview
4. Be able to screen for organic mental disorders with appropriate historical, physical, and laboratory data
5. Understand and be able to begin rapid tranquilization
6. Recognize that the symptoms of psychosis frequently require psychiatric consultation and probably hospitalization

Rapid tranquilization

The technique of rapid tranquilization or rapid neuroleptization is one in which rather large dosages of major neuroleptic agents are given to psychotic patients over a short period of time to eliminate their psychotic symptoms rapidly. Anderson and Kuehnle[5] deserve credit for stressing that psychosis is similar in urgency to any acute, serious medical conditions; that psychosis is intensely painful to the patient; and that specific antipsychotic therapy is available for terminating psychosis that is "a neurochemically medicated deficit in information processing."[6]

The essential feature of rapid tranquilization consists of the early administration of intramuscular, high-potency antipsychotic medication. The agent of choice is haloperidol (Haldol). Haloperidol has less chance of causing hypotension and fewer anticholinergic side effects than other major neuroleptics. Chlorpromazine (Thorazine) is generally avoided for this purpose, since it can cause a profound orthostatic hypotension when given in high doses.[7]

Rapid tranquilization begins with 5 to 10 mg of haloperidol given intramuscularly. Peak blood levels are reached 30 to 60 minutes after the initial dose, and the patient must be evaluated at these intervals to determine the results of therapy. If the signs of psychosis persist, another 5 to 10 mg of haloperidol is given. This process is continued at 30- or 60-minute intervals until the psychotic behavior and thought have disappeared or until a total of 50 mg has been given. Most patients should respond when total dosages of 15 to 35 mg are given within 3 hours.

Drug side effects. Acute dystonia is the most common side effect of rapid tranquilization with haloperidol. The features of dystonia may include a writhing of the arms or hands, acute torticollis or turning of the neck to one side, and inability to speak clearly or to withdraw the tongue back into the mouth. Patients who have been treated in the past with major antipsychotic agents recognize these symptoms themselves and are sometimes able to alert the clinician to their onset early in their development. More serious dystonias can impair swallowing or create upper airway obstruction.

The dystonias can be prevented by treating the patient with 1 to 2 mg of benztropine (Cogentin) intramuscularly with the first dose of haloperidol and to administer benztropine or diphenhydramine (Benadryl) when subsequent dystonia develops.

Anticholinergic effects like dry mouth, tachycardia, and visual blurring can occur with haloperidol. When the patient has a psychosis actually caused by anticholinergic poisoning, the administration of haloperidol may possibly worsen the overall clinical picture. When the patient's condition worsens after haloperidol is given, a previously undetected anticholinergic poisoning should be suspected.

Tardive dyskinesia may develop with long-term antipsychotic medications and is generally considered to be one of the concerns of the psychiatrist who assumes the patient's subsequent care.

The essential idea of rapid tranquilization is careful patient monitoring for both improvement and the development of unwarranted side effects. The analogy of the anesthesiologist closely monitoring his surgical patient[8] has been used to emphasize the careful monitoring and titration used in rapid tranquilization. This should be quite easy to accomplish in the emergency department.

SUMMARY

Though it is extremely important to rule out organic conditions as the cause of psychosis, rapid tranquilization with haloperidol should improve symptoms to some degree in all forms of psychosis except those caused by anticholinergic poisoning and perhaps those associated with factitious disorders like malingering.

In institutions where psychiatric consultation is easily available, it is sufficient for the emergency physician to recognize psychosis, rule out organic causes, and obtain consultation. Where such assistance is not immediately available, rapid tranquilization provides prompt and effective treatment for a painful and potentially dangerous psychosis.

REFERENCES

1. American Psychiatric Association. *Diagnostic and statistical manual of mental disorders* (3rd ed.). Washington, D.C.: The Association, 1980.
2. Wilkinson, DG. The suicide rate in schizophrenia. *British Journal of Psychiatry,* 1982, *140,* 138-141.
3. Kaplan, H, Freedman, A, and Sadock, B (Eds.). *Comprehensive textbook of psychiatry* (3rd ed.). Baltimore: The Williams & Wilkins Co., 1980.
4. Summers, WK, Rund, DA, and Levin, M. Psychiatric illness in a general urban emergency room: daytime versus nighttime population. *Journal of Clinical Psychiatry,* 1979, *40*(8), 340-343.
5. Anderson, WH, and Kuehnle, JC. Dosage of antipsychotic drugs. *New England Journal of Medicine,* 1976, *294,* 670.
6. Anderson, WH, Kuehnle, JC, and Catanzano, DM. Rapid treatment of acute psychosis. *American Journal of Psychiatry,* 1976, *133,* 1076-1078.
7. Donlon, PT, Hopkin, J, and Tupin, JP. Overview: efficacy and safety of rapid neuroleptigation method with injectable haloperidol. *American Journal of Psychiatry,* 1979, *136*(3), 273-278.
8. Mason, AS, and Granacher, RP. *Clinical handbook of antipsychotic drug therapy.* New York: Brunner/Mazel, Publishers, 1980.

5 SUICIDE

The annual number of completed suicides in the United States is approximately 40,000. This figure does not include completed suicides that appear to be accidental, such as single victim automobile accidents, hunting accidents, fatal industrial injuries, and apparently accidental poisoning. The problem of suicide is a particularly serious threat to the normally healthy life of young people. The Division of Vital Statistics of the U.S. Public Health Service reported close to a doubling of suicide rates in the white population between ages 15 and 24 years from the mid-1960s to the mid-1970s. Suicide is the second most common cause of death in the college-age population and the most common cause of death among young black women.[1]

Only a small percentage of known suicide attempts are successful. The ratio of suicide attempts to completed suicides is estimated at 39:1.[2] The percentage of emergency visits that involve a suicide attempt has been estimated to range from 0.3% to 1.0% of all patients seen.[3]

The suicide attempt is an acute medical event that generally involves evaluation and management in the emergency department. Since the magnitude of the problem is great, suicide attempts provide a steady flow of patients to nearly all emergency facilities. Because the problem is a common one and the results of poor assessment and treatment may result in abrupt and untimely death, the management of the patient who has attempted suicide represents a fundamental skill for all emergency physicians.

The traditional moans and groans of disgust and derision toward the suicide patient by the emergency staff must subside as these practitioners accept the suicide attempt as a legitimate emergency. They also need to accept behavioral disorders, in general, as problems that can be evaluated methodically and treated competently and effectively.

EMERGENCY STAFF ATTITUDE

The attitude of the emergency department staff should be supportive, not punitive. This is usually a surprisingly difficult goal to achieve. Ramon and coworkers[4] reported negative attitudes of physicians and nurses toward self-poisoned patients. It appeared that physicians and nurses showed less sympathy for patients who they believed to have taken overdoses for manipulative reasons than they did for patients who they judged to have done the same thing for depressive reasons. A study comparing the attitudes of emergency physicians toward victims of overdose was carried out by Ghodse.[5] It seemed that all clinicians demonstrated negative attitudes toward patients who took drug overdoses in the course of addictive behavior. Attitudes were somewhat more benign in cases in which the overdose was clearly perceived as a suicide attempt and were still more benign in cases in which the overdose seemed to be accidental. Goldney and others[6] studied the attitudes of house staff members toward those who attempt suicide. They found that house officers, of all physicians studied, exhibited the most unsympathetic attitudes toward the suicidal patient and that medical students tended to progressively develop more negative attitudes as they proceeded through the clinical years. This is understandable, since the house staff members are the most immediate role models for medical students. It was found in other studies that psychiatrists have the most empathic attitudes of all physicians toward the patient who attempts suicide.[7]

The busy, stressed emergency staff and paraprofessional care team in charge of the patient before he arrives at the emergency department often see the victim or his self-inflicted harm as a nuisance. Since the patient inflicted harm on himself (so the reasoning goes), he is less deserving of treatment than the victim of a medical illness or accident. The reasoning continues that if the treatment is harsh enough, it will "teach the patient a lesson." While these attitudes are perhaps understandable, they do not provide optimal professional treatment for the patient. The individual who experiences so much emotional pain that the only option out is self-destruction deserves some measure of positive emotional support from the emergency staff. Punishment or ridicule is neither therapeutic nor proper conduct for medical professionals. Such an unsupportive attitude may actually increase the risk of a subsequent attempt.

The reasoning that underlies the observation that a punitive attitude is counterproductive involves the ambivalence patients feel about making a suicide attempt. Ambivalence is an important aspect in the thinking and feeling processes of the person who attempts suicide.[8] The patient wishes both to die and to live. This is one explanation of why two thirds of those who complete suicide communicate the thought to their physicians before the attempt. The ambivalence that the suicide patient feels is perhaps the most compelling argument for establishing an empathic, nonjudgmental acceptance by those giving care before hospital admittance and those in the emergency department. A punitive, hostile approach amplifies the patient's self-destructive tendencies. When a respected authority figure like the physician rejects the patient, the patient's own feelings of diminished self-worth are reinforced and the chances of another attempt are increased. Data and experiences regarding this assertion are derived primarily from the personal experiences of psychiatrists in the treatment of such patients.[9]

The basic steps of management for the person who attempts suicide include maintenance of a supportive, accepting, nonjudgmental attitude; management of the medical or surgical problem created by the attempt; assessment of the patient's mental state; assessment of the patient's feelings; and determination of appropriate consultation, admission, or discharge.

MEDICAL MANAGEMENT

Medical management of the suicide-attempt victim generally precedes psychiatric evaluation. As mentioned previously, drug overdose, the most common method of attempted suicide, has increased dramatically over the past 20 years, particularly in young persons. The medical problems associated with drug ingestion become increasingly complex as multiple drug ingestions and drug-alcohol combination ingestions become more common. The standard emergency approach to the drug-overdose victim involves maintaining the airway, giving circulatory support, promoting gastric emptying, decreasing drug absorption, hastening drug elimination, and administering appropriate antidotes.

Carbon monoxide inhalation is basically treated with oxygen and ventilatory support when needed. Injuries from cuts or stabs are appropriately evaluated, and the wounds are surgically repaired in the customary fashion.

More violent methods of suicide include shooting, hanging, or jumping from heights. In general the severity of injury from these methods parallels the seriousness of the suicide intent or ''lethality.'' These seriously ill or injured patients may require extensive medical-surgical treatment and hospital admission. Psychiatric evaluation must be obtained in these cases before the patient is discharged.

Restraint

Some victims of intentional suicide may refuse medical care or violently refuse medical or surgical treatment. The physician's judgment in these cases is critical. If the physician decides that the medical or psychiatric condition of the patient poses a clear danger to the patient's life, the patient may need to be restrained for proper evaluation and treatment.

MEDICAL CLEARANCE

The person who attempts suicide should be ''cleared'' medically before an effort is made to evaluate intent, motives, and psychiatric status. This may require a period of observation in the emergency department or hospitalization on a medical or surgical service.

Drugs or alcohol may diminish the patient's concentration so significantly that a meaningful interview cannot be conducted until the effects of the drugs subside and the patient is fully awake.

A drug toxicology screen, including measurement of the blood alcohol level that shows drug types and blood concentration, is usually required to accurately assess the degree of drug intoxication. This allows the examiner to assess whether the patient's decreased affect or concentration are a part of an underlying psychiatric condition or the result of the effects of the drug. It also directs subsequent medical therapy.

In addition to the effects of the drugs, the patient may have metabolic abnormalities such as an acidosis associated with salicylate or methanol poisoning or hypoglycemia caused by insulin overdose.

It is inappropriate to hospitalize the patient on a nonmedical psychiatric service if there is danger of a deterioration in medical status caused by poisoning, metabolic derangement, or hypovolemia.

SUICIDE PRECAUTIONS

Because some suicidal patients have been able to repeat the attempt while in the emergency department or the hospital, suicide precautions are necessary. Suicide precautions include keeping the patient under close observation and removing any dangerous objects from the patient and the area. Needles and scalpels are obviously dangerous objects. Patients can create cutting instruments from intravenous bottles or drinking glasses; they can fashion a hanging rope from clothing or bed sheets. Suicidal patients should have all their clothing removed and searched for pills or instruments that could be used for self-injury. Even though most suicide attempts do not seriously threaten the patient's life, suicide precautions prevent further self-harm within the hospital. The best precautions are taken when the patient is under constant observation and accompanied everywhere by medical staff. The patient should not be placed in isolation or allowed to wander about unaccompanied until a thorough assessment of suicide potential has been completed.

PSYCHIATRIC DIAGNOSIS AND THE SUICIDE ATTEMPT

Establishing a tentative psychiatric diagnosis according to the DSM-III criteria is of value in assessing the patient who attempts suicide because certain diagnoses like schizophrenia and major depression usually signify a much greater suicide risk than other diagnoses like personality or adjustment disorder. A psychiatric diagnosis also allows the establishment of operational definitions that guide both acute and subsequent care. As clinicians learn to use a standard nomenclature, they should be able to aggregate their experience and gather data regarding the epidemiology, prevention, detection, and management of suicide attempts. Table 5-1 presents major categories of the DSM-III diagnoses, listed according to their frequency and derived from a sample of those who attempted suicide in at least one emergency department.[10]

Adjustment disorders

Previous studies have examined the relationship of psychiatric diagnosis to suicide attempt.[11,12] In these studies common diagnoses have included depression, personality disorders, and alcoholism. In most studies a significant group of patients have had insufficient criteria for any specific diagnosis but have had major life stress or "disturbed life circumstances" to which they responded by attempting self-harm. In the latest DSM-III terminology, these patients who respond in potentially harmful ways to a major life stress are diagnosed as having "adjustment disorders." When the patient's mood is a major manifestation of the clinical disorder, the modifiers can be introduced in the diagnoses, for example, "Adjustment disorder with depressed mood" or "Adjustment disorder with anxiety."

Results of studies conducted before the establishment of the DSM-III diagnostic classifications demonstrated a significant incidence of patients with conditions that would now be classified as adjustment disorders. In a study by McHugh[13] 15% of the patients were assigned to a category labeled *disturbed life circumstances*. Parker[14] con-

TABLE 5-1. Underlying psychiatric diagnoses in suicide attempts seen in emergency departments presented in order of relative frequency based on work in progress at the Ohio State University

Diagnosis	*Characteristics* (DSM-III)
Adjustment disorder	Maladaptive reaction to an identifiable stressor that occurs within 3 months of the onset of the stress; reaction impairs social and/or occupational functioning; symptoms are in excess of a normal reaction to the stressor
Major depressive episode	Depressed or sad mood; four of eight symptoms present every day for at least 2 weeks—appetite change, sleep disturbance, psychomotor activity changes, loss of interest, fatigue, guilt, decreased concentration, suicide ideation
Personality disorder	Enduring maladaptive patterns of perceiving, relating to, and thinking about the environment or self; significant impairment in social and/or occupational functioning or subjective emotional distress
Alcoholism and other substance use disorders	Undesirable behavioral changes associated with regular use of substances that affect the central nervous system; impairment in social and/or occupational functioning; inability to control or stop use of the substance; development of serious withdrawal symptoms after cessation or reduction of use
Schizophrenic disorders	Bizarre delusions, auditory hallucinations, incoherence, abnormal affect, and/or other grossly disorganized behavior; signs of the illness present for at least 6 months before the diagnosis can be made; prodromal phase characterized by odd or bizarre behavior, social isolation, and impairment of functioning

From Rund, DA, Saunders, AF, and Hutzler, JC. The suicide attempt. *Emergency Medicine Survey,* 1982, *1*(2), 53-60.

structed an analytic grid for assessing the patient's perceptions of suicide. Patients with low suicide intent did not see an attempt as equivalent to *dying*. Rather they considered it a way of reacting to a problem, equivalent to getting drunk, easing tension, talking to a friend, or being alone and crying. Such patients react to stress in such a maladaptive way that they qualify for the adjustment disorder category.

Depression

A major depressive episode is marked by the patient's sad, depressed mood and specific symptoms that last at least 2 weeks. Symptoms in four of the following categories are required for the diagnosis of major depression: appetite change, sleep disturbance, poor concentration, loss of interest, guilt, psychomotor activity changes, fatigue, recurrent thoughts of death, suicidal ideation or an expressed wish to kill oneself.

Although retrospective studies show that depression is the foremost psychiatric condition associated with completed suicide, it is not the predominate illness of those who attempt suicide. Patients who are depressed, however, make more serious suicide attempts than those with other underlying causes.[15] Thus they are most likely to require intensive management and admission to a medical-surgical service. The depressed patient who attempts suicide tends to show higher scores on the Beck Suicide Intent Scale.[16] This scale provides a measure of the patient's true intention of killing himself, based on responses to questions answered similarly by patients who have made the most serious suicide attempts. As a group, depressed patients plan their suicide attempts more carefully and continue to wish to die when saved. Such persons also often demonstrate their intent by leaving suicide notes and taking serious risks with little expectation or likelihood of rescue.

The traditional demographic and other epidemiological factors associated with suicide risk apply particularly to depressed patients. Such patients are more likely to be older, male, divorced, or widowed. Feelings of hopelessness, helplessness, and exhaustion signify particular risk in this population.[17]

Personality disorder

Our personalities are distinguished by enduring traits that characterize our view of the world and ourselves and the ways in which we react to situations and other persons. When these traits interfere with effective occupational or social functioning or when they result in emotional discomfort or pain, they are termed personality disorders.

Urwin and Gibbons[11] administered a standardized psychiatric examination to 539 overdose patients who were initially in an emergency department. They identified personality disorders in 26% of the men and 11% of the women. McHugh and Goodell[13] examined patients admitted to a neurology-psychiatry service after suicide attempts with sedative overdoses. They found a diagnosis of personality disorder in 63% of the patients. They also assessed the medical severity of each attempt and concluded that the patients with personality disorders made less serious attempts than patients with other underlying diagnoses.

Data from nonserious suicide attempt cases were reviewed by Pallis and Birtchnell.[18] Such patients showed greater deviance on the personality scores of the Minnesota Multiphasic Personality Inventory (MMPI) than did those who made serious attempt. The characteristics of personality showing the most marked deviation of this inventory were dependency, hostility, and unconventionality.

Alcoholism and other substance abuse

Alcoholism was the primary diagnosis in 18% of the men and 3% of the women in the study by Urwin and Gibbons.[11] Alcoholics have a suicide rate that is 50 times higher than the norm, and some have estimated that 25% of all successful suicides are associated with alcohol.[19]

Other substance abuse increases the risk of a suicide attempt. However, not every drug overdose is a suicide attempt, and the data are thus somewhat confounded. The abuser may take an overdose of drugs by accident or to achieve or maintain a "high." Nonetheless, such behaviors pose major risks of death by overdose and thus should put alcohol or substance abuse in a high-risk category, despite medical personnel biases about them.

Schizophrenia

Schizophrenia is not a prominent diagnosis in the overall sample of those who attempt suicide. Only 2% of such patients were schizophrenic in one study,[20,21] and the overall rate of schizophrenia in the general population is estimated at about 1%. Schizophrenics, however, do have a high suicide rate. As discussed later, the person attempting suicide who is schizophrenic requires psychiatric care and hospitalization.

ESTIMATION OF SUICIDE POTENTIAL

Most suicide attempts do not seriously threaten the patient's life. An estimated 15% of all patients who have taken drug overdoses are admitted to the hospital.[22] Nevertheless, in the early stages of emergency assessment, the suicidal patient should be regarded as a person with a psychiatric illness that may cause sudden death if untreated. This *potential* lethality makes the suicidal patient a true psychiatric emergency. With proper emergency evaluation, however, the emergency physician should discover that many victims of a suicide attempt are *low* risks for a subsequent attempt and may be discharged from the emergency department after a careful interview.

For most patients the moment of crisis will have passed and a repeated suicide attempt is not an immediate danger. Other authors have estimated that 99% of those who attempt suicide and are released from the hospital are alive 1 year following discharge.[23] Provisions must be made for adequate referral and outpatient psychiatric evaluation if the patient is discharged from the emergency department. The decision to hospitalize or discharge the patient depends on his psychiatric condition, attitude, and future plans. Some of the more important indicators are included in the following list:

Absolute indication (involuntary if necessary)
- Psychosis
- Violent, near lethal, preplanned attempt
- Continued suicidal ideation (with or without a plan)

Relative indication (may require involuntary hospitalization)
- Age over 45 (especially if no history of a manipulative attempt)
- High risk-rescue ratio
- Medical illness
- Alcoholism
- Drug addiction
- Living alone, poor social support
- Hopelessness, helplessness, or exhaustion
- Definite plans for repeated attempt

Psychosis

One of the absolute indications for hospitalization of the suicidal patient is the presence of psychosis. The psychotic patient who has attempted suicide or who plans suicide *must* be hospitalized, against his will if necessary. These patients may experience hallucinations that tell them they must destroy themselves or that cause them to act in a way that places them in grave danger.

Because their thoughts and delusions are unrelated to reality, they may impulsively obey an internal, unpredictable stimulus to kill themselves at any time. As noted in Chapter 4, 10% of all schizophrenics eventually kill themselves. The risk factors apply to patients with psychosis caused by an organic disorder and certainly to psychosis caused by an affective disorder like major depression. The treatment of psychotic patients must include antipsychotic medication, constant supervision, hospitalization (against the patient's will if necessary), and in some cases, treatment with antidepressant medication in the hospital. Most psychoses can and should be treated rapidly.

Depression

The patient with a major depression who attempts suicide nearly always requires hospitalization. The depressed patient probably has ambivalance about living or dying and has an excellent chance of being helped by inpatient treatment and antidepressant medication.

Risk-rescue ratio

The risk-rescue rating has definite value in assessing suicide potential. It may be calculated intuitively or numerically, according to the preestablished criteria of Weisman and Worden.[24] Table 5-2 shows the risk-rescue scoring form and lists various risk factors, rescue factors, and a method of calculating a risk-rescue score from the variables. Lower risk-rescue ratios indicate a lower suicide risk. An intuitive calculation is usually sufficient when the risk or likelihood of rescue is extreme. The rejected girlfriend who makes superficial slashes in her wrists or takes a few codeine pills in front of her boyfriend, for instance, has a low risk of dying and has a high likelihood of rescue. The chances of repeating this suicide attempt immediately are unlikely, and the patient has a lower overall suicide risk. On the other hand, a high risk-rescue ratio is estimated if the same patient attempts to hang herself in a lonely motel room or shoot herself in the head when no one is at home.

The method of the attempt has always been widely accepted as an indicator of overall suicide risk. Gunshot wounds or jumps from high places are more likely to kill and indicate higher risk than drug ingestion or skin lacerations, although each case must be assessed individually. In general the more often suicide is seriously attempted, the more likely successful completion will occur.

When calculating a formal risk-rescue rating, the risk factors include the agent used, impairment of consciousness, toxicity and extent of lesions, reversibility, and treatment required. The rescue factors include the location of the attempt, the person initiating the rescue, the probability of discovery, the accessibility to rescue, and the delay until discovery. As the risk to the patient increases under each category, the score increases from 1 to 3. As the likelihood of being rescued increases, the score increases from 1 to 3 under each category. The final score is computed according to the following formula:

$$\frac{\text{Risk score}}{\text{Risk score} + \text{rescue score}} \times 100 = \text{Risk-rescue rating}$$

TABLE 5-2. Risk-rescue factors and score computation

Risk factors

1. Agent used:
________ 1 Ingestion, cutting, stabbing
________ 2 Drowning, asphyxiation, strangulation
________ 3 Jumping, shooting

2. Impaired consciousness:
________ 1 None in evidence
________ 2 Confusion, semicoma
________ 3 Coma, deep coma

3. Lesions/toxicity:
________ 1 Mild
________ 2 Moderate
________ 3 Severe

4. Reversibility:
________ 1 Good, complete recovery expected
________ 2 Fair, recovery expected with time
________ 3 Poor, residuals expected, if recovery

5. Treatment required:
________ 1 First aid, emergency department care
________ 2 House admission, routine treatment
________ 3 Intensive care, special treatment

Total risk points ________

Risk score

5. High risk	(13-15 risk points)
4. High moderate	(11-12 risk points)
3. Moderate	(9-10 risk points)
2. Low moderate	(7-8 risk points)
1. Low risk	(5-6 risk points)

Rescue factors

1. Location:
________ 3 Familiar
________ 2 Nonfamiliar, nonremote
________ 1 Remote

2. Person initiating rescue*:
________ 3 Key person
________ 2 Professional
________ 1 Passerby

3. Probability of discovery by any rescuer:
________ 3 High, almost certain
________ 2 Uncertain discovery
________ 1 Accidental discovery

4. Accessibility to rescue:
________ 3 Asks for help
________ 2 Drops clues
________ 1 Does not ask for help

5. Delay until discovery:
________ 3 Immediate, 1 hour
________ 2 Less than 4 hours
________ 1 Greater than 4 hours

Total risk points ________

Rescue score†

1. Least rescuable	(5-7 rescue points)
2. Low moderate	(8-9 rescue points)
3. Moderate	(10-11 rescue points)
4. High moderate	(12-13 rescue points)
5. Most rescuable	(14-15 rescue points)

From Weisman, AD, and Jorden, JW. *Archives of General Psychiatry,* 1972, *26,* 555. Copyright 1972, American Medical Association.
*Self-rescue automatically yields a rescue score of 5.
†If there is undue delay in obtaining treatment after discovery, reduce the final rescue score by 1 point.

The possible lethality ratings range from 17 (indicating the lowest risk score of 1 and a high rescue score of 5) to 83 (indicating a high risk score of 5 and a low rescue score of 1).

The risk-rescue rating, whether estimated or calculated, should be valuable in determining the patient's lethality, need for psychiatric hospitalization, and perhaps overall prognosis.

Secondary gain

The attempt may have been made to achieve some secondary gains like increased attention from parents, friends, or paramours. When the goal has been achieved, the risk of an immediate repeated attempt is lessened.

In some attempts the plea for attention and the secondary gain are obvious. The rejected girlfriend who slashes her wrists in her boyfriend's home or the daughter who takes a handful of sleeping pills in her bathroom and then informs her mother of the act represents fairly common examples of suicide attempts in which the expected gain is obvious. The patient receives concerned attention from those close to her and is rushed to the hospital for continued treatment. For these patients the gain has been achieved, and an immediate repeated attempt is unlikely. They can usually be sent home safely with a psychiatric outpatient appointment. Early psychiatric follow-up provides intervention that can change these behaviors and reduce subsequent repetitions.

In attempts where there is no expected gain, other than death, the potential for a repeated attempt is great. The 60-year-old man who is exhausted and tired may look only for the relief from a lifelong struggle, perhaps against incurable illness. This patient obviously has a much higher lethality and needs psychiatric evaluation and probably inhospital treatment with antidepressant medication.

Social support system

Patients who are single, divorced, separated, widowed, or unemployed generally have a higher risk of suicide. A sense of loneliness or despair may be the overwhelming motive to complete a successful suicide. Psychosocial support systems include family and community resources and must be assessed when deciding to hospitalize the patient. If, for instance, the elderly man returns unaccompanied to his lonely apartment after leaving the emergency department, the subsequent risk of suicide is high. The patient who returns to a supportive, concerned family, on the other hand, has a much reduced risk of repeated suicide attempts.

Physical illness

Suicidal patients with medical illness, especially a painful, incurable one, must be taken seriously. The helplessness, despair, and unrelenting pain understandably drive these patients to seek "a way out." The ultimate management of these patients presents a difficult ethical dilemma for the physician. The immediate management, however, should be a fairly thorough medical and psychiatric assessment to detect any reversible or palliative factors that may make life more bearable for these patients.

Age and sex

Older individuals, particularly older men, are statistically more likely to complete suicide than younger patients. The person who attempts suicide and is over the age of 45 should be hospitalized unless there is a long history of frequent minor manipulative suicide attempts and a previous psychiatric evaluation that reveals the patient does not have a significant suicide risk.

Women attempt suicide more often than men (3:1), and men successfully complete suicide more often than women (3:1). Younger women are therefore usually considered to be at lower risk, according to these age-sex risk factors.

Alcohol

Alcoholism is a widely recognized risk factor for suicide. The alcoholic may have underlying depression and/or alcohol withdrawal depression. The alcoholic may be attempting to treat his own depression by drinking ethanol and experiencing a transient euphoria followed by a decreased awareness of his surroundings in general. The intoxicated patient has diminished emotional control and may commit suicide on impulse. Some patients only become suicidal when intoxicated; their inhibitions are lessened, and they can proceed with a suicidal act (Fig. 5-1). The diminished inhibition may also allow the underlying feelings of depression to emerge and become predominant in the alcoholic's thinking.

Drug abuse

A history of chronic drug use and abuse may be obtained from the patient, family members, or friends. Though the risk of suicide is high in incidence in this population,

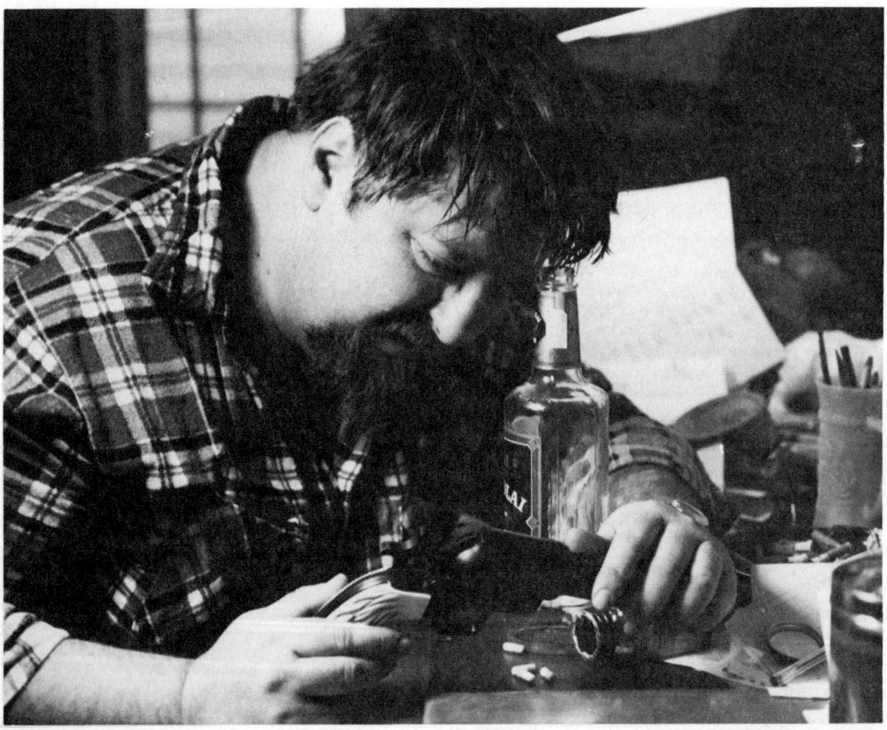

FIG. 5-1. Alcohol and drugs taken separately or in combination greatly increase the risk of suicide for someone likely to make an attempt.

it is difficult to determine because of the possibility of accidental lethal overdose. Similarly the patient with drug intoxication may relate a history of "just wanting to get high" or "sleep for a while." If these patients deny that they were attempting suicide, it is helpful to obtain additional history from family and friends about the patient's pattern of drug use, symptoms of depression, or previous comments or conversations about suicide. It is usually not enough to completely accept the story provided by the patient.

Drug users are accustomed to recreational drug use and probably have a ready supply of drugs that can be used for suicidal purposes. Underlying depression and diminished impulse control, while taking drugs, predispose the drug abuser to the same increased risk of suicide as the alcoholic.

Thoughts and feelings of those who attempt suicide

One of the most important aspects of patient evaluation, over and above medical assessment, assigning diagnoses, and determining risk-rescue ratings, is understanding how the patient was *feeling* and what he was *thinking* at the time of the attempt.

Certain patients, especially those with personality disorders, act on impulse. In one study,[25] 40% of the patients in two large series reported that they acted impulsively (with less than 5 minutes of premeditation) when they took an overdose. In a patient with drug overdose, the information about feelings immediately preceding the attempt is usually obtainable by simply asking the patient, "What were you feeling when you took the pills?" Hopelessness, despair, anger, guilt, and anxiety may coexist in the suicidal patient. Schneidman attempts to explain the interplay of these emotions by proposing that the patient first experiences heightened self-anger (inimicality), then increased emotional chaos (perturbation), increased constriction of intellectual focus or narrowing of the mind's content, and finally the idea of cessation—"the insight that it is possible to stop consciousness and put an end to suffering." That final idea is the "igniting element that explodes the mixture."[26] When the patient reaches an emotional crisis and "explodes" in the form of a suicide attempt, there may be a discharge of tension and even an emotional catharsis followed by a period of relative calm. During this period the emergency physician may mistake this apparent calm as indicating that the patient is no longer suicidal and, therefore, discharge the patient prematurely. Actually the patient's defenses may diminish at this stage, and it may be the best time to begin psychotherapy or at least to establish rapport that can be of help in subsequent treatment. Studies that have evaluated a special team approach to the management of suicide attempts have found that the patient is much more likely to keep a follow-up psychiatric appointment if he is to see a person with whom he established rapport immediately after the attempt.[27]

Attitude and affect

The patient's attitude and affect following the attempt are helpful in assessing lethality and the likelihood of a subsequent attempt. Patients who have attempted suicide because of feelings of hopelessness, helplessness, loneliness, and exhaustion have the highest suicide risk. The patient who sits quietly with eyes cast to the floor may answer questions slowly and express overall feelings of failure and fatigue. He may claim that he "just can't go on." His affect is clearly one of depression and fatique.

An opposite extreme is the patient who sulks angrily and expresses hostility toward parents, spouse, or friend. The patient who attempts suicide because of anger or in an effort to gain revenge has a far better prognosis than one who feels hopeless or helpless.

In general a low risk is present if the patient is embarrassed, angry, or remorseful; a higher risk is present if the patient appears sad, quiet, fatigued, or apathetic.

Future plans

Patients who relate a detailed plan for a repeated suicide attempt must be taken seriously, especially if the plan outlines a violent mode of death. The patient who says that he has a revolver at home and plans to lock himself in the bathroom and kill himself requires hospitalization. In general the more specific and detailed the plan, the more serious is the suicide threat.

Previous attempts

Patients who have made previous suicide attempts, especially serious ones, have a greater risk of trying suicide again. A possible exception to this general rule is the manipulative patient who makes repeated minor attempts to achieve some clear secondary gain.

Family history

Patients with a family history of suicide, alcoholism, or depression have a much higher suicide risk than patients without this type of family history.

Self-mutilation

The typical case of self-mutilation seen in the emergency department is the "wrist slasher." The patient is usually a young female who has a history of trouble with the police, family members, or school authorities. The underlying dynamic in this patient is thought to be a desire to gain attention combined with a difficulty in verbal communication. The patient may fear the withdrawal of affection from someone and cut her wrists to prevent the loss.

These patients may be institutionalized, and the daring label "slasher" or "cutter" becomes one that provides self-esteem. In institutional settings, slashing may reach epidemic proportions when the cutting behavior is learned in the institution or hospital and the behavior is reinforced by the other patients or the staff.

In the emergency management of these patients, the wounds should receive adequate but not overly elaborate medical attention. Superficial dermal scratches require only cleaning and a sterile dressing. Deeper lacerations should be repaired appropriately. These patients are then returned to their homes or institutions with proper guidelines and instructions to return to the normal routine as soon as possible. This approach provides minimal reinforcement of such behavior.

TREATMENT

The emergency treatment of a patient who attempted suicide includes medical management, suicide precautions, and psychiatric treatment. If it is easily available, psychiatric consultation can be obtained for all patients who survive a suicide attempt. If psychiatric resources are sparse, the emergency physician must identify patients who require hospitalization and discharge the others. In general, patients who may return home are nonpsychotic, younger patients whose attempts involve low risk, high likelihood of rescue, and high manipulative intent. The discharged patient should have adequate follow-up and a good social support system. These patients should always be discharged with someone who will stay with and observe them.

Contract

One technique of managing those who attempt suicide as outpatients involves the notion of a "contract." The contract is an agreement between the physician and the patient and states that the patient will not attempt suicide again until he calls the physician or some other source of help. Since some member of the emergency department staff is available 24 hours a day, arrangements could be made for the patient to call that number to talk to someone. An alternative would be a suicide prevention "hot line" to provide support when needed. The most effective contract, however, is one between the patient and the treating physician or a specific individual whom the patient met in the emergency department while undergoing treatment.

Medication

The patient may request a refill of medication. The patient with a seizure disorder may have taken all his phenytoin and phenobarbital in the suicide attempt, or the depressed patient may have taken his supply of tricyclic antidepressants. In most cases it is best to withhold all outpatient medication until the patient has a follow-up appointment with the appropriate physician. In one study, half of the cases of successful suicides occurred in patients who had received full lethal quantities of medication from a physician.[28] If medications like anticonvulsants are deemed necessary, only a small, nonlethal amount should be prescribed. A 2- to 3-day supply should be adequate to provide interim treatment.

Follow-up care

The most important feature for the management of those patients who attempt suicide and are discharged from the emergency department is the adequacy of referral for subsequent psychiatric care. The importance of even a minor suicide attempt must not be overlooked. The attempt is a sign that the patient definitely requires psychiatric evaluation and treatment even though the moment of crisis has passed and the patient is no longer suicidal. The emergency staff must emphasize the importance of the psychiatric follow-up appointment. The appointment should be scheduled within 48 to 72 hours after the attempt. A longer wait encourages the patient to minimize the event and never obtain proper treatment.

SUMMARY

The suicide attempt is an event that provides a steady flow of patients to the emergency department. The early management involves medical stabilization, a supportive attitude by the staff, and suicide precautions. Suicide risk should then be assessed. Psychotic patients require hospitalization. Severely depressed patients should be hospitalized.

When psychiatric resources are available 24 hours a day, all patients can be evaluated when they are awake and alert. When the emergency physician must decide who needs hospitalization, the guidelines for high suicide risk should be used. Patients who are discharged should make a "contract" with the physician and receive only a minimal quantity of medication.

REFERENCES

1. Kiev, A. Crisis intervention and suicide prevention. In Schneidman, ES (Ed.), *Suicidology: contemporary developments. Seminar in psychiatry series.* New York: Grune & Stratton, 1976.
2. O'Brien, J. Increase in suicide attempts by drug ingestion. *Archives of General Psychiatry,* 1977, *34*(10), 1165-1169.
3. Weisman, M, et al. Suicide attempts in an urban community. *Social Psychiatry,* 1973, *8,* 82-91.
4. Ramon, S, Bancroft, JHJ, and Skrimshire, AM. Attitudes towards self-poisoning among physicians and nurses in a general hospital. *British Journal of Psychiatry,* 1975, *127,* 257-264.
5. Ghodse, AH. The attitudes of casualty staff and ambulance personnel towards patients who take overdoses. *Social Science and Medicare,* 1978, *12,* 541-546.
6. Goldney, R, and Bottrill, A. Attitudes to patients who attempt suicide. *Medical Journal of Australia,* 1980, *2,* 717-720.
7. Hawton, K, Marsack, P, and Fagg, J. The attitudes of psychiatrists to self-poisoning: comparisons with physicians and nurses. *British Journal of Medical Psychology,* 1981, *54,* 341-348.
8. Morgan, HG. Point of view, management of suicide behavior. *British Journal of Psychiatry,* 1981, *138,* 259-260.
9. Bloom, V. An analysis of suicide at a training center. *American Journal of Psychiatry,* 1967, *123*(8) 918-925.
10. Rund, DA, Saunders, AF, and Hutzler, JC. The suicide attempt. *Emergency Medicine Survey,* 1982, *1*(2), 53-60.
11. Urwin, P, and Gibbons, JL. Psychiatric diagnosis in self-poisoning patients. *Psychological Medicine,* Aug. 1979, *9*(3), 501-507.
12. Gardner, R, et al. Psychological and social evaluation in cases of deliberate self-poisoning admitted to a general hospital. *British Medical Journal,* 1977, *2,* 1567-1570.
13. McHugh, PR, and Goodell, M. Suicidal behavior: a distinction in sedative poisoning seen in patients in a general hospital. *Archives of General Psychiatry,* 1971, *25,* 456-464.
14. Parker, A. The meaning of attempted suicide to young parasuicides: a repertory grid study. *British Journal of Psychiatry,* 1981, *139,* 306-312.
15. Stengel, E. A survey of follow-up examinations of attempted suicides. In Waldenstrom, J, Larsson, T, and Ljungstedt, N (Eds.), *Suicide and attempted suicide.* Stockholm: Nordiska Vokhandelns Forlag, 1972.
16. Beck, AT, Schuyler, D, and Herman, I. Development of suicide intent scales. In Beck, AT, Resnik, HLP, and Lettren, D (Eds.), *The prediction of suicide.* Bowie, Md.: Charles Press, 1974.
17. Beck, AT, Kovacs, M, and Weisman, A. Hopelessness and suicidal behavior: an overview. *Journal of the American Medical Association,* 1975, *234*(11), 1145-1149.
18. Pallis, DJ, and Birtchnell, J. Seriousness of suicide attempt in relation to personality. *British Journal of Psychiatry,* March 1977, *130,* 253-259.
19. Tomb, DA. *Psychiatry for the houseofficer.* Baltimore; The Williams & Wilkins Co., 1981.
20. Wilkinson, D. The suicide rate in schizophrenics. *British Journal of Psychiatry,* 1982, *140,* 138-141.

21. Miles, CP. Conditions predisposing to suicide: a review. *Nervous and Mental Disease*, 1977, *164*, 231-246.
22. Stewart, RB, et al. Epidemiology of acute drug intoxications: patient characteristics, drugs, and medical complications. *Clinical Toxicology*, 1974, *7*(5), 513-530.
23. Williams, C, et al. Impulsive suicidal behavior. *Journal of Clinical Psychology*, Jan. 1980, *36*(1), 90-93.
24. Weisman, AD, and Worden, JW. Risk-rescue rating in suicide assessment. *Archives of General Psychiatry*, June 1972, *26*, 553-560.
25. Williams, CL, Davidson, JA, and Montgomery, I. Impulsive suicidal behavior, *Journal of Clinical Psychology*, 1980, *36*(1), 90-94.
26. Schneidman, E. Psychological theory of suicide. *Suicide and Life Threatening Behavior*, Winter 1981, *11*(4), 221-231.
27. Hawton, K, et al. Management of attempted suicide in Oxford. *British Medical Journal*, 1979, *2*, 1040-1042.
28. Murphy, GE. The physician's responsibility for suicide. II. Errors of omission. *Annals of Internal Medicine*, 1975, *82*(3), 305-309.

6 VIOLENCE

Anyone in touch with current events realizes that violence is widespread and predictable in our society. Violent deaths (including accidents) are the third largest cause of death in our population, and in the United States most citizens perceive that the prevalence of violent crime is at its highest level in the nation's history.[1]

In many ways emergency departments act as "safety valves" in our health care system. They must respond to wide fluctuations in patient demand for care. When violent patients are encountered by police or emergency medical service (EMS) personnel, they may be brought to the emergency department for care of physical injuries sustained during a violent encounter, detoxification, or psychiatric assessment. Other patients may enter the emergency department voluntarily because of a frightening impulse to "kill someone."

Whether the patient is brought in by the authorities or self-referred, the violent or potentially violent patient can completely disrupt the normal working of the emergency department. Effective evaluation and treatment of the violent patient requires that the emergency staff use a systematized approach to the problem and bear in mind certain priorities of management.[2]

The first priority is the protection of other patients and emergency personnel and the overall stabilization of the situation.[3] This may require early physical or chemical restraint. The second priority is an assessment of the patient, which requires a patient interview and an alertness for an organic mental disorder caused by underlying medical ailments, drug abuse, or alcohol intoxication or withdrawal states. The third step of management is an attempt to make a preliminary diagnosis of the patient and institute proper treatment. This may require rapid tranquilization, psychiatric consultation, medical consultation, hospitalization, or incarceration.

PROTECTING THE SCENE

Whether the patient exhibits violent behavior (Fig 6-1), has been observed to be violent, has threatened to be violent, or is considered potentially violent, the physician's first obligation is to protect other patients and the hospital staff. For the clearly hostile, assaultive patient, adequate protection requires the summoning of adequate force. If police officers deliver a struggling, combative patient, they should be asked to remain until the patient can be restrained. If the patient arrives in restraints, they should not be removed until a thorough patient assessment is completed. If the patient arrives alone

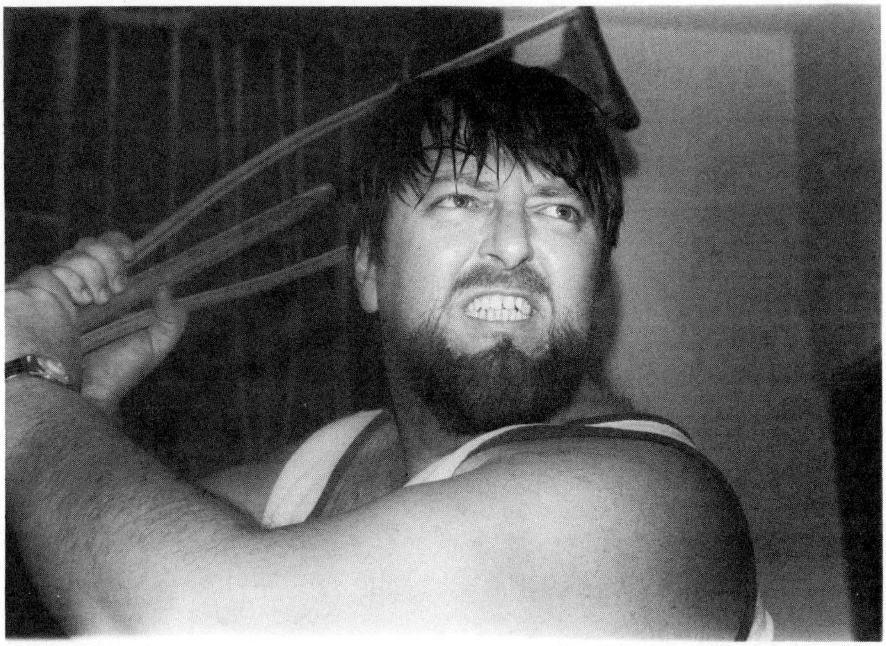

FIG. 6-1. Actively violent patient can pose a significant threat for emergency staff and other patients.

and then becomes violent, the hospital security force must be summoned or a plan should be made for restraint by a coordinated and united team of medical staff. The worst mistake the physician or nurse can commit is to try to physically subdue the patient singlehandedly or with inadequate force (Fig. 6-2). These ineffective measures always make the situation more unstable. The patient's anxiety and belligerence increase because he recognizes that he is out of control and unmanageable. Such a patient becomes increasingly anxious and belligerent. In such a state, he may harm other patients or bystanders. Responses to *actively* violent patients brought to the emergency department include the following:

1. Have others leave the examining room
2. Do not sit between the patient and the door
3. Have force available
4. Maintain a submissive posture
5. Do not try to physically stop the patient
6. Allow the patient to ventilate feelings

Adequate force

The physical restraint of a violent patient should be swift and certain but not brutal. Adequate restraint requires that the patient be subdued with an overwhelming and co-

A

B

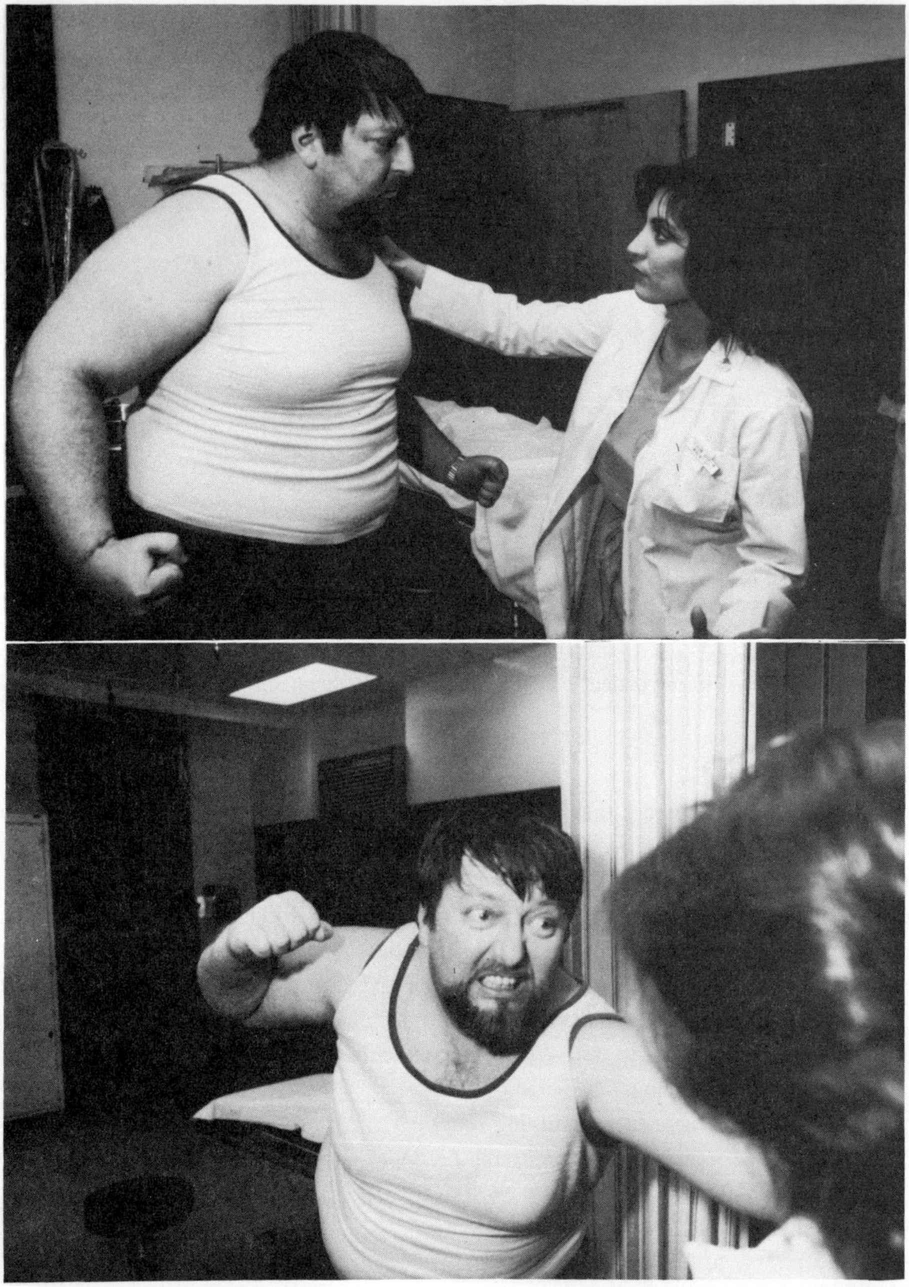

FIG. 6-2. A, Single-handed attempts to subdue obviously violent patient should be avoided. Ineffective physical contact should also be avoided. Paranoid patients perceive this as threat or intrusion. **B,** Such single-handed attempts to subdue patient can result in serious injury to hospital staff.

ordinated force. The most widely recommended tactic requires that one security officer or aide be available for each limb. The officers are assigned a limb beforehand, and at a given time, they grab and immobilize the designated limbs at the major joint (knee or elbow) simultaneously. The team then maneuvers the patient to a cart for further restraint (Fig. 6-3).

When the hospital does not have a special security force, the emergency department staff can be coordinated to subdue the patient as a united team.[4] To show the patient

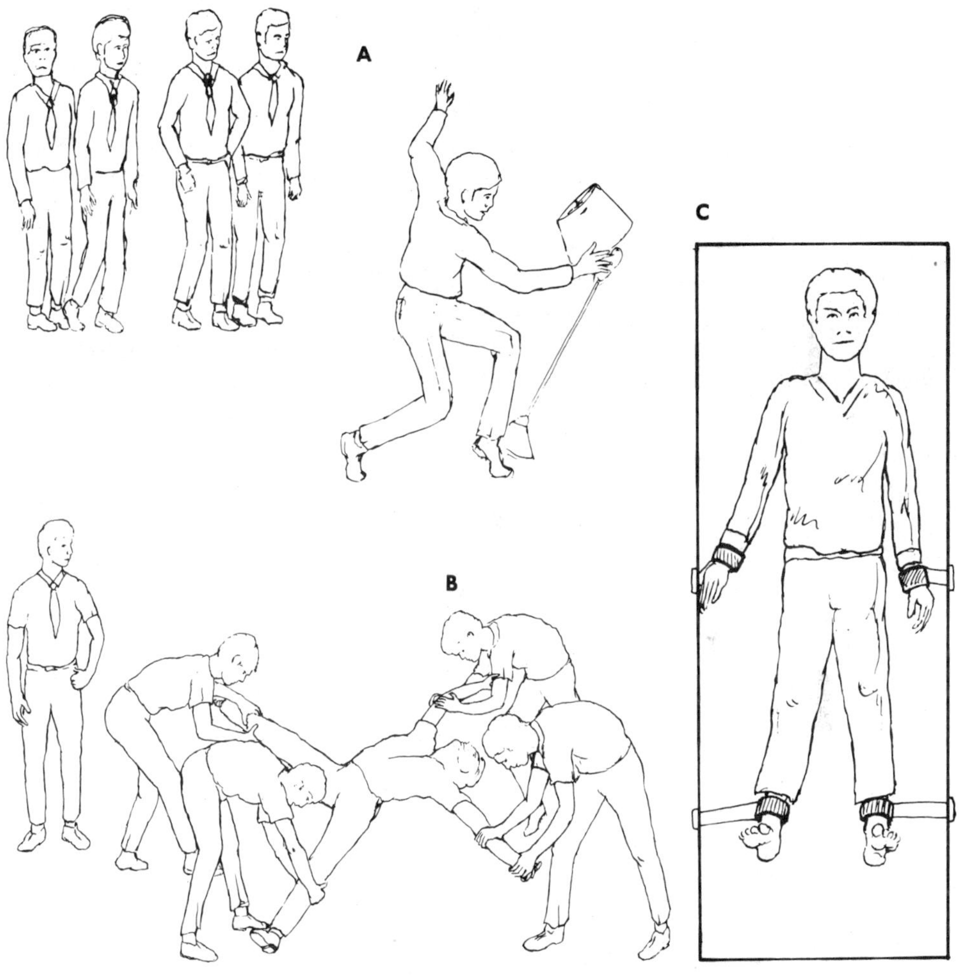

FIG. 6-3. A, Show of force with at least four persons and one additional team leader may be enough to subdue violent patient. Team should be spaced apart and stand about 20 feet away from patient when possible. **B,** Effective means of restraining patient is for each team member to grab one limb at major joint (knee or elbow). **C,** Four-point restraint generally immobilizes patient. Under certain circumstances chest restraint can be used, and under other circumstances patient should be restrained in prone or side position.

that the staff can indeed restore order, a single individual should assume leadership. This person should be knowledgeable about these situations. The charge nurse, for instance, may be better able to coordinate the team than a physician. The team should include four persons and a leader. Other persons can be asked to leave the immediate vicinity. When the staff appears strong, coordinated, and determined, the patient may yield without force; a staff that seems disorganized may cause the patient to become more anxious, agitated, and violent. The staff should position themselves about 20 feet from the patient, if possible. This distance minimizes the patient's fear of immediate attack and decreases his perceived need to retaliate.

The leader should speak calmly and inform the patient that his violent behavior is inappropriate in a hospital and will not be tolerated. If the patient remains violent, the team can approach him from all sides; each team member grabs the previously assigned limb at the major joint, and the leader remains in control. This approach minimizes the danger of fracture and allows even four or five small persons to subdue a larger and stronger person.

An alternate method, useful when the patient has a knife or club, requires the use of a mattress as a shield for four or five security officers or emergency staff members. The advancing mattress gradually forces the patient against the wall where he can be disarmed. Two mattresses held at each end work equally well to sandwich a menacing patient in the middle. The show of plenty of force may be sufficient to quiet the violent individual and permit the physician to evaluate him before proceeding with chemical tranquilization.

If violent behavior is expected but has not been observed, the physician or emergency staff should summon sufficient force in advance to stand by as the patient is evaluated. This group should be nearby but out of sight. Responses to patients who *become* violent after arriving in the emergency department include the following:

1. Listen
2. Promise the patient anything
3. Maintain a submissive posture
4. Do not stand between the patient and the exit
5. Be decisive

Restraint

Physical restraint involves some risk to the patient and a small probability that the restraint will increase the patient's anxiety and belligerence. In most cases, however, the patient should become calmer after restraint. The patient knows that someone else is in charge and that he need no longer fear his uncontrollable impulses. Four-point restraints that leave the patient "spread-eagled" on a cart carry the risk of aspiration if the patient would lose consciousness or vomit. Restraining the patient on his side or in a prone position reduces the risk, but the only sure protective mechanism is to place the restrained patient under continuous supervision. This precaution has the added advantage that someone is able to talk to the patient in an attempt to soothe and reassure him. Padded leather restraints or those made with sheets or blankets usually provide the safest and most effective ones used, and an additional ''belt'' restraint around the chest may be needed (Fig. 6-4). When a chest restraint is used, the emergency staff must ensure that the restraint does not seriously impair respiration.

Physical restraints should only be used temporarily to protect the patient and the staff and allow a medical evaluation. Appropriate pharmacological treatment may begin when evaluation is completed so that the restraints can be removed as soon as possible.

Following restraint, the patient may plead for release, promising to be calm if the restraints are removed. The patient must be informed that the restraints need to be left in place until an adequate medical evaluation can be conducted.

Weapon search. The restrained patient must be searched for weapons. Knives and guns must be removed and locked away before the patient can be released. An effective weapon policy may be needed in some emergency departments. Security guards may have to search all suspicious persons before they enter the department.

When the disruptive situation and the condition of the combative patient are stabilized, the emergency staff can once again attend to other patients; the flow of activity proceeds smoothly, and the once threatening patient can be evaluated methodically.

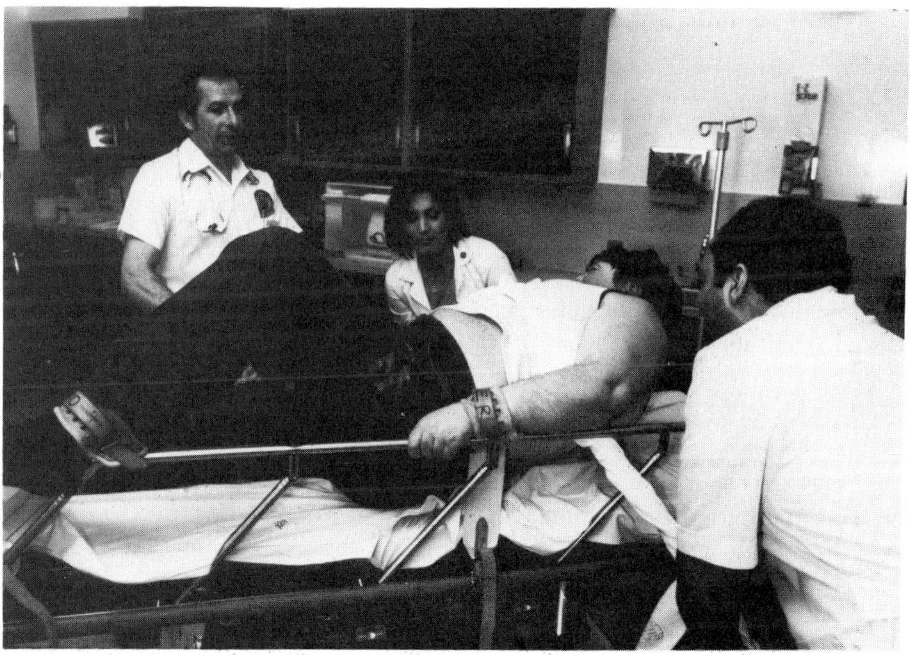

FIG. 6-4. Adequate patient restraint with leather cuffs, including chest restraint.

Evaluation

The setting. If the patient is securely restrained, the physician may want to interview the patient in a quiet place. Everyone who brought the patient in may be asked to leave the room because combative patients tend to be more belligerent when confronted by a crowd. A curious emergency department staff should not peer into the room intermittently during the interview. If the restraints are removed early, the room should be stripped of dangerous objects, and it needs to be large enough for the patient and physician to sit comfortably apart.

General appearance and vital signs. The general appearance of the patient may provide a clue to a lifethreatening medical disorder that needs immediate attention. The violent patient may have been stabbed, shot, or beaten before his arrival. Hypoxia and hypovolemia make the victim even more agitated. When these wounds go undetected, the results can be disasterous. There are recorded cases of patients who were initially restrained in the emergency department and soon died because of massive blood loss from an undetected stab wound. The physician must therefore examine the restrained patient from ''head to toe'' and measure vital signs. If the patient is unrestrained and it is felt that the physical contact of an examination might precipitate a violent response, the physician may scan the patient quickly for pallor, diaphoresis, cyanosis, or other clear signs of injury or organic illness, while a rapport is established that will permit a subsequent examination.

Interview. If the patient is not in immediate danger, the initial evaluation begins with an interview. As indicated previously, the ideal interview begins with a question something like, ''What started all this?'' The patient is then given approximately 3 minutes to answer the question, while the physician should sit calmly, listening and observing.

It is during this open-ended period that the physician listens for indicators of psychosis and observes the patient's overall behavior and appearance. Signs of organic mental disorder like diaphoresis or nystagmus can be detected during this period. The second phase of the interview requires that more specific information be obtained about the patient's illness, and the third phase includes an explanation to the patient about further examination and treatment.

INTERVIEWING THE UNRESTRAINED PATIENT

The self-referred patient who has violent impulses and is ''afraid of hurting someone'' may not require restraints but should be interviewed in a manner that adheres to the basic principles discussed in the following paragraphs.

Keep physical assistance nearby

When restraint has been accomplished or when the threat of violence has passed, the physician should ask all but one or two people to leave the room but remain nearby in case the patient becomes violent.

Maintain an open exit

If at all possible, the physician should not sit or stand in a location that blocks the patient's exit and the door should *remain open*. Leaving the exit open allays the patient's fears of being trapped and allows and provides an unencumbered egress if the patient decides to jump up and leave the room. The violent patient should not feel the need to go ''through'' the physician to get out. When the patient bolts out of the room, the physician must not try to intervene. The patient's recapture and restraint should be left to the police. An ideal interview setting is one that also permits the physician an easy way out of the interview area.

Maintain adequate distance

The physician should not offer to shake hands or reach toward the patient and should stand at least 8 feet away. Maintaining adequate ''distance'' protects the physician and avoids ''pressuring'' the hostile patient. The physician may move nearer as rapport is established but should not touch the patient until the physician explains the examination, describes precisely how it will proceed, and receives verbal permission from the patient.

Listen and sympathize

The sympathetic listening mode allows the patient to ventilate anger and frustration verbally instead of physically. It allows the physician to determine whether the violence is directed toward a person or institution, what kind of disorder the patient has, and whether it is a psychosis or an organic mental disorder. The experienced physician frequently nods in agreement and uses a low, calm, soothing tone of voice.

Promise anything

If the behavior becomes more agitated or violence erupts before adequate force is at hand, the physician may promise the patient anything he wants—drugs, release from the hospital, or admission to a medical ward. This may distract or defuse the patient temporarily until adequate force is available.

Avoid eye contact

Looking another person or any animal directly in the eye represents a personal challenge or threat (Fig. 6-5). This knowledge formed the basis for the ''Irish Dragoon Rule'' years ago when British soliders were instructed to keep their eyes downcast or straight ahead when marching through a conquered Irish village to avoid needlessly arousing the hostility of the villagers.

Maintain a submissive posture

Since the hostile patient is likely to respond violently to a challenge, the physician who adopts a rather submissive body posture may reduce the perceived challenge and likelihood of violence. A slightly slouched posture, turned somewhat away from the

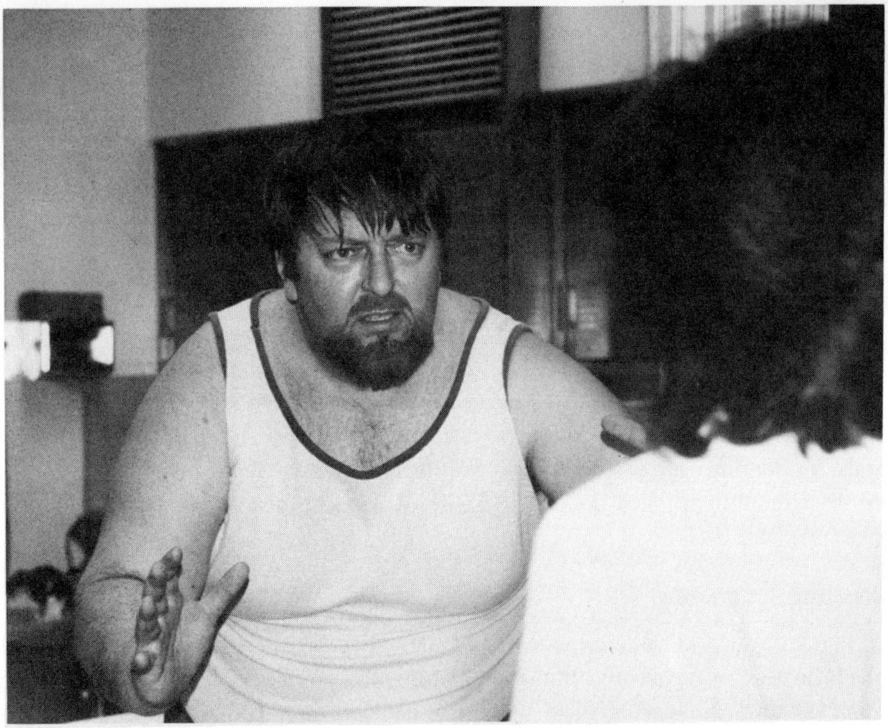

FIG. 6-5. Direct eye contact with potentially violent patient may precipitate aggressive outburst.

patient may be effective. In some ways this posture is like the submissive posture adopted by a conquered male wolf when approaching the leader of the pack. It signifies that there is no threat of aggression.

Be decisive

Decisiveness and swift action are appropriate when adequate resources are available to bring the situation under control. When indicated, appropriate medication should be given immediately. Violent patients are generally best managed by swift restraint, rapid medical evaluation, and the request for psychiatric consultation.

VIOLENT PATIENTS—CATEGORIES AND CAUSES

Several types of patients are likely to become violent. They end up being the same way (violent), but they have significant differences and their treatment depends on the cause or underlying disorder (Tables 6-1 and 6-2).

The intoxicated patient

Alcohol or drug intoxication causes most organic mental disorders in emergency patients and is most likely to cause violent behavior in this group. When possible, blood

TABLE 6-1. Violent patients: the symptoms

Diagnostic categories	*Clear sensorium*	*Delusions*	*Violent history*	*Grandiosity*	*Remorse*	*Overreaction to stressor within previous 3 months*
Self-referred, violent	+	−	−	−	+	+
Borderline	+	±	±	−	+	+
Psychotic with paranoid delusions	±	+	−	±	−	−
Intoxicated	−	−	±	±	±	−
Adjustment disorder	+	−	−	−	+	+
Personality disorder	+	−	+	−	−	−
Depression	+	−	−	−	+	−
Intermittent explosive disorder	+	−	+	−	+ +	+
Akathisia	+	−	−	−	+	−
Organic or postictal disorder	−	±	−	−	−	−

for toxicological testing should be drawn on every violent patient. Such a procedure is usually refused initially by the violent combatant. When calm, however, the patient may submit to a venipuncture. A urine sample may be the only fluid sample the patient provides, since taking blood may again be interpreted as an assault.

A patient who appears intoxicated should ideally be given no medication. Most intoxicated patients can be placed in a room with subdued lighting and attended by someone who speaks in a calm, reassuring manner. The patient can be assured that his condition will improve within a few hours. The intoxicated patient can almost invariably be "talked down" from his delirium. Small doses of phencyclidine cause an intoxication that responds best to a "minimum stimulation" regimen that may include medication with diazepam (Valium) for violent behavior. If the cause of psychosis is a hallucinogen like lysergic acid diethylamide (LSD) and it is absolutely clear that there is another process causing hallucinations and delusions, haloperidol (Haldol) generally quiets the patient and gradually restores his previous level of thinking and behavior.

Barbiturates are associated with the most dangerous and violent behavior in intoxicated patients. Barbiturates evidently cause a disinhibiting effect that allows belligerent and hostile behavior to surface easily. Contrary to popular opinion, the amphetamines do not normally produce dangerous behavior, although amphetamine intoxication can sometimes cause violent, agitated types of action. Generally speaking, "downers," like

TABLE 6-2. Violent patients: their treatment and disposition

Diagnostic categories	*Physical restraints*	*Chemical restraint*		*Problem solving*	*Outpatient medical treatment*	*Admission*
		Intramuscularly	*Orally*			
Self-referred	−	−	−	+	−	±
Borderline	−	−	−	+	−	±
Psychotic with paranoid delusions	±	±	+	−	+	+
Intoxicated	±	−	−	−	−	±
Adjustment disorder	−	−	± (Minor tranquilizer)	+ +	−	−
Personality disorder	±	−	−	+	−	−
Depression	±	−	−	+	+	±
Intermittent explosive disorder	±	−	−	+	+	−
Akathisia	−	+ (benztropine)	+ (benztropine)	−	+	−
Organic or postictal disorder	±	±	−	−	−	+

barbiturates, are associated with assaultive and violent behavior far more often than other kinds of medications. Use of the hallucinogens rarely results in violent behavior. When it does, it is because of a perceived threat associated with hallucinations. Alcohol intoxication results in more frequent episodes of violent behavior than abuses of other substances.

Any patient who appears to be intoxicated from alcohol should be at least passingly evaluated for mania. The presence of grandiosity, pressured speech, and euphoria suggests mania. Many people who are "high" because of a manic episode become involved in substance abuse and become intoxicated.

A disease state of *pathological intoxication* occurs when a patient becomes severely intoxicated on as small an amount as 2 to 4 ounces of alcohol. The patient may be amnestic for the period of intoxication. He should be hospitalized, observed, and allowed to "sleep it off," a process that may take many hours. An episode of pathological intoxication rarely lasts for more than a few hours.

The patient who has been abusing alcohol must be evaluated for the alcohol withdrawal syndrome. Since withdrawal syndromes can be fatal, hospitalization is indicated in many of these cases.

The patient could have sustained a head injury during the violent behavior and may require further neurological investigation. The intoxicated patient need not be restrained unless absolutely necessary, can usually be "talked down," and should unquestionably be held in the emergency department until sober. Many underlying organic or pathological features, obscured by intoxication, lend themselves to substance abuse and subsequent intoxication.

When it is suspected that the violent behavior is a result of drug or alcohol intoxication, medication is usually withheld initially even though a loud and belligerent patient creates a difficult problem in the emergency department. In the initial phase of management, the patient can be placed in a room with a staff member who works well with excited people. Usually the patient can be "talked down," and a thorough history can be obtained from the family, friends, or the patient himself.

Intoxicated patients may be admitted to a general medical service for diagnostic evaluation when the nature of the intoxication is unclear. Psychiatric consultation can be obtained for these hospitalized patients. If a detoxification unit is available and the patient seems to genuinely want to stop using drugs or alcohol, it is best to refer him to such a unit when he is sober.

Patients who come to the emergency department in an intoxicated state should always be given a referral to an appropriate agency that deals with drug or alcohol abuse. Even a "one-time drunk" may be a sign of an underlying pattern of some form of chemical abuse. While in the emergency department, the patient is still somewhat "shocked," his emotional defense mechanisms are lowered, and he is more likely to accept and follow straightforward, professionally given advice that explains the referral and answers his questions about his condition.

The adjustment disorder patient

The essential feature of an adjustment disorder is a maladaptive reaction to an identifiable stressor. The reaction occurs within 3 months after the onset of the stressor. Patients with this disorder overreact to a life event but not necessarily in any regular pattern. This type of disorder occasionally results in violent behavior. When it does, the stressor must be identified immediately. Since such a patient has already begun calming down by the time he gets to the emergency department, a sense of competent tranquility aids in his ability to be attentive to the examination.

By definition, the disturbance should begin within 3 months of the onset of the stressor. A history should uncover the events of the last 3 months. The examiner must ask about discrete events such as the loss of a job, a divorce, a separation from a loved one or spouse, the sudden discovery of a physical illness, or the death of a relative. When this information is obtained, a problem-solving activity can begin.

Focusing on a specific problem is in itself therapeutic. It is the *backbone of crisis intervention therapy*. After the stressor has been identified, the patient can begin working with the physician, examining alternate ways of handling it. This not only calms the patient, distracting him from his sense of anxiety or rage, but it also models problem-solving behavior. When the crisis passes, the physician can begin to search for a preexisting personality disorder or organic mental disorder. These two disorders predispose the patient to developing an adjustment disorder.

Once it is clear that the patient is overreacting to a life event, the focus of the interview is concentrated on the event itself. The patient should be encouraged to think of two or three alternate ways to deal with the stress, other than the method he is currently using. The patient may even be left alone with a pencil and paper and asked to write them down. It is important that the patient develop these alternatives rather than having them suggested to him. The patient usually sees the physician as a powerful person with a high level of education. This is important because adjustment disorders often occur after a rejection by an important loved person. The emergency department personnel, particularly the physician must therefore be acutely aware that the patient is highly sensitive to rejection. Approaching the patient with some warmth and a concerned appearance and tone of voice does a great deal to prevent furthering the sense of despair. This also deescalates belligerence or impending violent behavior. Reacting to the patient coldly or aloofly may precipitate increasingly hostile behavior.

Medication is not necessary. The patient's condition, if treated appropriately with this brief kind of psychotherapy, will improve. In addition, the patient may need no further psychiatric evaluation, particularly if he does not feel a need for such a referral. He may even be invited to return to the physician the next day to talk for 10 to 15 minutes. When the patient knows that someone is sympathetic to him and is available, he feels relieved. Other professionals in the community, such as a minister, priest, or rabbi, may be the most appropriate source for consultation to help the patient with problem-solving behavior.

The personality disorder patient

The belligerent or violent patient who has had problems on and off throughout his life should be evaluated for a personality disorder. We all have personality traits, which are ways of interpreting our world and ways of interacting with our environment and other people. It is only when these traits "get in the way" of the normal progress of life that they are pathological. If certain types of personality traits interfere with occupational or social functioning or cause subjective distress, they constitute a personality disorder. These disorders are generally recognized at the beginning of adolescence and may continue throughout the life of the individual unless intervention is attempted.

Differentiation of a personality disorder from an adjustment disorder (an overreaction to a stressor) is important because the patient with a personality disorder who is violent is likely to have had a history of belligerent or combative behavior. He is also likely to continue this behavior pattern in the future. Thus the differentiation between these two diagnoses has important implications for prognosis and preventive intervention.

Types of personality disorders

Paranoid personality disorder. The most typical personality disorder seen in violent patients is a *paranoid personality disorder*. This patient feels an all-present and unwarranted suspiciousness concerning other people. He has a narrow emotional life and is hypersensitive to criticism or perceived rejection. He is constantly looking around him to confirm his expectation that he is being manipulated or "used" by others. Usually these patients find some kernel of truth to their beliefs, and this gives rise to the concept of a "self-fulfilling prophesy"; what the patient believes to be true will become true, if he only looks hard enough. These people are often argumentative and appear tense. They often counterattack whenever they perceive a threat. Their misperception of the world around them, however, never reaches delusional proportions. The disorder is more often seen in men. They may get into a fight in a bar or other social gathering where they feel that they are being laughed at, stared at, or in some way ridiculed. They react violently to these perceived threats and provoke a fight. The fight validates their view that others are out to "get them."

Antisocial personality. Another commonly diagnosed personality disorder in patients who become violent is the *antisocial personality*. These patients have a history of trampling over the rights of others. This pattern of behavior persists from childhood into adult life. The symptoms begin before the age of 15. There is usually an early history of truancy or setting fires. The older patient exhibits failure to maintain a job, drunkenness, and marital chaos. These patients typically have a history of lying, stealing, cheating, defying authority, childhood aggression, precocious sexual behavior, excessive drinking, and substance abuse.

They may be charming, although superficial in their interaction with others, and they do not appear particularly anxious. They may enjoy frightening others and wielding their fearlessness with obvious enjoyment. They are, nonetheless, potentially violent and lack remorse for their actions. Since these patients are not always as anxious as those around them during the violent behavior, their actions may be particularly methodical.

Patients with antisocial personality disorder often complain of feeling tense and have many somatic complaints. They are frequently bored and depressed and do not have any long-term relationships. These patients have difficulty becoming self-sustaining adults and may be in constant conflict with the law. Substance abuse and aggressive behavior are the most common complications of the disorder. After the age of 30, the more flagrant aspects of this disorder tend to diminish; if the antisocial personality disorder is going to improve, it does so between the ages of 30 and 40. No known psychiatric treatment at the present time is useful in treating this disorder.

This disorder begins before the age of 15 by definition. A similar picture occurring clearly after the age of 15 should give rise to consideration of other diagnoses, including organic mental disorder or an adjustment disorder.

Borderline personality disorder. Patients with the borderline personality disorder have severe problems in interpersonal relationships. These relationships are usually marred by intense and stormy outbursts. Borderline patients are generally unpredictable and have sudden outbursts of intense anger stimulated by relatively trivial circumstances. They can become intensely angry, often at members of the family or close friends. They frequently have severe problems in their sense of self-identity, and it is typical for them to feel chronically empty and bored. They often consider themselves "odd" or eccentric, are "loners," and may be perceived as "strange" by others.

These patients are unpredictable and labile. They alternate between being extremely dependent on others and very independent and assertive. Under severe stress they may shows signs of reality distortion, depression, and a clinical picture resembling psychosis. These patients usually have had great difficulty maintaining their jobs and rarely have long-term, satisfying personal relationships. Their history is usually one of the tumultuous occupational and interpersonal failures.

The diagnosis of borderline personality appears to be becoming more common, as it is called to the attention of more clinicians. The disorder is far more common among men than women. This diagnosis should not be made in a patient younger than 18 years.

Histrionic personality. Patients with histrionic personalities are usually female, overly dramatic, reactive, and intensely expressive. They have severe disturbances in interpersonal relationships. A typical onset of violent behavior may occur after drinking. The patient abruptly becomes agitated or excited over some trivial argument. Suddenly the patient is expansive, dramatic, and angry. The attention this attracts escalates the angry behavior and may result in violence. This patient is often brought to the emergency department as the center of a great deal of attention. It is notable that the more people who are watching the patient, the more likely it is that the patient's behavior will escalate.

These patients should be removed from the center of attention. They should be seen by only one person at a time, and this person should preferably be a male if the patient is a female. The patient then tends to thrive on the one-to-one relationship and tries to meet the expectations of a powerful authority figure. Usually this calms the patient almost immediately. She should ideally be listened to at some length without interruption and can generally be sent home after this period of listening.

Treatment for the personality disorder. Once the diagnosis of a personality disorder has been made, certain steps can be taken. The patient will probably not respond to hospitalization in any dramatic or meaningful way. He should only be hospitalized if the situation to which he is to return is explosive. For instance, if there is an ongoing family conflict, sending the patient back into it is asking for trouble. The same is true of a troubled marriage, severe difficulties with children, or problems with the parents of these patients. A 1- to 5-day hospitalization may be indicated in these situations. During the hospitalization, therapy can be started with crisis intervention techniques, and the patient can be prepared for continued psychiatric treatment after hospitalization.

Most patients with a personality disorder do not respond to inpatient treatment except on a long-term basis. Therefore the appropriate referral source should be to an outpatient setting where the patient can receive ongoing psychotherapy or counseling. No medication should be given to these patients, despite their request for it. Patients with personality disorders often seek external treatment for ongoing internal conflicts. They tend to perceive the world as out of step, rather than their own behavior as the problem. Therefore it is important, as soon as the patient is seen in the emergency department, to get him to reflect on the idea that he may have some difficulties in his style of relating to others. The patient should realize that the problem can be investigated and that help is available. The physician should point out that many people have such difficulties, and it is not a weakness to talk it over with a trained professional. An appointment should be made as close as possible to the time that the patient is seen in the emergency department. This is because these patients tend to react defensively against intervention, since they perceive that the causes of their problems are often individuals or circumstances, rather than their own behavior.

The self-referred violent patient

A common complaint in the emergency department by patients is that they feel they might kill someone, they are going to kill their spouse or they want to hurt someone for no reason. A variation on this theme is the common complaint of a young mother who becomes afraid of knives or other dangerous objects because she is fearful that she may use them on her infant child.[5]

Such a patient may already have acted violently or belligerently. More often, however, these patients feel that they are on the verge of doing so. These self-referred patients should not be falsely reassured. They require careful evaluation, and the physician should believe them. It is important to assure these patients that they will not be allowed to act in a dangerous way. This can be done by alerting the staff to assemble a security force to stand by. This does not frighten the patient but should, in fact, lessen anxiety. These patients are actually afraid of losing control. A strong security force represents an external control force to assure that the patient will be brought under control if internal restraints are eroded.

The decision to hospitalize depends on what the patient says. The patient who is afraid of losing control of his impulses should probably be hospitalized. These patients should always be taken seriously, even if the physician has doubts that the patient will carry through his threats. If the patient requests hospitalization, arrangements must be made for admission. If a transfer to a psychiatric hospital is necessary, an ambulance team and attendants should transport the patient.

Neurological disorders may cause certain fears. The patient may experience headaches, odd sensations, altered states of consciousness, or auras. He may experience odd compulsions, alien to his own life-style. Since complex partial (or temporal lobe) seizures can cause these signs, the physician should ask about appropriate symptoms. Relatives or friends should also be questioned about recent personality change, and a family history of neurological disorders such as epilepsy or recent head trauma should be obtained to screen for the possibility of intracranial infection or neoplasm. The physician should listen carefully to the patient who feels that he is losing control and should avoid a quick reassurance.

The patient who seems to feel better after ventilating feelings to an understanding person could be given a small dose of haloperidol or thioridazine (Mellaril) and sent home with instructions to return for a psychiatric appointment. Two or three tablets of haloperidol (2 mg) or thioridazine (10 or 25 mg) should be sufficient. Minor tranquilizers such as diazepam or chlordiazepoxide (Librium) may occasionally cause a paradoxical reaction, including hyperactivity or agitation. The patient should experience a feeling of control if he takes the medication when he feels that it is necessary over the following 24 hours. The emergency staff should give the patient a number he may call the next morning for an appointment, and they should instruct him to return to the emergency department if he feels the same violent impulse again. The patient who claims that he cannot control his impulses or who requests hospitalization should be admitted at least until psychiatric evaluation can be completed.

Psychotic patients with paranoid delusions

If the interview reveals that the patient holds a delusional belief that violence is only a defense against people who are trying to cause harm, there is no need to disagree. In fact, the examining physician should try to become the patient's ally and agree with the delusional system. Statements such as "I'm on your side" make the patient more comfortable and communicative. Once the patient includes the emergency department personnel in his paranoid delusional system and feels that they too are against him, all forms of treatment become more difficult.

The patient with a paranoid delusional system is most dangerous, since he is extremely unpredictable. The patient is responding to internal stimuli, rather than real events. "Voices" may be telling him to hurt or kill others, or because of his complete reality distortion, he may misinterpret the actions of others and react as though they are attacking him. Once it is established that the patient is suffering from a paranoid delusional system, treatment should begin. Sensory overstimulation produced by loud noises, bright lights, and rapid movement or speech create anxiety and may precipitate violence.

Oral medication is preferred to intramuscular medication if the patient will accept it. An intramuscular injection may be perceived as a physical assault by the psychotic patient. He should be approached calmly and told that he is going to receive some medication that will help him calm down and be able to handle the situation more easily. The patient can be given some water to help him swallow the medication.

Oral medication is not as quickly absorbed as an intramuscular dose, but the time difference is not great (often as little as 15 minutes), and even the suggestion of intramuscular medication may precipitate violent behavior. Furthermore, a psychotic patient is likely to misinterpret the meaning of "the needle" and continue to distort this later.

The depressed patient

Sometimes people who are becoming severely depressed also may become enraged and angry. These patients direct their rage outwardly and may become violent, rather than acting on themselves, as in the case of a suicide. These patients are intensely angry and are enraged at a primitive level. They feel they have little to lose and may even be seeking out punishment or self-destructive responses to their actions. They may goad a policeman or other authority to shoot them or in some way attack them. When these patients are brought to the emergency department, they continue this sort of behavior. They invite rejection, punishment, and abuse. Within a brief period of time of interacting with these patients, it becomes evident that they are severely depressed.

Any show of concern on the part of the physician usually results in the patient bursting into tears and having difficulty controlling his tearfulness. This is cathartic and therapeutic and should be encouraged with such statements as, "I know how you must feel. It's all right to cry. This will help you." Once this step has been taken, spending some time with the patient or having one of the emergency department personnel spend time with him is the best treatment. This person does not require treatment of any sort at this time. Setting up a firm follow-up appointment with the specific time and place for the next day is helpful. The appointment should be one with a psychiatrist or other physician who can begin antidepressant medication. Giving the patient a sleeping medication for one night helps him through to the next day. Making sure that the patient does not feel suicidal at the time and giving him a telephone number that he can call at any time until his appointment is most important. The patient should go home with someone he trusts and knows, rather than going home by himself.

Intermittent explosive disorder

The intermittent explosive disorder is both puzzling to the examining physician and the patient. This patient is calm by the time the physician sees him. The short episode of violence during which the patient exploded and became belligerent or violent has passed. The explosive behavior, however, may have resulted in a serious injury or destruction of property. Apparently these patients have no real provocation and react grossly out of proportion to any stress. They frequently refer to their "attacks" or "fits." The major hallmark of this disorder is the tremendous amount of remorse and guilt that the patient feels. The expression of grief includes a great deal of tearfulness and sorrow for any damage done.

These people are often overly self-controlled and somewhat too conscientious between episodes. They do not show signs of general impulsivity or lack of control. Their behavior is usually a surprise to those around them. They feel that an irresistible force has pushed them into such behavior. They may have some amnesia for the events precipitating the explosion.

Sometimes these patients have nonspecific electroencephalogram (EEG) abnormalities or minor neurological signs and symptoms, thought to reflect subcortical or limbic system dysfunction. Epilepsy is more common in these individuals than in those without the disorder. The history often reveals childhood hyperactivity and proneness to accidents. With more than one or two of these episodes, the patient is shunned to some extent. Social and occupational impairment may result. Any condition conducive to organic brain dysfunction or the use of substances such as alcohol may precipitate the explosive disorder.

Patients with an intermittent explosive disorder should be referred to a psychiatrist who can do a reasonable neurological evaluation and consider various forms of medication. It can be indicated to them that they may have an unusual condition that requires further medical and psychiatric attention. No medication should be given. Consideration of the use of antiseizure medications may be made after further evaluation, but it is not worthwhile in the initial management.

Akathisia

Akathisia is an extrapyramidal disorder caused by phenothiazines. The major feature of akathisia is that the patient feels agitated and experiences the uncontrollable desire to move about. Akathisia is a subjective desire to be in constant motion, with a feeling of inner agitation and muscle tension. The patient typically cannot sit still and paces constantly. It is possible that after using fairly high doses of neuroleptic medication on an acute or chronic basis, a patient may develop akathisia. The patient feels a tremendous need to walk or pace and move constantly. If the patient is already quite anxious, has had some recent stresses, or has been feeling angry, this sensation reinforces his need to act in a hostile and angry fashion. The patient becomes increasingly agitated and feels more tense; he may be given more neuroleptic medication either orally or parenterally. The additional medication accentuates the feeling of a need to act out his muscular tension. This may eventually result in explosive, violent behavior in the emergency department and should be thought of when a patient becomes paradoxically worse while receiving neuroleptic medication for high levels of tension or anger.[6]

The treatment for akathisia is benztropine (Cogentin). Since the half-life of haloperidol is about 24 hours, the patient is given an initial dose of 2 mg benztropine (orally or intramuscularly) and is given 2 mg twice a day for 2 days.

The organic postictal patient

The patient who has an organic deficit or has recently had a seizure can be violent. He is misperceiving the world around him because of metabolic derangements and transient dysfunction of the central nervous system. Because these patients become confused, they may distort reality, become frightened, and ultimately become belligerent. They may strike out against others. Most organic disorders require attention to the underlying cause. The postictal patient can be treated with verbal reassurance in a quiet room that has subdued lighting. Physical restraints are avoided when possible. Occasionally it is helpful to invite a family member or familiar person to be with the patient.

Generally, medication should be withheld until there is some certainty about the cause of the underlying organic disorder. However, if the patient is combative, violent, and unwilling to cooperate with any investigative procedures, it may be necessary to treat him with chemical restraint. Intravenous, fast-acting barbiturates for rapid treatment of postictal violence may be useful for this purpose. Since some phenothiazines lower the seizure threshhold, they should be used with caution in the postictal patient.

RAPID TRANQUILIZATION

If the patient has become violent and has required physical restraint, intramuscular neuroleptic medication such as haloperidol (5 mg) is indicated. In many ways chemical restraint is more humane for brief periods of time than physical restraints. It is probably also safer for the patient. A technique called *rapid tranquilization* is highly effective in controlling delusions and hallucinations within 1 to 3 hours.

Rapid tranquilization is accomplished by administering 5 to 10 mg of haloperidol intramuscularly every 30 to 60 minutes up to a total 24-hour dosage of 50 mg or until the symptoms of psychosis subside (Fig. 6-6). When the patient is no longer violent, the oral form of the medication may be given.

The antipsychotic medications like haloperidol are also effective in certain organic psychoses. The major exception is psychosis caused by anticholinergic poisoning. The anticholinergic properties of the antipsychotic may increase the overall toxicity and aggravate the symptoms.

The violent patient must be watched closely during the period of rapid tranquilization. Vital signs should be monitored, and the patient should be watched for dystonia. Restraints may be left in place until the psychosis is controlled and the patient is nonviolent.

The use of minor tranquilizers is contraindicated in the management of the violent patient. Minor tranquilizers may lower the patient's inhibition and cause a paradoxical response, and the patient may become more agitated. Minor tranquilizers do not affect psychotic symptoms such as hallucination or delusions.

The psychotic violent patient probably suffers from schizophrenia or mania, although as usual, organic disorders must be carefully excluded. These patients usually require psychiatric hospitalization and appropriate treatment. Schizophrenics require neuroleptic drugs administered in the hospital, and patients with affective disorders may require lithium therapy as well. The physician may fear that enforced hospitalization

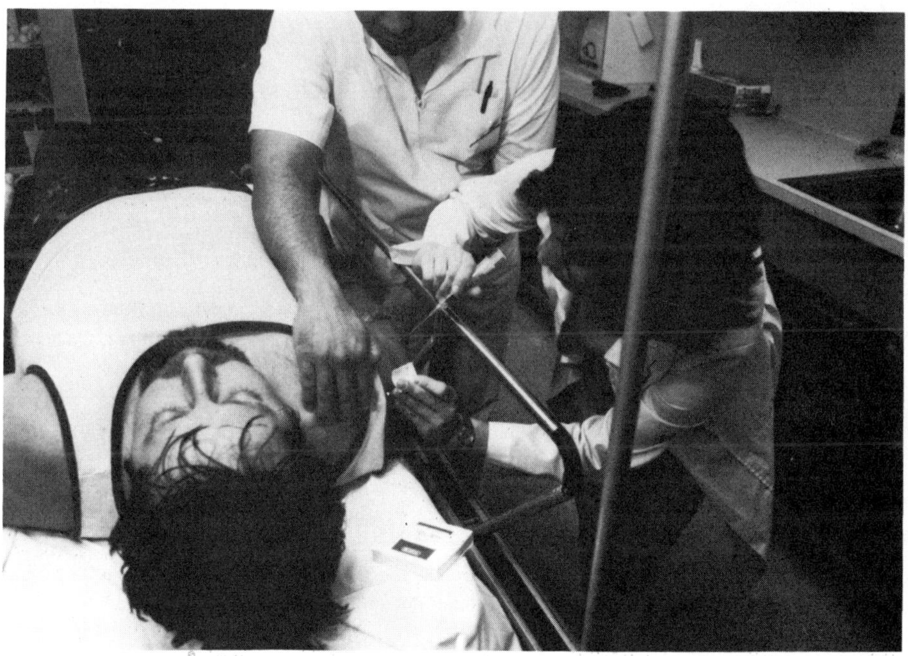

FIG. 6-6. Intramuscular haloperidol provides means of rapid tranquilization for violent patient.

may result in retaliation. This fear is completely unfounded. The patient, in retrospect, is thankful for the treatment he has received and indeed feels better almost immediately on being told he requires hospitalization because he knows his potentially violent behavior is going to be controlled. It is always important to remember that the patient is as frightened by his loss of control as those witnessing it. Occasionally psychiatric assessment may result in a patient being sent home with appropriate medication and a follow-up appointment. When in doubt, admission is the best course.

PATIENT CONSENT

A fundamental medical-legal principle is that the patient must consent to diagnostic or treatment procedures performed by medical personnel. Under certain circumstances, however, the patient may either be incapable of making a rational decision, or he may be an immediate danger to others. In these cases the physician has a duty to follow proper procedures for dealing with the patient's management without his consent. The fundamental process for proceeding against the patient's will is a determination by the court that the patient is incompetent to make the decision to refuse treatment (boxed material on this page).[7]

Early steps

When such a determination is necessary, the physician must begin to gather and document information related to competence. Evidence of psychosis includes the patient's hallucinations, delusions, loose associations, and bizarre thought content. The

PROCEDURES TO FOLLOW WHEN THE VIOLENT OR SEVERELY DISTURBED PATIENT REFUSES TREATMENT

1. Gather and document information related to competence and/or threats toward others.
2. Contact the patient's family, appropriate hospital administrator, and hospital attorney.
3. Contact probate court or judicial authority responsible for civil commitment.
4. Begin court action to have the patient declared incompetent.
5. Proceed with medical treatment against the patient's will:
   a. If the condition poses an immediate, significant, and irreversible loss of physical or mental health to the patient or to another person, *and*
   b. If the loss will occur before a competency hearing can be arranged, *and*
   c. If a medical treatment is available to prevent the loss, *and*
   d. If the court will most likely consider the person incompetent
6. Arrange for police arrest if the condition is not a medical emergency, if the person is competent, and if the hospital administrator and judicial officials so decide.

Adapted from Perry, SW, and Gilmore, MM. The disruptive patient or visitor. *Journal of the American Medical Association*, 1981, *245*(7), 755-757.

best pieces of evidence for making a determination of incompetence are sometimes the patient's own words; statements that he makes in front of witnesses can be documented and used later if substantiation of incompetence needed. Statements like, "the psyches are after me, and I need to fight back," indicate a serious paranoid delusional system, bizarre thought content, and probably hallucinations. The emergency physician should not hesitate to declare the psychotic violent patient incompetent.

The patient's witnessed actions provide good evidence for incompetence and/or danger to others. Violent actions or bizarre gestures support the declaration of incompetence. A clear history of bizarre or totally inappropriate behavior, obtained from the police or EMS personnel, is generally good evidence of at least temporary incompetence, especially in the violent patient. The physician or nursing staff then contacts the patient's family, the appropriate hospital administrator, and the hospital attorney.

The next step involves contacting the probate court or appropriate judicial agency for civil commitment. When the judge or his designee is contacted, the physician must explain the reason for proceeding with evaluation and treatment against the patient's will, and a temporary court order must be obtained. Most states have provisions in their law that allow a physician to detain a patient against his will if he is incompetent to make a rational decision about his health that is likely to result in harm to himself or others. The clinician is on safest ground, however, when these decisions are made in concert with administrative authorities, attorneys, and judicial officials experienced in such matters. When it is not possible to contact such persons, the physician must proceed in a way that benefits the patient even though charges of assault and battery can follow. Failing to act on the patient's behalf can result in injury to the patient and charges of negligence.

If the physician must pick one person to notify about the proceedings, it should be the patient's closest relative. When possible, the relative should give written permission for the treatment on behalf of the patient.

Documentation

Adequate documentation about the necessity for proceeding with evaluation and treatment against the patient's expressed wishes helps protect the physician and hospital from subsequent legal liability. The emergency department's record should show the following features of the patient's behavior when applicable:

1. Statements in the patient's own words about himself wanting to or planning to hurt others
2. A description of how the patient looks and acts
3. Historical and/or physical evidence suggesting the presence of medical or psychiatric conditions severe enough that withholding treatment may cause imminent significant, possibly permanent, damage to the person's physical or mental health

INVOLUNTARY COMMITMENT

The two major historical legal bases for involuntary civil commitment statutes for the mentally ill are the doctrine that the state has an obligation to care for those who cannot care for themselves *(parens patriae)* and the obligation of the state to keep the peace.[7] Most states have civil commitment statutes that are based on these historical tenets.

The *California Civil Commitment Statute,* for instance, provides time-limited involuntary treatment of individuals who need psychiatric care but are unwilling or unable to accept it. This statute states that such a person can be committed to medical psychiatric care if evaluation by a police officer, authorized medical professional, or court official reveals that the patient is probably a danger to others, a danger to himself, or gravely disabled. If there is continued impairment, the initial commitment can be extended by 14 days.

Since each state has its own specific statute regarding involuntary commitment, each department's policy for managing these patients should be tailored to the specific requirements of the law. In general, however, the initiation of treatment should proceed, while the physician attempts to obtain a court order to evaluate or treat a patient against his will. The prediction of violent behavior from clinical data obtained in the emergency department requires further research and has been the focus of recent investigations.

Generally, whenever the emergency physician wishes to commit the patient to involuntary psychiatric hospitalization because of dangerous behavior, disability, or psychiatric impairment, it is most helpful to have the benefit of a psychiatric consultation to support these conclusions. The psychiatrist can make a tentative diagnosis and set the tone for subsequent treatment before hospitalization. The psychiatric testimony may also be important in any subsequent legal proceedings.

When psychiatric consultation is not available, however, the emergency physician must act in the patient's best interests, with the assistance of the patient's family, the hospital administration, and the court.

Once the patient has been formally committed for evaluation and treatment, the physician may use the degree of force necessary to hold him in custody, including police restraint and transportation, if needed.

The violent patient who escapes

When the violent or potentially violent patient escapes, the emergency staff has the obligation to document the proceedings and notify the police. The problem of the violent person then becomes one covered by the general doctrine that the state must keep the peace.

PHYSICIAN LIABILITY

Physicians are generally concerned about legal constraints in treating the violent patient. It may be an oversimplification, but it should be remembered that physicians can be sued for assault and battery if they treat a patient against his will. However, they can also be sued for negligence if they fail to treat a patient who is in dire need of available aid. Generally the physician should use good judgment, document it well on the chart, and do what must be done to prevent the patient from endangering himself or others. Legal battles are held later and often depend on chart documentation. The physician's statement on the chart should not be too cold or clinical since this does not sound empathetic when subsequently reviewed by a jury or other professionals.

SUMMARY

Though the violent patient is dramatic and frightening, he must be understood so that proper treatment can be initiated. Although the immediate approach to all types of violent patients may include physical or chemical restraints, the emergency physician must look further into the cause of the symptoms of violence. There are very few causes of violent behavior. In all but one (antisocial personality disorder), treatment can begin immediately. Treatment is generally straight-forward, is specific, and has implications for the prevention of further violence. Thus it is very likely that the emergency physician can become instrumental in reducing the number of assaults, murders, and other violent behaviors in our society. Just as clinicians do not panic over severe trauma or cardiac arrest, they need not feel at a loss in the treatment of the violent patient.

One of the most important issues that can be addressed by the emergency physician is in-service training for the staff concerning the diagnosis and treatment of violent behavior. Every emergency department should have a specific plan for dealing with the violent patient. Alarm systems should be checked out periodically. ''Dry runs'' should be tried to test the system. Role playing and discussing fantasies about violent patients should be part of emergency staff training. It also helps to demystify the frightening concept of the violent patient.

REFERENCES

1. Kaplan, HI, Freedman, AM, and Sadock, BJ. *Comprehensive textbook of psychiatry* (3rd ed.). Baltimore: The Williams & Wilkins Co., 1980.
2. Rada, RT. The violent patient: rapid assessment and management. *Psychosomatics,* 1981, *27*(2), 101-109.
3. Rund, DA. Psychiatric emergencies. In *Essentials of emergency medicine,* Norwalk, Conn.: Appleton-Century-Crofts, 1982.
4. Perry, SW, Gilmore, MM. The disruptive patient or visitor. *Journal of the American Medical Association,* 1981, *243*(7), 755-757.
5. Lion, JR, Rach-y-Rita, G, and Ervin, FR. The self-referred violent patient. *Journal of the American Medical Association,* 1968, *205,* 91-93.
6. Keckich, WA. Violence as a manifestation of akathisia. *Journal of the American Medical Association,* 1978, *240,* 2185.
7. Yesavage, JA, et al. Short-term civil commitment and the violent patient. *The American Journal of Psychiatry,* 1982, *139*(9), 1145-1149.
8. Monahan, J. Prediction research and the emergency commitment of dangerous mentally ill persons: a reconsideration. *American Journal of Psychiatry,* 1978, *135,* 198-201.
9. Monahan, J. Strategies for an empirical analysis of the prediction of violence in emergency civil commitment. *Law and Human Behavior,* 1977, *1,* 363-371.
10. American Psychiatric Association. *Task force report 8: clinical aspects of the violent individual.* Washington, D.C.: The Association, 1974.
11. Rofman, ES, Askinazi, C, and Fant, E. The prediction of dangerous behavior in emergency civil commitment. *American Journal of Psychiatry,* 1980, *137,* 1061-1064.
12. Yesavage, JA, et al. Inpatient evaluation of aggression in psychiatric patients. *Journal of Nervous and Mental Disease,* 1981, *169,* 299-302.

7 SUBSTANCE USE DISORDERS

Even the novice emergency physician soon realizes that a large portion of emergency patients have disorders that are somehow related to the use of alcohol or drugs; these patients seem to appear more frequently in the nighttime population in urban hospitals. They may be intoxicated, in states of withdrawal, or suffering from illness or injury created by drug or alcohol abuse. Intoxicated patients may be brought in by the police for "medical clearance" before being incarcerated, or the patient may request help for a drug problem. Some may be trying to feign illness to obtain drugs.

The appearance of these patients may be overtly unappealing. The malodorous, ataxic, unkempt, unshaven inebriate who staggers into the emergency department and retches in the reception area creates an easily discernible and quite unpopular clinical portrait. By contrast, the appearance may be subtle. The patient may be a well-dressed housewife or business executive who, when deprived of the customary alcohol or barbiturate intake for several days, experiences irritability, palpitations, diaphoresis, depression, or a full-blown withdrawal syndrome.

Alcohol and drug use disorders are clearly contributors in many cases of "accidental" trauma and violence,[1] and they produce secondary medical and psychiatric illnesses that require treatment. The most predictable reactions of the emergency staff to these patients are ones of revulsion, disgust, and anger. This easily understood and quite human response is not the most therapeutic one, however, and it may lead to a violent confrontation or missed diagnosis of a serious medical problem.

This chapter focuses on diagnostic criteria that pertain to substance abuse proposed by the American Psychiatric Association in the DSM-III. Where appropriate, a few basic strategies of management are considered. The detailed management of acute and chronic intoxication for each individual substance can be found in other references.[2,3]

SUBSTANCE USE, ABUSE, AND DEPENDENCE

Recognizing that caffeine, tobacco, alcohol, and, to a lesser extent, other recreational drug use is widespread in our society, the American Psychiatric Association has conceptualized the substance *user* as one without a mental disorder and the substance *abuser* as an individual with a mental disorder. The DSM-III thus distinguishes the nonpathological substance user who takes drugs for recreational or medical purposes from the substance abuser. The patient with substance dependence abuses drugs and also manifests tolerance to increasing doses of a drug or a withdrawal syndrome that develops when the patient stops taking the drug. All these patterns of substance use are

TABLE 7-1. Characteristics of substance use, abuse, and dependence

	Substance use	*Substance abuse*	*Substance dependence*
Substance use	+	+	+
Pattern of pathological use		+	+
Impairment of social function as a result of substance use		+	+
Impairment of occupational functioning as a result of substance use		+	+
Duration of disturbance for at least 1 month		+	+
Tolerance			+
Withdrawal			+

defined in the DSM-III, which describes the use of substances that modify mood or behavior: substance use, abuse, and dependence. The basic characteristics of these patterns are shown in Table 7-1.

Substance use

Substance use means that the patient ingests or smokes a substance that alters mood or behavior. Substance use ranges from the widely practiced use of coffee, tobacco, and alcohol to the occasional use of minor tranquilizers or cannabis. Patients included in this category do not have major impairment in social or occupational function and do not exhibit a pattern of pathological use. Since most adults occasionally use some sort of substance for stimulation or relaxation (e.g., caffeine, tobacco, or alcohol), the category carries no pathological significance but is used primarily for research purposes and to provide a fuller clinical portrait of patients with other psychiatric disorders.

Substance abuse

Pathological use of the substance is determined when the abuser consumes an amount far in excess of that used for recreational or medical needs, when the patient feels he cannot function without the substance, and when unsafe preparation of the substances is injected in a desperate attempt to "get high." The specific patterns of pathological use of alcohol and drugs are outlined in the discussion regarding each disorder. Alcohol syndromes are considered in Chapter 8.

A diagnosis of substance abuse requires three criteria, as shown in the box on page 98.[4]

Substance dependence

A diagnosis of substance dependence relies on the presence of tolerance or withdrawal in addition to certain symptoms. Tolerance means that as time progresses the

A. *Pattern of pathological use:* inability to cut down or stop use; intoxication throughout the day; frequent use of the equivalent of 600 mg or more of secobarbital or 60 mg or more of diazepam; amnesic periods for events that occurred while intoxicated.
B. *Impairment in social or occupational functioning due to substance use:* e.g., fights, loss of friends, absence from work, loss of job, or legal difficulties (other than a single arrest due to possession, purchase, or sale of the substance).
C. Duration of disturbance of at least 1 month.

From American Psychiatric Association. *Diagnostic and statistical manual of mental disorders* (3rd ed.). Washington, D.C.: The Association, 1980.

Tolerance: Need for markedly increased amounts of the substance to achieve the desired effect, or markedly diminished effect with regular use of the same amount.

Withdrawal: Development of Barbiturate or Similarly Acting Sedative or Hypnotic Withdrawal after cessation of or reduction in substance use.

From American Psychiatric Association. *Diagnostic and statistical manual of mental disorders* (3rd ed.). Washington, D.C.: The Association, 1980.

patient must take greater amounts of the substance to achieve the desired effect. Another way of viewing this is the observation that the patient remains relatively asymptomatic at blood levels of alcohol or drugs that would severely impair the nondependent individual.

Cessation of drug or alcohol intake for 12 to 72 hours in substance-dependent patients produces a withdrawal syndrome specific to the substance. The presence of these withdrawal symptoms confirms the diagnosis of substance dependence.

Five classes of substances are associated with abuse and dependence. They are the following:

1. Alcohol
2. Barbiturates
3. Opioids
4. Amphetamines
5. Cannabis

Drugs that are similar in action to barbiturates and amphetamines are included under their respective headings. Cocaine, phencyclidine (PCP), and hallucinogens do not produce tolerance or withdrawal; they are substances that create drug abuse but not drug dependence.

Alcohol. Alcohol syndromes are so common in emergency practice that they are considered separately in Chapter 8.

Sedative-hypnotic agents. The patterns of sedative-hypnotic abuse and dependence are like those for similarly acting drugs such as the benzodiazepines (diazepam and chlordiazepoxide), ethchlorvynol (Placidyl), glutethimide (Doriden), methaqualone (Quaalude, Sopor), and barbiturates. The overall discussion of diagnosis for abuse and withdrawal of these agents is similar in many respects to that of barbiturates.

The benzodiazepines are considered by many to be the "safest" of all the hypnotics because, when used alone in large doses, (e.g., taken in a suicide attempt) they rarely cause death.[5] When taken in combination with other substances like alcohol.[6] however, they can precipitate severe central nervous system (CNS) depression and death.

Other sedative-hypnotics like ethclorvynol, glutethimide, and methaqualone can cause severe toxicity when taken in overdoses and are involved in cases when single or multiple substances are taken for their psychotropic effects.

Barbiturates. Barbiturates are discussed as the prototype of this class of agents in the DSM-III, perhaps because both acute and chronic toxicity are so dangerous and because, unlike alcohol or opioids, the lethal dose level of barbiturates does not increase as tolerance develops. The barbiturate user may thus rapidly approach the lethal range with steady increases in daily dose. The barbiturate-dependent patient is therefore at greater risk for sudden, possibly inadvertent overdose, causing respiratory depression, coma, and death when he takes only a small amount of drugs in excess of the customary daily dose.

Patients with barbiturate abuse seem to fall into two patterns: young patients in the teens or twenties who use barbiturates "to get high" and older patients who typically begin their barbiturate use legally for medical purposes with hypnotics prescribed by a physician to temporarily relieve insomnia. The latter patients eventually use greater and greater quantities throughout the day to ease the tensions and relieve the stress of daily living and may eventually become dependent.

The diagnosis of barbiturate intoxication is suspected when the patient is noted to be ataxic and dysarthric without the accompanying odor of alcohol. A toxicology screen of the blood shows toxic barbiturate levels and confirms the diagnosis.

Barbiturate abuse can be diagnosed when criteria similar to those for alcohol abuse are present: a pattern of pathological use, impairment in social or occupational functioning as a result of barbiturate use, and a duration of use greater than 1 month.

Barbiturate dependence is diagnosed when tolerance or withdrawal are observed. Tolerance occurs when greater amounts of the drug are required to produce the same level of euphoria or clinical intoxication. As mentioned previously, this phenomenon causes the abuser to gradually increase the daily ingestion and come dangerously close to a lethal dose.

Barbiturate withdrawal. Barbiturate withdrawal may be more severe and potentially lethal than other withdrawal syndromes. Grand mal seizures, delirium, and cardiovascular collapse are the most serious components of barbiturate withdrawal and usually occur around the third day of abstinence. Milder clinical features include anxiety, insomnia, weakness, and diaphoresis. A previous habitual dose of 600 mg per day may be enough to produce a serious withdrawal illness.

Tolerance: need for markedly increased amounts of opioid to achieve the desired effect, or markedly diminished effect with regular use of the same amount.

Withdrawal: development of Opioid Withdrawal after cessation of or reduction in substance use.

From American Psychiatric Association. *Diagnostic and statistical manual of mental disorders* (3rd ed.). Washington, D.C.: The Association, 1980.

The patient may show signs of psychosis. Hallucinations are commonly visual but may be auditory as well. Barbiturate withdrawal is clearly part of the differential diagnosis when a psychotic patient is encountered in the emergency department.

The patient with barbiturate dependence clearly needs supervised detoxification because of the tremendous lethality of tolerance and withdrawal. Detoxification usually consists of a program in which the patient is started on a dose of barbiturates near the normal daily dose, and it is gradually tapered over days or weeks. Phenobarbital, a longer-acting barbiturate, is often used for this purpose; about 30 mg of phenobarbital is substituted for each 100 mg of pentobarbital or secobarbital ordinarily taken by the patient.

Barbiturate amnestic disorder is similar to that associated with alcohol. In barbiturate amnestic disorder, the patient retains no memory of events that occurred while intoxicated, even though he appeared to be conscious and aware during that period. The disorder usually lasts a few hours to a few days and is generally associated with full recovery.

Opioids (narcotics). The opioids include morphine, heroin, meperidine, opium, and hydromorphone (Dilaudid). Both the intravenous and oral routes are used by opioid abusers. The diagnosis of opioid abuse and dependence are made according to the DSM-III criteria, which are quite similar to those for sedative-hypnotic abuse and dependence.

Opioid-dependent patients typically create dilemmas for the emergency physician in at least three ways: they simulate physical illness (like a kidney stone) to obtain narcotics; they are brought to the department as a case of drug overdose; or they have real illness or injury that is complicated by concurrent narcotic intoxication or withdrawal.

Patients who want to obtain narcotics frequently simulate physical illnesses that commonly cause great pain. The "ideal" illnesses for this purpose, like ureterolithiasis and migraine headache, produce few confirming physical findings. More sophisticated schemes involve an alleged out-of-state physician calling in for his patient, who supposedly suffers from a malignant neoplasm, and asking the emergency physician to prescribe narcotics. The police should probably be involved in these complex schemes. Some drug addicts readily admit their addiction and request enough drug to get them through the night or to get them home where they can obtain help. Patients with these drug demands are best treated by briefly evaluating them for physical illness (vital signs, physical examination) and referring them to a drug rehabilitation center, *without prescribing or administering narcotics*. This is sometimes extremely difficult because the sophisticated drug user can be highly manipulative.

Another difficult situation arises when the patient with a previously established painful disease like sickle cell disease or hemophilia becomes dependent on opioids. Most emergency physicians treat these patients with opioids for their pain during the first several visits but become increasingly suspicious and reluctant as the frequency of visits increases. The management plan for these patients is ideally carried out in conjunction with the patient's own physician, who is responsible for management of the underlying disease.

The problem that the opioid addict creates for the emergency physician reflects the enormity of the problem for our society in general and opioid treatment programs in particular. In the decade of the 70s it was estimated that there were at least 500,000 opioid addicts in the United States and that 2% to 3% of young adults had tried heroin at some point in their lives.[7] The Viet Nam conflict produced a large group of drug veterans who reported experiences with or addiction to narcotics.

Though the problem of drug addiction is substantial, the psychiatric explanations are inadequate. The concept of an ''addictive personality'' has given way to the notion that the problem of drug addiction cuts across many psychiatric diagnoses, involves complex social and economic factors, and may well be associated with biochemical explanations that are as yet incompletely understood.[8]

Although there is no addictive personality classification in the DSM-III, studies have repeatedly demonstrated that drug addicts have definable psychiatric disorders and that in some cases their drug use is an attempt to treat their underlying psychiatric disorder themselves.

The prevalence of depression in compulsive drug users is particularly high. In one study, depression was found in at least 70% of compulsive drug addicts, anxiety disorders in 15%, and antisocial personality disorder in 41% of the patients. In this sample, schizotypal personality disorders, schizoid disorders, and paranoid disorders were present in 13% of the patients.[9] Anxiety disorders and antisocial personality disorders are also common diagnoses in the drug-using population. The treatment of these patients, therefore, can be quite complex. It involves careful psychiatric assessment and specific treatment, according to the patient's diagnosis and other individualized considerations. Psychotherapy is ideally performed when the patient is abstaining from drugs. It is only during these drug-free periods that he is able to bring the greatest insight to the problem and is able to focus his attention on therapy.

Among the most effective programs for opioid addicts, however, are those that provide legal sources of opioids (methadone for addicted patients) and those that emphasize group support and reward for abstinence from narcotics.

Because the problem is complex and the treatment specialized, the emergency physician can be most effective in the patient's management by getting him involved in a drug rehabilitation program as soon as possible. Most states have some resources available for such patients, and the emergency department should have procedures for providing the addicted patients with these services.

Convincing the opioid abuser or addict to accept such treatment can certainly be difficult. The patient has learned to maintain his habit partially through the manipulation of others, and he is likely to be highly skilled in getting physicians and others to provide opioids. Perhaps the most honest and humane approach to the opioid abuser is to empathize with his difficulties and try to explain that he needs specialized treatment, the support of others, and may even need to be maintained on methadone to be able to lead a useful and happy life. Though the patient typically proposes reasons he still requires opioids temporarily, the physician should be able to withhold narcotics from the abuser and endure the verbal abuse that may follow.

By contrast, when the physician can tell that the patient does have genuine pain from a real physical illness, there is little to be gained by withholding proper dosages of analgesic agents, including opioids, when they are truly needed.

Opioid intoxication. Severe opioid (narcotic) intoxication is suspected when the unconscious patient with pinpoint pupils and shallow respiration arrives in the emergency department. Intravenous naloxone (Narcan) is the narcotic antagonist of choice for reversal of the depressant effects of opioid intoxication. Naloxone rapidly displaces the opioid from receptors in the central nervous system and, in the case of intoxication with a single agent like heroin, caused a rapid return of consciousness and normal respiration. A single dose of 0.4 to 0.8 mg should be effective in cases where a single opioid like heroin has been taken. In mixed overdoses, however, larger doses of naloxone are required, particularly with those that involve propoxyphene (Darvon), pentazocine (Talwin), or large doses of other narcotics. Naloxone has essentially no depressant effect of its own and may thus be used safely in these doses.

Two protocols using larger doses of naloxone have been proposed.[10] One protocol provides an initial intravenous bolus of 2.0 mg (5 ampules) for both children and adults. If this dose is ineffective in a few minutes, a repeat intravenous bolus of 2 to 4 mg may be given. When the naloxone is effective, it must be administered every 20 to 60 min-

A. *Pattern of pathological use:* inability to reduce or stop use; intoxication throughout the day; use of opioids nearly every day for at least a month; episodes of opioid overdose (intoxication so severe that respiration and consciousness are impaired).
B. *Impairment in social or occupational functioning due to opioid use:* e.g., fights, loss of friends, absence from work, loss of job, or legal difficulties (other than due to a single arrest for possession, purchase, or sale of the substance).
C. Duration of disturbance of at least 1 month.

From American Psychiatric Association. *Diagnostic and statistical manual of mental disorders* (3rd ed.). Washington, D.C.: The Association, 1980.

utes because most narcotics have a longer half-life than naloxone. A second protocol uses a continuous intravenous infusion method; the patient receives a continuous infusion of 0.4 mg or larger per hour for 10 to 12 hours if residual effects of the narcotic return when the infusion is stopped.

The patient with serious CNS respiratory and/or circulatory compromise requires appropriate immediate interventions, including maintenance of adequate ventilation and blood pressure. Naloxone may precipitate abrupt opioid withdrawal, and the physicians may then be confronted with a new clinical problem.

Opioid withdrawal. The opioid-dependent patient experiences opioid withdrawal as early as 6 hours after the cessation of opioid use. The intensity of withdrawal symptoms typically reaches a peak on the second or third day after stopping the drug. When the opioid is morphine or heroin, symptoms typically occur within 8 to 12 hours after cessation of use; when it is meperidine, they may occur within 3 hours; and when it is methadone, the symptoms do not develop until 24 to 48 hours after cessation of use. The symptoms of withdrawal for the methadone-dependent patient develop more slowly and are less intense than those of the heroin- or morphine-dependent patient.

When the effects of the opioid are reversed with naloxone, the withdrawal syndrome typically develops within minutes and reaches peak intensity within 30 minutes. The withdrawal syndrome precipitated by naloxone is more intense than that associated with cessation of drug use.

The total withdrawal syndrome includes both purposive, goal-seeking behavior and nonpurposive symptoms and signs of withdrawal.[7] The purposive phenomena are exaggerated when the patient feels he is being observed and they are directed toward the goal of getting more narcotic drugs. These purposive phenomena include moans, groans, complaints, repeated shouting, writhing, simulated pain, self-induced vomiting, pleading, or other attempts to manipulate the medical staff in ways that are as varied as the imagination of the drug user.

The signs that are not goal directed are more reliable clinically for determining opioid withdrawal. The following symptoms and signs have been traditionally associated with opioid withdrawal.

Early signs (8 to 12 hours)
- Restless sleep
- Piloerection (''gooseflesh'')
- Tremor
- Loss of appetite
- Irritability

Signs during peak intensity (may last several days)
- Yawning
- Sneezing
- Lacrimation
- Rhinorrhea
- Abdominal cramps
- Nausea

Vomiting
Diarrhea
Fever
Chills
Sweating
Muscle spasms
Hypertension
Tachycardia

Protracted abstinence syndrome

Irritability
Inability to tolerate pain
Poor self-image

Several hours after discontinuing opioids, the patient may fall into a fitful restless sleep. When he awakens, he appears restless and irritable. The skin may show piloerection or gooseflesh that resembles the skin of a newly plucked foul (''cold turkey''). Dilated pupils signify sympathetic stimulation. The syndrome progresses to its greatest intensity within the next 2 to 3 days. During its peak, opioid withdrawal can produce dramatic uncontrollable yawning, prolonged severe sneezing, rhinorrhea, abdominal cramps, nausea, vomiting, diarrhea, fever, chills, sweats, muscle spasms, hypertension, and tachycardia.

If the history of narcotic withdrawal is not provided and the emergency physician has not had the opportunity to observe the total syndrome over several days, the patient may appear to have one or several physical illnesses. The watery eyes, running nose (''sniffles''), and sneezing resemble the common cold, influenza or seasonal allergy. Abdominal cramps, nausea, and vomiting could create the impression that the patient has a serious intraabdominal process or gastroenteritis. The presence of fever may stimulate a search for an infectious process and make the associated symptoms seem more ominous. Elevated blood pressure and racing pulse make the process seem more severe when physical illness is suspected. Involuntary muscle spasms that cause abrupt jerking of arms and legs (''kicking the habit'') confuse the clinical picture when narcotic withdrawal is not suspected.

Opioid withdrawal is dramatic but is rarely lethal, provided that the patient's fluid and electrolyte balance is maintained. The anorexia, nausea, and vomiting associated with opioid withdrawal can cause hypovolemia, acid-base disturbances, ketosis, and electrolyte imbalance. When the patient is provided with appropriate fluids or nutrients, the opioid withdrawal syndrome runs its course and subsides in 7 to 10 days. The syndrome can be abruptly reversed by giving opioids at any point along its course. This fact forms the basis for its most effective treatment: detoxification.

Detoxification. The standard treatment of the opioid withdrawal syndrome involves substitution of the long-acting narcotic methadone for the patient's previous opioid. The detoxification should be done only in the hospital or in a properly licensed detoxification center.

The initial dose of methadone to be given rarely exceeds 20 mg. The total daily dose is usually calculated to be one half the patient's habitual daily intravenous dose of heroin or one fourth of his daily dose of morphine. The dose can be adjusted upward or downward as needed. This effective dose of methadone is then reduced by 20% every 1 to 2 days until the patient is symptom free. The detoxification process should be completed in 10 days.

When the patient has associated physical illnss or injury that requires medical maintenance or hospitalization, methadone may be started at 10 to 30 mg per day as a temporary measure, while the medical or surgical condition is still acute. The medication can and should be given by mouth and should not need to be given more than twice a day. The use of methadone in this setting is best accomplished in cooperation with psychiatric or social service consultation to provide liaison with a detoxification program. Methadone is indicated in the emergency department for acute opioid withdrawal when there is assurance that the patient will continue with the detoxification over the next 10 days. When the patient refuses specialized consultation and treatment by a detoxification service, there is nothing to be gained by temporarily relieving the withdrawal syndrome in the emergency department.

Other agents may be effective in the opioid withdrawal syndrome. Clonidine, a centrally acting alpha adrenergic agent, has been effective in suppressing the opioid withdrawal syndrome and has been recommended for this purpose.[12,13]

Long-term methadone maintenance may be the only effective way to treat one who is dependent on opioids. By legalizing access to methadone, the patient has a way to avoid illegal activities and lead a productive life. Methadone maintenance reduces the patient's need for other narcotics and limits or abolishes the euphoric "rush." Methadone maintenance must be carried out by a special treatment center licensed for this purpose.

Cocaine. Cocaine is second only to marijuana in popularity, and some believe it is fast becoming "American's recreational drug of choice."[14] The use of cocaine by athletes, prominent politicians, and media celebrities is well publicized. The white, crystalline cocaine, also called *toot, snow, blow, gold dust,* or the *Cadillac of drugs,* may be sniffed into the nasal passages ("snorted"), smoked, or dissolved and injected intravenously. When mixed with heroin, the concoction is injected as a "speed ball." An extremely dangerous method of cocaine use is "free-basing." Using a simple ether extraction technique, cocaine hydrochloride can be converted to the sulfate form or "free-base." The resulting preparation is volatile yet heat stable and can be smoked in a cigarette or water pipe. This method is dangerous because the user is unable to titrate the dose and large amounts of cocaine may be inhaled. By contrast, with intranasal use the vessels in the nasal mucous membranes constrict in response to the topical cocaine, and the absorption is reduced.

Cocaine's predominant effect is stimulation. Peruvian Indians have chewed it for centuries to enable them to work longer at high altitudes and achieve a sense of well-being. In many respects cocaine's stimulating effect is similar to that produced by amphetamines. Cocaine also generates a feeling of euphoria. The user typically arranges some cocaine powder in a small straight line and inhales it through a hollow tube into the nasal passages. The user thus snorts a "line" of cocaine, experiences a "high," and becomes garrulous, euphoric, and animated. This effect typically lasts 1 or 2 hours. As the user "comes down," he may experience the urge to take additional "hits" of cocaine to prolong the euphoric sensation.

Cocaine has enjoyed waves of popularity in the past.[15] The Incas used coca leaves in religious ceremonies and a cocaine saliva mixture as a topical anesthetic. In 1860 Niemann purified the coca alkaloid and named it *cocaine*. In the mid-nineteenth century, cocaine was mixed with red wine to produce something called *Vin Mariani,* which was a favorite beverage of Queen Victoria. Sigmund Freud experimented with this drug and used it to combat his own depressive moods. Cocaine was a principal ingredient of Coca Cola from its creation in 1886 until it was removed in 1906.

The current diagnosis of cocaine abuse requires a pattern of pathological use, an impairment of social or occupational functioning as a result of cocaine use, and a disturbance duration of at least 1 month. Pathological use includes factors such as the inability to stop using cocaine, intoxication throughout the day, and cocaine overdose severe enough to cause hallucinations and delusions. Cocaine hallucinations typically consist of an object seen in a flash of light in the peripheral field of vision. Well-formed, complex hallucinations are unusual. Chronic mydriasis also may cause altered vision. Tactile hallucinations, like the sensation of insects crawling over the skin (formication), may be present. As with hallucinations caused by other organic disorders, the patient recognizes that the insects are not really there but reacts as if they were by scratching or squirming to become comfortable. Olfactory and gustatory hallucinations have also been reported.

Delusions experienced by the cocaine abuser are frequently paranoid. The patient believes that others are against him or out to get him. The patient may try to escape from his imagined danger or confront it head on, in which case there may be violent behavior. A full-blown paranoid psychosis associated with cocaine is virtually indistinguishable from that associated with amphetamines.

The patient who abuses cocaine has periods of induced elation and euphoria that alternate with drug-free periods of apathy, depression, and even suicidal ideation. When the patient first arrives at the emergency department, therefore, the cocaine abuser can be mistakenly diagnosed as having schizophrenia or bipolar affective disorder (manic-depressive illness). Other bizarre behavior associated with cocaine use includes meticulous attention to details, ritualistic behavior, and repetitive actions similar to the patient with obsessive compulsive personality disorder.

Even a cursory physical examination should provide the clues to cocaine intoxication. Among the most consistent clues are signs of adrenergic hyperactivity, dilated pupils, tachycardia, and hypertension. The duration of these effects is typically short—1 or 2 hours, in contrast to the more prolonged duration of similar signs associated with amphetamines or PCP. Nasal septal ulcerations, perforations, epistaxis, and/or atrophic nasal septum suggest chronic nasal inhalation of cocaine. Vertical nystagmus may accompany mydriasis. The patient may have an arrhythmia. In young patients with frequent premature ventricular contractions (PVCs) unresponsive to lidocaine, cocaine intoxication may be the underlying cause.

Cocaine has not been positvely shown to cause dependence because cocaine withdrawal or tolerance has not been definitively demonstrated, even though short-term tolerance to the euphoric effect as well as that to the convulsant and cardiorespiratory effects has been reported.[16] Prolonged cocaine use can lead to periods of severe depression when the patient does not use the substance. In this sense, perhaps there is a withdrawal pattern, but in our present classification scheme it is not sufficient to warrant a diagnosis of cocaine dependence, according to the DSM-III.

Amphetamines. Amphetamines offer the user effects that are similar to those obtained with the use of cocaine. Following the ingestion of amphetamines, the user feels increased energy, diminished appetite, diminished need for sleep, increased capacity for repetitive routine work, and euphoria. Amphetamine or speed may be used as an occasional recreational drug by persons who wish to lose weight or by those who must stay awake to perform their jobs, like truckers who drive throughout the night. Amphetamines are commonly taken by mouth but are also injected intravenously or intraarterially.

The diagnosis of amphetamine abuse requires a pattern of pathological use for at least 1 month that impairs the patient's social or occupational functioning. Patterns of pathological use include intravenous or intraarterial injections or taking amphetamines daily for 1 or 2 weeks in a "run" of continued use. The run is usually followed by a "crash" that generally includes fatigue and significant depression.

Amphetamine abuse is also diagnosed when the patient exhibits the amphetamine delusional disorder or amphetamine delirium. Amphetamine delusional disorder is characterized by a paranoid psychosis with features that are virtually indistinguishable from paranoid schizophrenia. The patient is suspicious and has delusions that others are against him and that he must protect himself. These patients may exhibit psychomotor agitation, hostility, aggression, and violent behavior. The delusional disorder may occur within 1 week of the beginning of amphetamine use. Amphetamine delirium is similar to delirium associated with other causes: impaired perceptions, memory disturbance, incoherent speech, psychomotor agitation or retardation, and other signs that indicate clouding of consciousness.

Amphetamine withdrawal is characterized by fatigue, disturbed sleep, and increased dreaming following a period of prolonged use of amphetamines or similar drugs. During the withdrawal period the patient may be severely depressed and even suicidal.

Acute amphetamine intoxication may be treated with the standard measures. Acidification of the urine enhances amphetamine excretion and may be a useful adjunct in therapy. The treatment of the substance abuse disorder requires psychiatric consultation or referral to the community facility responsible for these treatment programs.

Phencyclidine (PCP) or similarly acting arylcyclohexylamine intoxication. Phencyclidine is the most widely used of a group of arylcyclohexylamines. Originally developed as an anesthetic agent, phencyclidine was quickly discontinued for human use because patients frequently experienced an uncomfortable delirium in the period following surgery. A related arylcyclohexylamine, ketamine, is still in clinical use as a "dissociative anesthetic." Such an agent allows the patient to remain conscious and responsive to verbal stimuli but blocks the sensation of discomfort from a normally painful procedure.

PCP, also called *crystal, angel dust,* or other names, can be sprinkled on marijuana and smoked ("crystal joint"), snorted into the nostrils, injected intravenously, or taken orally. A usual dose for recreational purposes varies from 1 to 5 mg. When taken in these doses, phencyclidine typically causes a sensation of numbness, euphoria, altered sense of time, and disturbance of sensory interpretation.

The patient may have slurred speech, ataxia, nystagmus, elevated blood pressure, and hypersalivation. The characteristic clinical portrait is the patient with a blank stare who is uncommunicative. By contrast, the patient may be agitated, excited, and experiencing visual, tactile, or auditory hallucinations. Pain preception is diminished, and the patient may injure himself when agitated. At a low level of intoxication, the patient is best managed by avoiding excessive stimulation. He can be left in a quiet atmosphere with subdued lighting, where he can be observed. Since most of the effects of a small dose of phencyclidine clear within 4 hours, by the time such a patient arrives in the emergency department, he should be returning to normal. When 5 to 20 mg of phencyclidine are taken, the patient shows the more severe symptoms of muscle rigidity, hypersalivation, flushing, diaphoresis, muteness, and responsiveness only to noxious stimuli.

In severe poisoning, when doses greater than 20 to 25 mg have been taken, coma, convulsions, and even death result. Patients with severe intoxication require more aggressive management, including support of vital signs, acidification of the urine, and, in some cases, beta blockade with propranolol.

When the organic psychosis precipitated by phencyclidine is severe, haloperidol is the antipsychotic agent of choice. The phencyclidine user may experience anxiety, confusion, depression, phencyclidine delirium, or phencyclidine organic mental disorder for up to 1 week following the acute intoxication.

The delirium can include disordered sensory interpretation, hallucinations, disturbed sleep, increased or decreased psychomotor activity, and memory impairment. The organic mental disorder is characterized by memory loss, impaired intellect, impaired judgment, and even disorientation.

The chronic treatment of the phencyclidine user requires an understanding of the reasons underlying the patient's urge to use the agent. As in the use of many drugs, the young patient may experience peer pressure to use the drug or curiosity about the drug's effects. Older patients may simply wish to alter their consciousness because they find it pleasurable or a relief from the misery or boredom of their daily lives. Many patients may be trying to treat their own underlying mental illness.

Cannabis organic mental disorders. Cannabis sativa or marijuana is widely used in this country as a recreational drug. Commonly smoked or eaten, its effects include euphoria, intensification of perceptions, a sensation of slowed time, and a sense of well-being or relaxation. Tachycardia and conjunctival hyperemia are easily recognized physical manifestations of cannabis intoxication.

Some patients develop disturbing psychiatric symptoms following the use of cannabis. These effects include paranoid ideation, paranoid delusions, panic attacks, or dysphoria (depression).

Cannabis abuse occurs whenever there is a pattern of pathological use (e.g., everyday, all day, for a month), when there is impairment of social or occupational functioning as a result of cannabis use, or when the patient repeatedly experiences a cannabis delusional disorder (e.g., really believing that the police are in the house somewhere).

Cannabis dependence can be diagnosed when the patient meets the criteria for cannabis abuse, yet develops tolerance for the drug. The patient thus begins using more of the drug to achieve the desired effect, or he experiences a diminished effect with the customary doses.

Tobacco. The mention of tobacco dependence is presented here only for completeness because it is included within the DSM-III categories of substance abuse.

SUMMARY

Substance abuse is common in emergency patients and can complicate diagnosis and treatment. It can be associated with other psychiatric diagnoses such as affective disorder, anxiety disorder, or antisocial personality disorder. An underlying contribution to the abuse of substances may be the user's attempt to treat his own mental or emotional discomfort. Substance abuse is also associated with concomitant medical problems or traumatic injuries. The diagnosis of substance abuse depends on establishing a pattern of pathological use, impaired social or occupational functioning, and duration of at least 1 month. Substance dependence is diagnosed when the patient exhibits tolerance or withdrawal.

Disposition of the substance abuser usually depends on the availability of detoxification facilities in the community, which should be listed at least in the emergency department's policy and procedure manual. Certain substance-dependent patients who require medical or surgical hospitalization need drug maintenance and psychiatric consultation during the acute phase of their illness.

REFERENCES

1. Hughes, JH, et al. Trauma in patients influenced by drugs and alcohol. *Annuals of Emergency Medicine,* Jan. 1980, *9*(1), 15-19.
2. Rumack, BH (Ed.). *Poisindex.* Rocky Mountain Poison Control Center, Englewood, Colo.: Micromedex, Inc., 1982.
3. Goldfrank, LR. *Toxicologic emergencies: a comprehensive handbook in problem solving* (2nd ed.). New York: Appleton-Century-Crofts, 1982.
4. American Psychiatric Association. *Diagnostic and statistical manual of mental disorders* (3rd ed.). Washington, D.C.: The Association, 1980.
5. Finkle, BS, McCloskey, KL, and Goodman, LS. Diazepam and drug associated deaths: a survey in the United States and Canada. *Journal of the American Medical Association,* 1979, *242,* 439-434.

6. Hayes, SL, et al.: Ethanol and oral diazepam absorption. *New England Journal of Medicine,* 1977, *296,* 186-189.
7. Jaffe, JH. Drug addiction and drug abuse. In Gilman, AG, Goodman, LS, and Gilman A (Eds.), *The pharmacological basis of therapeutics* (6th ed.). New York: Macmillan Publishing Co. 1980.
8. Lion, JR. *Addictive personalities, personality disorders,* Baltimore: The Williams and Wilkins Co., 1982.
9. Treece, C, and Nicholson, B. DSM-III personality type and dose levels in methadone maintenance patients, *Journal of Nervous and Mental Disease,* 1980, *168*(10), 621-628.
10. Goldfrank, LR, and Bresnitz, EA. Opioids. In Goldfrank, LR (Ed.), *Toxicologic emergencies: a comprehensive handbook in problem solving* (2nd ed.). New York:, Appleton-Century-Crofts, 1982.
12. Gold, MS, Pottash, ALC, and Extein, I. Clonidine: inpatient studies from 1978 to 1981. *Journal of Clinical Psychiatry,* 1982, *43*(6), 35-38.
13. Washton, A, and Resnick, RB. Outpatient opiate detoxification with clonidine. *Journal of Clinical Psychiatry,* 1982, *43*(6), 39-41.
14. Haddad, LM. 1978: Cocaine in perspective. *Journal of the American College of Emergency Physicians,* 1979, *8,* 374-376.
15. Anderson, RJ. Illicit drug and substance abuse: cocaine and phencyclidine, In Rund, DA, and Walcott, BW (Eds.), *Emergency Medicine Annual: 1983.* Norwalk, Conn: Appleton-Century-Crofts, 1983.
16. Matsuzaki, M. Alteration in patterns of EEG activities and convulsant effect of cocaine following chronic administration in the rhesus monkey. *Electroencephalography and Clinical Neurophysiology,* 1978, *45,* 1-5.

8 ALCOHOL SYNDROMES

From the most ancient times man has learned to ferment fruit, grain, or potatoes to create an intoxicating alcoholic beverage. Excluding tobacco, alcohol is the most widely abused substance in our society; it is estimated that up to 10% of Americans are alcoholic. Of all the psychoactive drugs, alcohol is the most toxic and damaging to individuals and to society.

Alcohol-related problems are common in emergency practice. At least 7% of emergency visits are directly caused by alcohol abuse,[1] and the percentage of alcoholic patients in the emergency department has been estimated between 12% and 36%.[2] A study using strict research diagnostic criteria demonstrated the prevalence of alcoholism in an emergency population of an urban hospital to be 20%, with an 11% prevalence in the daytime and 29% in the nighttime population.[3] Alcohol is often associated with violence, depression, suicide attempt, nonspecific complaints, acute gastrointestinal disorders, inability to care for oneself, and a generally unsalubrious life-style (Fig. 8-1).

Trauma is particularly influenced by alcohol.[4] At least 50% of automobile accidents involve one intoxicated person.

The DSM-III recognizes the following nine syndromes associated with the use and abuse of alcohol:

Alcohol intoxication
Alcohol idiosyncratic intoxication
Alcohol withdrawal
Alcohol withdrawal delirium (delirium tremens)
Alcohol hallucinosis
Alcohol amnestic disorder (Korsakoff's disease)
Dementia associated with alcoholism
Alcohol abuse
Alcohol dependence

ALCOHOL INTOXICATION

In general the severity of intoxication increases as the blood alcohol level rises. The average person feels an initial disinhibition and stimulation in the earliest phase of drinking. The first signs of intoxication may be seen at blood levels as low as 20 to 30 mg/dl. These early signs may be increased sociability, talkativeness, and a sense of well-being or mild euphoria. For the average-size person, 44 gm of alcohol, about 4

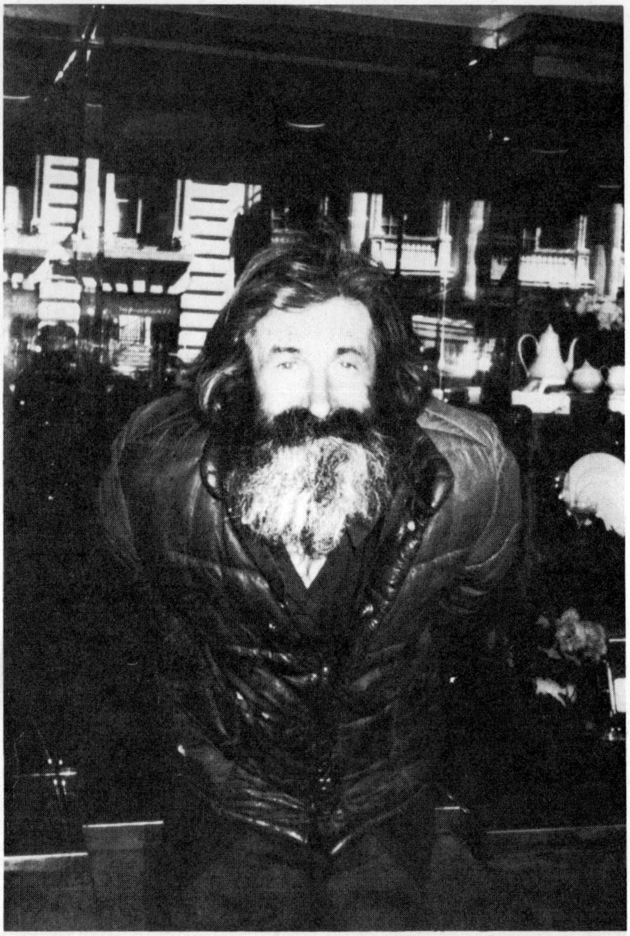

FIG. 8-1. Intoxicated alcoholic patient presents familiar picture to emergency physician. Medical or psychiatric disorders can be complex and difficult to unravel in such patients.

ounces of 86-proof whiskey, should result in a blood alcohol level of 60 to 90 mg/dl. A standard drink contains about 1½ ounces of hard liquor. The alcohol content in one of these drinks is approximately as much as is in a 12-ounce can of beer or a 5-ounce glass of wine. Thus three to four standard drinks, cans of beer, or glasses of wine consumed over a short time or on an empty stomach can raise the blood level to nearly 100 mg/dl. When food is present in the stomach, alcohol absorption is slowed. The same amount of ingested alcohol results in a blood concentration of 30 to 60 ml/dl.

For most persons the intoxication associated with a blood level of 100 mg/dl is sufficient to impair reaction time and judgment enough that the person should not be operating a motor vehicle (Table 8-1). This is usually the blood level that supports the legal definition of intoxication. At this level the average person may show signs of mild

TABLE 8-1. Relationship of blood ethanol level to clinical evidence of motor reaction

Blood ethanol mg/dl (mg%)	*Effect*
100	Mild intoxication, judgment often impaired, reaction time diminished (legal baseline in most states for diagnosis of intoxication), relaxation, disinhibition
200	Mild to moderate intoxication, slurred speech, unsteady gait, may have flushed face or nystagmus, nausea, mood changes of loquacity and euphoria or irritability, may have hostility, desire to fight
300	Marked intoxication, incoherent speech, stupor, markedly impaired judgment and motor skills, vomiting may occur (All patients with a blood alcohol level of 300% are alcoholic.)
400	Stupor, deep sleep or coma, difficult or impossible to arouse with vigorous stimulation (Some tolerant alcoholics are not so severely affected.)
500	Death can occur at these and higher blood alcohol levels

Adapted from Rund, DA. *Essentials of emergency medicine*. New York: Appleton-Century Crofts, 1982.

incoordination, some slurring of speech, and decreased ability to perform complex tasks. At 200 mg/dl most nonalcohol-tolerant persons are severely intoxicated. They usually exhibit slurred speech, ataxic gait incoordination, and markedly decreased ability to perform difficult intellectual or motor tasks. Flushed face or nystagmus may be present. Mood changes that accompany this level of intoxication range from euphoria, loquaciousness, and "good will toward all" to marked irritability, hostility, and the desire to fight. At levels of 300 mg/dl, the nontolerant patient is markedly intoxicated. When the blood alcohol level increases above 300 mg/dl, there is increased risk of severe respiratory depression and death. The central nervous system (CNS) becomes severely depressed at levels of 400 mg/dl, and most persons are then comatose. Levels greater than 500 mg/dl are usually lethal. At levels of 300 to 600 mg/dl, the risk of aspiration of vomitus, food, or other secretions is significantly increased. Aspiration may be either the immediate or ultimate cause of death in an alcoholic.

Tolerance

The alcohol levels and effects just cited are those expected for an average person. The phenomenon of tolerance is well known to emergency personnel. Persons who chronically ingest large amounts of alcohol are able to tolerate much higher levels and perform with less obvious impairment than those not accustomed to drinking large amounts every day. The levels that predict impaired behavior and judgment in moderate drinkers do not apply to these patients. The alcoholic with a blood level of 250 mg/dl may walk into the department, converse with personnel, exhibit only slightly slurred speech, and appear to function rather well.

A short-term tolerance to alcohol in the nonalcoholic is also well known. After several hours of drinking, some can appear less intoxicated than after a short period of drinking.

Metabolism

In the normal person about 10 to 15 ml of pure 100% alcohol or about one drink is metabolized per hour. This means that the person who drinks only one "drink" per hour may not become intoxicated at all. By contrast, the person who ingests a large amount of alcohol requires a certain period of time for the metabolism of the ingested alcohol. This feature is important for predicting the duration of intoxication or its course in a patient admitted to the emergency department. A useful rule is to assume that each drink in a 70 kg person increases the blood alcohol level by 25 mg/dl. The constant rate of metabolism for alcohol is approximately the same, one drink should be metabolized per hour, and the blood alcohol level should fall at a rate of 10 to 20 mg/dl per hour. The usual rate is about 15 mg/dl per hour. The emergency physician can then predict the patient's length of stay in the department from an initial blood alcohol measurement. Most patients can be safely discharged with levels between 50 and 100 mg/dl.

Other phenomena associated with alcohol intoxication

Some intoxicated individuals may appear suspicious. If they become markedly paranoid with delusions that they are being controlled or watched, consideration for hospitalization should be given to rule out organic mental disorders, including alcoholism, other chemical dependence, or an acute psychosis. *Blackouts* may occur when the patient is amnestic for the events that occurred during the last several hours of intoxication. Blackouts are difficult to predict when the patient is intoxicated because, even while "blacked out," he appears to be able to carry on superficial social discussions. It is only after the event that the patient remembers nothing of his trip to the emergency department. This is something that the family or friends should be warned about; they should be encouraged to keep their resolve strong to get this patient to a treatment program within a very few hours.

The intoxicated patient may express suicidal ideation. Suicide-prone persons are more likely to commit suicide when their inhibitions are diminished by alcohol. Suicide is very common among alcoholics. One quarter of all suicides occur when the individual is drinking. The alcoholic who also ruminates about suicide is possibly at a very high risk and should be evaluated by a psychiatrist before discharge when possible.

Management

The initial management of the intoxicated patient must focus on the patient's medical problem or any acute injury responsible for the emergency visit. Hypoglycemia, dehydration, hypothermia, and metabolic acidosis[5] are rather common metabolic problems in the alcoholic population. Gastrointestinal hemorrhage results from gastritis or peptic ulcer disease in these people. Occult head injury may produce a subdural hematoma that accounts for the patient's diminished consciousness. Most alcoholics have depleted thiamine stores and require an intramuscular injection of 100 mg of thiamine.

The staff should maintain an "objective therapeutic attitude"[6] toward the intoxicated person. The maintenance of such an attitude results in a supportive, nonpunitive, calm

TABLE 8-2. Alcohol-related organic mental disorders

	Ataxia	*Tremor*	*Autonomic hyperactivity (sweating, tachycardia, hypertension)*	*Delirium*	*Hallucinations*	*Seizures*	*Short- and long-term memory loss*
Intoxication	+						
Withdrawal		+	+				
Withdrawal delirium		+	+	+	+		
Withdrawal seizures						+	
Hallucinosis		±			+		
Amnestic disorder	±						+

approach to the patient. The intoxicated person has some sort of problem that requires attention by the emergency staff (Table 8-2). There is little to be gained and much harm to be done when the staff begins to preach to the alcoholic about what he is doing to himself, his family, and his career. This approach only intensifies the alcoholic's shame and guilt. Similarly, an angry attitude may cause the patient to respond in kind or to try to walk out. Rather than argue with the intoxicated person, the staff should ask the patient to cooperate with the evaluation (e.g., "Please lie down on the cart," or "Sorry, you may not smoke in this area"). The patient often responds dramatically to being treated as a distressed person with a treatable problem. When sober, the patient is most grateful for caring, thoughtful treatment provided by the emergency staff.

ALCOHOL IDIOSYNCRATIC INTOXICATION

An idiosyncratic reaction is diagnosed when the patient drinks a relatively small amount of alcohol (often as few as three to six drinks) and becomes extremely agitated, becomes belligerent, and appears to be severely intoxicated. The patient is often amnestic for this event and may need to be allowed to "sleep it off" for up to 12 to 15 hours. Patients with such reactions should be told about their idiosyncratic reaction to alcohol so that they have the opportunity to remedy the situation. The reaction should be noted on the patient's chart, and the fact that he has been told that alcohol produces this reaction in him must be noted. Idiosyncratic reaction is also known as *pathological intoxication*. Patients with this disorder have often been mild-mannered, shy, and retiring while sober, but when they begin to drink a very small amount of alcohol, they may become assaultive, belligerent, and extremely loud. This behavior is markedly different from the patient's normal behavior. These patients are usually alcoholics and should be started in a suitable treatment program.

Some individuals with this disorder have been reported to have temporal lobe spikes

DIAGNOSTIC CRITERIA FOR ALCOHOL IDIOSYNCRATIC INTOXICATION

A. Marked behavioral change, e.g., aggressive or assaultive behavior that is due to the recent ingestion of an amount of alcohol insufficient to induce intoxication in most people.
B. The behavior is atypical of the person when not drinking.
C. Not due to any other physical or mental disorder.

From American Psychiatirc Association. *Diagnostic and statistical manual of mental disorders* (3rd ed.). Washington, D.C.: The Association, 1980.

on an electroencephalogram (EEG) taken after receiving small amounts of alcohol. It is possible that people with subclinical or clinical brain damage lose tolerance for alcohol and behave abnormally after drinking. People who have had trauma or encephalitis may become intolerant to alcohol, and patients with debilitating physical illnesses may also have a low tolerance. Borderline personality disorders may be present in these patients. The concomitant use of other substances must also be suspected when this diagnosis is considered. Some patients take sedatives and alcohol concurrently to increase the effect of each. Other patients may drink while taking a prescription medication like diphenhydramine that adds to the sedative effect of alcohol. Medications like flurazepam (Dalmane) or diazepam (Valium), with metabolites that produce effects for several days, may predispose the patient to increased intoxication after drinking a small amount of alcohol 12 to 24 hours after taking the medication.

ALCOHOL WITHDRAWAL

Alcohol withdrawal results when the alcoholic stops drinking or markedly reduces the amount he has drunk regularly to produce intoxication. Even though the patient still drinks, he is at risk for alcohol withdrawal even if his consumption decreases just a small amount from normal. The first symptoms of alcohol withdrawal occur about 8 to 17 hours after the cessation of a prolonged period of chronic, heavy drinking or after a 1- or 2-week "binge" of persistent, daily alcohol intoxication (Table 8-3). The first sign usually noted on the patient's arrival at the department is tremulousness. This somewhat fast, irregular, and coarse intention tremor may be noted as early as 6 hours after cessation of or reduction in drinking. The tremulousness may be accompanied by nausea, weakness, anxiety, and diaphoresis. The tremor may be rather mild or may be so severe that the patient has trouble getting dressed or eating without assistance.

Other features of this early alcohol withdrawal syndrome include irritability, agitation, and signs of autonomic hyperactivity (tachycardia and hypertension). The patient may be inattentive or depressed, but orientation and alertness are typically preserved.

Occasionally the patient with early alcohol withdrawal does not resemble the classic picture. The patient may be nontremulous and have far more subtle signs, such as a

DIAGNOSTIC CRITERIA FOR ALCOHOL WITHDRAWAL

A. Cessation of or reduction in heavy prolonged (several days or longer) ingestion of alcohol, followed within several hours by coarse tremor of hands, tongue, and eyelids and at least one of the following:
   1. Nausea and vomiting
   2. Malaise or weakness
   3. Autonomic hyperactivity, e.g., tachycardia, sweating, elevated blood pressure
   4. Anxiety
   5. Depressed mood or irritability
   6. Orthostatic hypotension

B. Not due to any other physical or mental disorder such as Alcohol Withdrawal Delirium.

From American Psychiatric Association. *Diagnostic and statistical manual of mental disorders* (3rd ed.). Washington, D.C.: The Association, 1980.

TABLE 8-3. Features of disorders associated with alcohol withdrawal in relation to hours of diminished alcohol intake preceding the onset of each specific stage

Stage	*Hours since diminished intake or cessation of drinking*	*Major manifestation*
1	6 to 8 hours	Tremulosis
2	24 hours	Hallucinosis
3	7 to 48 hours	Alcohol withdrawal seizures
4	3 to 5 days	Withdrawal delirium

mild tachycardia and confusion, elicited only by a careful mental status examination. This is particularly true of some elderly patients. The first clue may be some unexpected bizarre gesture associated with hallucinosis, like brushing nonexistent material or creatures off the bed sheets. Alcoholism is so common in emergency patients that alcohol-related disorders should be an early and primary consideration in the evaluation of any organic mental disorder.

ALCOHOL WITHDRAWAL DELIRIUM

When untreated, the early features of withdrawal may become more prominent and intensify over the next several days. Alcohol withdrawal delirium typically reaches maximum intensity 72 hours after the last drink. The term *alcohol withdrawal delirium* replaces the older, traditional term *delirium tremens*. The essential feature of the syndrome is delirium with impaired perception, hallucinations, incoherence, and clouding of consciousness.

The typical picture of a patient with alcohol withdrawal delirium is the characteristic

DIAGNOSTIC CRITERIA FOR ALCOHOL WITHDRAWAL DELIRIUM

A. Delirium occurs within 1 week after cessation of or reduction in heavy alcohol ingestion.
B. Autonomic hyperactivity, e.g., tachycardia, sweating, elevated blood pressure.
C. Not due to any other physical or mental disorder.

From American Psychiatric Association. *Diagnostic and statistical manual of mental disorders* (3rd ed.). Washington, D.C.: The Association, 1980.

wild-eyed, tremulous person who sees snakes crawling on the wall. The picture may be far more subtle, however, and may be clouded by concomitant physical illness. Tremor of the hands, tongue, and eyelids is part of the typical portrait. Vomiting causes severe dehydration. Weakness and malaise are usually present.

Autonomic activity is manifested by tachycardia, sweating, and increased blood pressure. Hypoglycemia, electrolyte imbalance, dehydration, and seizures are among the most lethal medical complications of the syndrome. A seizure may occur apart from the delirium; this may happen in up to 10% of withdrawing alcoholics.

Hallucinations are typically visual and may be frightening to the patient. Auditory and tactile hallucinations do occur, however. Tactile hallucinations, like the sensation of insects crawling on the skin, may be associated with peripheral neuritis. Olfactory hallucinations and vestibular disturbances (like the floor moving beneath the feet) may be present. When hallucinations occur in a withdrawing alcoholic who does not show delirium, the condition is labeled alcohol hallucinosis.

The syndrome rarely lasts longer than 7 days if untreated but as mentioned, may be quite lethal. Seizures, aspiration pneumonia, hypoglycemia, and severe electrolyte disorders are some of the medical risks in alcohol withdrawal delirium. It has been estimated that up to 10% of patients who have an alcohol withdrawal delirium die. A much higher percentage (25%) of patients who have an alcoholic withdrawal syndrome and have complicating medical or surgical factors die.

The full-blown syndrome of alcohol withdrawal delirium may be regarded as an emergency and always requires inpatient treatment. For active delirium, a rapidly acting sedative is most helpful. Intravenous diazepam is probably the most appropriate medication in this setting. A dosage of 5 mg intravenously can be given every 5 to 15 minutes after the initial dose until the patient becomes calm. This treatment clearly requires constant patient monitoring and close medical supervision. Chlordiazepoxide (Librium) is probably the most commonly used medication for this disorder. The dosage given is 50 to 100 mg orally every hour until the patient becomes calm. A dosage of 50 mg may be given orally every 6 hours thereafter. Chlordiazepoxide should not be given intramuscularly because it is absorbed erratically from an intramuscular site.

If the patient does not respond to this regimen, haloperidol (Haldol) can be prescribed (10 to 20 mg orally four times a day). This is also especially appropriate when some underlying psychosis may be present. Phenothiazines like chlorpromazine (Thorazine) have been used in this stage of the patient's treatment; they lower the patient's seizure threshold and may thus increase the patient's likelihood of having a seizure. They also carry the complication of severe orthostatic hypotension. This is a particularly worrisome problem in the agitated alcoholic who may become hypotensive and syncopal when he stands up. Thiamine (50 to 100 mg intravenously) should be given immediately before the patient has any other food or intravenous glucose. Since thiamine is a cofactor in the metabolism of glucose, it is consumed when the patient eats or metabolizes glucose. The poorly nourished alcoholic often has thiamine deficiency as a result of his poor diet, and the sudden metabolism of glucose provided in food or intravenous fluid will deplete the patient's thiamine stores, including those in the central nervous sytem (CNS), even further. This depletion of thiamine precipitates Wernicke's encephalopathy, characterized by confusion, ataxia, and impaired eye movement. Such a patient may demonstrate paresis of upward gaze, for instance. Magnesium sulfate in a 5% sterile solution should be given as a 1 gm dose intravenously for several days to prevent seizures and replace magnesium.

Alcohol withdrawal syndromes, including hallucinations, may be subtle, and this is described in the following case example.

CASE EXAMPLE 1

A 64-year-old woman was brought to the emergency department by her family because she was "not thinking right." She seemed confused and pulled nonexistent hair off her hairless legs and handed it to the examiner. Her pulse was 120 beats per minute, and her respirations were 36 per minute. An initial diagnosis of hyperthyroidism was made until the family was interviewed. They related that the patient customarily drank at least a pint of liquor a day, but had run out of both money and liquor about 3 days ago.

Alcohol withdrawal syndromes, including delirium, can occur at any age. Sometimes an illness that results in hospitalization cuts off the patient's customary intake of alcohol and precipitates alcohol withdrawal delirium within 12 to 72 hours.

ALCOHOL HALLUCINOSIS

Alcohol hallucinosis is a specific syndrome associated with alcohol withdrawal in which vivid auditory (and possibly visual) hallucinations are the major abnormality. The syndrome typically begins 24 to 48 hours following cessation of or reduction in alcohol ingestion by an individual who has alcohol dependence. The most prominent early feature of the syndrome is the occurrence of auditory hallucinations despite an otherwise clear sensorium; these patients do not demonstrate clouding of consciousness, disorientation, memory loss, confusion, or decreased level of consciousness. In this major respect, the syndrome is distinct from alcohol withdrawal delirium.

DIAGNOSTIC CRITERIA FOR ALCOHOL HALLUCINOSIS

A. Organic Hallucinosis with vivid auditory hallucinations developing shortly (usually within 48 hours) after cessation of or reduction in heavy ingestion of alcohol in an individual who apparently has Alcohol Dependence.
B. Response to the hallucinations appropriate to their content, e.g., anxiety in response to hallucinatory threats.
C. No clouding of consciousness, as in Delirium.
D. Not due to any other physical or mental disorder.

From American Psychiatric Association. *Diagnostic and statistical manual of mental disorders* (3rd ed.). Washington, D.C.: The Association, 1980.

The hallucinations are usually voices but may be musical sounds (tones or low-pitched chants) or unformed sounds like hissing, buzzing, or clicking. When the patient hears voices, they are generally perceived to be from family or friends discussing him in the third person as though he were not present. The content of the conversations is generally derogatory, disturbing, or threatening. In the early stages of the disorder, the patient with alcohol hallucinosis may interpret these unpleasant hallucinations as real and react to perceived threats by calling the police or barricading the door. The presumed source of the hallucinations is typically hidden from the patient; the voices seem to come from behind a door, from another room, or through the wall. The hallucinations rarely command the patient to act in a certain way; rather the patient reacts to threatening or derogatory hallucinations as though they were real and in a way that shows an attempt to avoid being injured, killed, or disgraced. Occasionally the hallucinations are neither threatening nor unpleasant to the patient, and he is able to remain relatively calm. The disorder generally resolves spontaneously after several days, although a chronic form has been described.

It has been suggested that if the voices are calling the patient "queer" or making other sexual remarks about him, he is protecting himself against underlying homosexual feelings. If this occurs in women, it is often the case that the voices accuse her of promiscuity. These hypotheses should not be used to search for an underlying cause of the patient's alcoholism. The alcoholism itself requires major therapeutic attention.

Alcohol hallucinosis usually occurs in male patients over 40 years of age. In most cases the syndrome is preceded by several years of heavy drinking. Schizophrenia is perhaps the most commonly mistaken diagnosis made when this syndrome occurs. In schizophrenia the age of onset is earlier, the hallucinations are more bizarre, and there is a variable history of alcohol intake.

Patients with alcohol hallucinosis usually should be admitted to the hospital and treated with chlordiazepoxide given orally and an adequate diet. Presumably the patient is not able to continue drinking alcohol in the hospital. The patient may be discharged when the hallucinations disappear and should be warned that they will recur if drinking is resumed.

ALCOHOL WITHDRAWAL SEIZURES AND THE POSTICTAL STATE

Alcohol withdrawal seizures, traditionally known as "rum fits," generally occur within 7 to 48 hours after reduction or cessation of alcohol intake in an alcohol-dependent individual. The seizures often occur independently of alcohol withdrawal delirium, but up to one third of the patients who develop seizures progress to the stage of alcohol withdrawal delirium. The seizures are generalized, are brief, and typically occur in rather rapid succession over several hours. Status epilepticus rarely occurs. If the seizures are focal, a specific CNS lesion must be suspected.

Following a seizure, the postictal period may suggest delirium. The patient typically remains unconscious for a short period, then gradually awakens but remains confused and disoriented for up to several hours. The clouding of consciousness usually clears, but in some patients the postictal confusion may merge with the onset of delirium.

The treatment of alcohol withdrawal seizures is controversial. The most widely accepted approach is to withhold anticonvulsant treatment for brief self-limited alcohol withdrawal seizures. The seizure disorder is not considered permanent, and the seizures should not recur if the patient enters alcoholism treatment and stops drinking.

When treatment is required, diazepam is probably the most effective agent for immediate control. Phenytoin (Dilantin) is not normally used for the control of brief, self-limited alcohol withdrawal seizures. If the patient resumes drinking, he will probably stop taking the phenytoin anyway. It can only be speculated that the resulting simultaneous withdrawal of anticonvulsants *and* alcohol in these noncompliant patients might even lead to increased likelihood of seizures. Phenytoin is indicated, however, in patients with a concomitant seizure disorder unrelated to alcohol withdrawal.

Since the use of phenytoin in alcohol withdrawal seizures is controversial, each physician's individual practice should perhaps be decided in cooperation with a consulting neurologist, psychiatrist, and/or alcoholism expert or specialist.

WERNICKE'S ENCEPHALOPATHY

Wernicke's encephalopathy has three prominent clinical features: ophthalmoplegia, ataxia, and mental changes (confusion and memory loss). The disease is caused by severe thiamine deficiency and is seen almost exclusively in alcoholics. As mentioned previously, rapid infusion of glucose in the alcoholic may use up thiamine in glucose metabolism and deplete already low thiamine stores in CNS even further. This causes the abrupt onset of Wernicke's encephalopathy. Treatment rests on the administration of thiamine; 50 to 100 mg can be given intravenously, and 50 mg can be given intramuscularly. As the patient's ocular gaze paresis and ataxia improve with hydration and B complex vitamins, a memory deficit may remain. When such a deficit persists, the diagnosis of alcohol amnestic disorder (Korsakoff's disease) applies.

ALCOHOL AMNESTIC DISORDER

Classically known as Korsakoff's disease, the alcohol amnestic disorder typically follows an episode of Wernicke's encephalopathy. The central features of the syndrome are deficits of both short- and long-term memory. Short-term memory loss is suspected

DIAGNOSTIC CRITERIA FOR ALCOHOL AMNESTIC DISORDER

A. Amnestic Syndrome following prolonged heavy ingestion of alcohol.
B. Not due to any other physical or mental disorder.

From American Psychiatric Association. *Diagnostic and statistical manual of mental disorders* (3rd ed.). Washington, D.C.: The Association, 1980.

when the patient cannot remember events in the immediate past. The patient may not know he is in the hospital or what the examiner asked or told him only a few minutes earlier. Short-term memory deficits are easily diagnosed when the examiner gives the patient several objects to remember for 5 minutes (e.g., a brown chair, a red flower, a blue book). If the patient cannot remember any of the objects or even any of the colors, a severe short-term memory deficit is present. The patient with long-term memory deficits cannot remember events of the intermediate or distant past like birthplace, schooling, or early employment. Thus the patient cannot remember either information he knew before the onset of the disease or that which he learned after the onset.

When the diagnosis of alcohol amnestic disorder is made, there should be no concomitant signs of delirium, like impaired consciousness or intellectual diminishment. The patient must be able to understand what others are saying, be able to make simple calculations, and be willing to try to remember. Confabulation is a characteristic clinical feature of the amnestic disorder. To make up for the deficit in memory, the confabulatory patient invents his own information. He ''recognizes'' the examiner when told they have met before or fabricates an account of other recent events in his life.

The treatment for the disorder includes avoidance of alcohol and early administration of thiamine at the first signs of encephalopathy. When well established, however, the deficit persists indefinitely, and the patient may need continuing custodial care. An unknown percentage of these patients may improve on high dosages of thiamine (e.g., 400 mg given orally four times a day with meals for up to 2 years).

DEMENTIA ASSOCIATED WITH ALCOHOLISM

Dementia associated with alcoholism cannot be diagnosed for at least 3 weeks following the cessation of alcohol intake. It should not be confused, therefore, with alcohol intoxication or alcohol withdrawal delirium. Dementia signifies a more severe cognitive deficit than the alcohol amnestic syndrome. The dementia individual has severe impairment in all areas of intellectual functioning including calculations, memory, judgment, and ability to understand speech or perform relatively simple motor functions. The presence of dementia implies that the individual has been heavily abusing alcohol for many years and has suffered nearly irreversible cerebral changes. The prognosis for recovery is poor and depends on abstinence from the use of alcohol. As is always the case, however, the clinician must consider reversible causes for the syndrome, like chronic subdural hematoma, before committing the patient to a course of chronic supportive care without further diagnostic evaluation. High dosages of thiamine, as mentioned previously, may occasionally be helpful.

ALCOHOL ABUSE

Diagnosis of alcohol abuse

The diagnostic criteria for alcohol abuse according to the DSM-III includes all of the following criteria:

1. Pattern of pathological use
2. Social or occupational impairment caused by alcohol abuse
3. Duration of at least 1 month

Previously published research criteria similar to those presented for alcoholics in the DSM-III are given in the box on this page. To establish the diagnosis of alcoholism with reasonable confidence, the examiner should receive a ''yes'' answer to three of the four questions.

Pathological use. Three main drinking patterns are seen in the alcohol abuser. The first pattern is continuous drinking. The second pattern is heavy drinking that takes place only on weekends. The third is severe, heavy binge drinking that lasts for days or weeks. These binges are interspersed with long periods of abstinence. Advanced stage pathological patterns of drinking include consumption of nonbeverage alcohol (e.g., canned heating fuel or rubbing alcohol) or persistent drinking, despite medical complications that worsen with alcohol ingestion.

Social or occupational impairment. The alcoholic employee who fails to perform well because of persistent intoxication or who has repeated absences from work because of drinking has occupational impairment and meets this criterion for the diagnosis. Social impairment includes divorce, separation, other family problems, and any major consistent disturbances in social settings as a result of alcohol.

The duration of pathological alcohol use should have been present for at least 1 month to justify the diagnosis of alcoholism. Shorter periods of alcohol use define the diagnosis of alcohol intoxication.

CRITERIA FOR DEFINITE DIAGNOSIS OF ALCOHOLISM*

A. Alcohol withdrawal, medical complication, binge drinking, alcoholic blackout
B. Cannot stop drinking, before breakfast drinking, nonbeverage alcohol consumption
C. Arrests, fights, or work trouble because of drinking
D. Patient's family or others think patient drinks too much

Adapted from Feighner, JP, et al. Diagnostic criteria for use in psychiatric research. *Archives of General Psychiatry*. Jan. 1972, *26*, 57-63.

*To establish a diagnosis of alcoholism, at least one item in three of four categories must apply to the patient.

DIAGNOSTIC CRITERIA FOR ALCOHOL ABUSE

A. *Pattern of pathological alcohol use:* need for daily use of alcohol for adequate functioning; inability to cut down or stop drinking; repeated efforts to control or reduce excess drinking by "going on the wagon" (periods of temporary abstinence) or restricting drinking to certain times of the day; binges (remaining intoxicated throughout the day for at least 2 days); occasional consumption of a fifth of spirits (or its equivalent in wine or beer); amnesic periods for events occurring while intoxicated (blackouts); continuation of drinking despite a serious physical disorder that the individual knows is exacerbated by alcohol use; drinking of nonbeverage alcohol.
B. *Impairment in social or occupational functioning due to alcohol use:* e.g., violence while intoxicated, absence from work, loss of job, legal difficulties (e.g., arrest for intoxicated behavior, traffic accidents while intoxicated), arguments or difficulties with family or friends because of excessive alcohol use.
C. Duration of disturbance of at least 1 month.

From American Psychiatric Association. *Diagnostic and statistical manual of mental disorders* (3rd ed.). Washington, D.C.: The Association, 1980.

BRIEF SCREENING QUESTIONS FOR ALCOHOLISM

A. Has your family ever objected to your drinking?
B. Did you ever think you drank too much in general?
C. Have others (such as friends, physicians, clergymen, etc.) ever said you drink too much for your own good?

Adapted from Woodruff, FA, et al. A brief method of screening for alcoholism. *Diseases of the Nervous System,* Aug. 1976, *37*(8), 434-435.

Screening for alcoholism

The high prevalence of alcoholism in emergency patients and the complexity of the associated problems provide a justification for somewhat routine screening for alcoholism in emergency patients. A rapid screening technique proven to be highly accurate is outlined in the above box. Three questions about whether the patient, the family, or others think the patient is drinking too much are asked. When these questions were tested on a study population, 96% of the alcoholic population answered "yes" to one of the questions. Only 11% of the nonalcoholics answered "yes" to one of these questions.[10] This rapid screening technique should sort out a group of patients who can be further evaluated for alcohol abuse or alcohol dependence.

TABLE 8-4. The brief MAST for alcoholism screening.*

Questions	*Circle correct answers*	
1. Do you feel you are a normal drinker?	Yes (0)	No (2)
2. Do friends or relatives think you are a normal drinker?	Yes (0)	No (2)
3. Have you ever attended a meeting of Alcoholics Anonymous (AA)?	Yes (5)	No (0)
4. Have you ever lost friends or girlfriends/boyfriends because of drinking?	Yes (2)	No (0)
5. Have you ever gotten into trouble at work because of drinking?	Yes (2)	No (0)
6. Have you ever neglected your obligations, your family, or your work for two or more days in a row because you were drinking?	Yes (2)	No (0)
7. Have you ever had delirium tremens (DTs), severe shaking, heard voices or seen things that weren't there after heavy drinking?	Yes (2)	No (0)
8. Have you ever gone to anyone for help about your drinking?	Yes (5)	No (0)
9. Have you ever been in a hospital because of drinking?	Yes (5)	No (0)
10. Have you ever been arrested for drunk driving or driving after drinking?	Yes (2)	No (0)

From Pokorny, AD, Miller, BA, and Kaplan, HB. The brief MAST: a shortened version of the Michigan Alcoholism Screening Test. *American Journal of Psychiatry,* 1972, *129*(3), 342-345.
*A score of 6 or more should raise suspicion that the patient suffers from alcoholism.

Other screening techniques include the CAGE mnemonic and the Michigan Alcoholism Screening Test (MAST). CAGE is a mnemonic, describing a simple test that attempts to ascertain the patient's control over drinking and feedback from others about his alcoholic habits. The examiner asks the patient about four areas.

1. Has he ever felt the need to Cut down on his drinking?
2. Is he Annoyed by criticism of his drinking?
3. Has he had Guilty feelings about drinking?
4. Has he ever taken a morning Eye opener?

The test does not focus on the amount the patient drinks but on the negative consequences of drinking. If all questions are answered positively, there is a high probability of alcoholism.[7]

The MAST asks 25 questions that distinguish the alcoholic from the nonalcoholic population.[8] The brief MAST[9] asks 10 of the most highly discriminating questions and may be useful for such screening in the emergency department. The brief MAST is reproduced in Table 8-4. A score of 6 or more should certainly raise the clinician's suspicion of alcoholism.

ALCOHOL DEPENDENCE

Alcohol dependence can be diagnosed in an alcohol abuser when the patient has impairment in social or occupational functioning, uses alcohol in a pathological way, and demonstrates either tolerance or withdrawal. Tolerance is the need for increasing the amounts of alcohol to achieve a desired or decreased effect with the usual doses.

DIAGNOSTIC CRITERIA FOR ALCOHOL DEPENDENCE

A. Either a pattern of pathological alcohol use or impairment in social or occupational functioning due to alcohol use:

Pattern of pathological alcohol use: Need for daily use of alcohol for adequate functioning; inability to cut down or stop drinking; repeated efforts to control or reduce excess drinking by "going on the wagon" (period of temporary abstinence) or restricting drinking to certain times of the day; binges (remaining intoxicated throughout the day for at least 2 days); occasional consumption of a fifth of spirits (or its equivalent in wine or beer); amnesic periods for events occurring while intoxicated (blackouts); continuation of drinking despite a serious physical disorder that the individual knows is exacerbated by alcohol use; drinking of nonbeverge alcohol.

Impairment in social or occupational functioning due to alcohol use: e.g., violence while intoxicated, absence from work, loss of job, legal difficulties (e.g., arrest for intoxicated behavior, traffic accidents while intoxicated), arguments or difficulties with family or friends because of excessive alcohol use.

B. Either tolerance or withdrawal:

Tolerance: Need for markedly increased amounts of alcohol to achieve the desired effect, or markedly diminished effect with regular use of the same amount.

Withdrawal: Development of Alcohol Withdrawal (e.g., morning "shakes" and malaise relieved by drinking) after cessation of or reduction in drinking.

From American Psychiatric Association. *Diagnostic and statistical manual of mental disorders* (3rd ed.). Washington, D.C.: The Association, 1980.

The alcohol withdrawal syndrome includes tremulousness, nausea, malaise, irritability, and increased autonomic activity (hypertension, tachycardia, diaphoresis) that is relieved by drinking.

SUMMARY

Alcohol-related problems comprise a prominent segment of emergency practice. Alcohol intoxication creates an increased risk that the patient will be injured or involved in some sort of social disruption that results in an emergency department admission. Alcoholism can be fairly easily diagnosed in the emergency department. When referral facilities are adequate, screening for alcoholism in the emergency population may be quite worthwhile.

REFERENCES

1. Krome, RL, Wilson, RF, and Walt, AJ. The organization of the modern emergency department. In Walt, AJ, and Wilson, RF (Eds), *Management of trauma: pitfalls and practice*. Philadelphia: Lea and Febiger, 1975.
2. Brown, JD, and Harvey, ML. Emergency services: psychiatric emergencies in the general hospital: a review. *Canadian Psychiatric Association Journal,* 1971, *16,* 105-109.

3. Rund, DA, Summers, W, and Levin, M. Alcohol use and psychiatric illness in emergency patients. *Journal of the American Medical Association,* 1981, *245*(12), 1240-1241.
4. Hughes, JH, et al. Trauma in patients influenced by drugs and alcohol. *Annuals of Emergency Medicine,* Jan. 1980, *9*(1), 15-19.
5. Goldfrank, LR, and Starke, CL. Metabolic acidosis in the alcoholic (the drunk). In Goldfrank, LR (Ed.), *Toxicologic emergencies: a comprehensive handbook, in problem solving* (2nd ed.). New York: Appleton-Century Crofts, 1982.
6. Barnardy, T, Whitfield, CL, and Becker, CE. The alcoholic patient in the emergency department. In *The patient with alcoholism and other drug problems*. Chicago: Year Book Publisher, in press.
7. Ewing, J, and Mayfield, D. CAGE. *American Journal of Psychiatry,* 1974, *131,* 1121-1122.
8. Selzer, ML. The Michigan Alcoholism Screening Test: the quest for a new diagnostic instrument. *American Journal of Psychiatry,* 1971, *127,* 1635-1658.
9. Pokorny, AD, Miller, BA, and Kaplan, HB. The Brief MAST: a shortened version of the Michigan Alcoholism Screening Test. *American Journal of Psychiatry,* 1972, *129*(3), 342-345.

9 ANXIETY DISORDERS

Patients who experience severe anxiety report it as a terrible sense of apprehension, fear, and impending doom. Anxiety is accompanied and partially defined by a constellation of symptoms that reflects intense autonomic activity and hyperventilation. These symptoms include palpitations, dry mouth, dizziness, paresthesia, faintness, and exhaustion.

Patients in the emergency department frequently show signs of anxiety. The illness or accident that brings them to the emergency department in the first place creates apprehension and uneasiness. These symptoms become linked to psychiatric disorders when, like many other ailments, they interfere with the patients' social, occupational, or interpersonal life. These symptoms cause such pain and emotional distress that the patients request help.

Some definitions of anxiety distinguish it from fear. These definitions describe fear as a conscious response to a real and known external danger. Fear is the response a person has when he is about to experience a head-on collision on the freeway or local infiltration of dental anesthesia and tooth extraction. Anxiety, by contrast, is a response to an unknown source of danger and includes the patient's self-doubt about how he will cope with the anticipated problem.

Anxiety states represent various groups of symptoms and signs that are manifestations of a number of underlying conditions. In a way they are like the symptoms and signs of fever. They produce discomfort, and reduction of the anxiety (like lowering of the fever) produces symptomatic relief but does not affect the underlying condition.[1]

ALERTNESS FOR MEDICAL DISORDERS

Various signs and symptoms of anxiety disorders are listed in Table 9-1. It is fairly well established that the emergency physician must be constantly vigilant for serious medical illnesses that produce signs and symptoms identical to those associated with anxiety disorders. It is not unheard of for a patient with a large pulmonary embolus, for instance, to be discharged with a diagnosis of ''hyperventilation syndrome'' or for a patient with a myocardial infarction, experiencing mild nausea, apprehension, and shortness of breath, to be misdiagnosed as ''panic attack'' and erroneously discharged.

CASE EXAMPLE 1

A 54-year-old obese man was admitted to the emergency department with a complaint of shortness of breath. His pulse was 120, and the respiratory rate was 24 per minute. The examination of his lungs revealed no rales or dullness, and the heart examination showed no murmurs or rubs. The patient was discharged with a diagnosis of hyperventilation syndrome. He returned several hours later with marked respiratory distress, cyanosis, and hypoxia. A pulmonary arteriogram revealed multiple large pulmonary emboli. The patient was admitted to the intensive care unit to receive anticoagulation treatment involving heparin.

The patient with a severe anxiety syndrome may present a portrait similar to the patient just described. The diagnosis of an anxiety disorder should be made only when the physician is convinced that a medical condition is not responsible for the symptoms.

TABLE 9-1. Abnormal symptoms and signs that may be associated with anxiety syndromes

Type of examination	*Symptoms and signs*
General appearance	Worried, anxious, pacing, breathless
Vital signs	Tachycardia, tachypnea
Cardiovascular	Heart racing, pounding, palpitations
Respiratory	Shortness of breath (can not catch breath)
Gastrointestinal	Dry mouth, dysphagia (lump in the throat) abdominal pain, diarrhea, nausea, loss of appetite
Neurological	Dizziness, headache, muscle tension, irritability, uneasiness, terror, worry, apprehension, tremor, mild diaphoresis

TABLE 9-2. Acute medical illnesses associated with symptoms and signs of anxiety disorders

Medical disorder	*Associated clinical feature*
Pulmonary embolus	Apprehension, hyperventilation
Myocardial infarction	Nausea, shortness of breath
Thyrotoxicosis	Nervousness, jitteriness, hyperventilation
Hypoglycemia	Diaphoresis, agitation
Hypoxia	Agitation, shortness of breath
Drug intoxication (e.g., amphetamine)	Agitation, tachycardia
Drug withdrawal	Tremulousness, agitation
Caffeine toxicity (usually greater than 1000 mg of caffeine or 7 to 10 cups of coffee)	Nervousness, jitteriness
Paroxysmal supraventricular tachycardia	Palpitation, tachycardia, apprehension
Mitral valve prolapse	Palpitation, apprehension
Metabolic acidosis	Hyperventilation

The physician must not misdiagnose paroxysmal supraventricular tachycardia or hypoglycemia as panic attack or anxiety disorder. Table 9-2 lists various acute medical conditions associated with signs and symptoms of anxiety disorders.

HISTORICAL FEATURES

The linkage of anxiety syndromes to disorders of the heart dates at least back to the Civil War when the stress of anticipating a battle or experiencing severe physical exertion rendered the soldiers incapacitated because of palpitations, dizziness, faintness, and shortness of breath. The "soldier's heart" syndrome was also labeled *Da Costa's syndrome, neurasthenia,* and *neurocirculatory asthenia.* By World War II this syndrome was called *anxiety neurosis.* The linkage of anxiety symptoms with cardiac pathology remains. Some anxiety syndromes have recently been shown to be associated with mitral valve prolapse (MVP).[2]

CLINICAL ASSESSMENT

As in the determination of psychosis, the emergency physician should be able to begin the evaluation of an anxious patient with a history and perhaps a simultaneous physical examination of the external appearance of the head as well as a check on vital

TABLE 9-3. Common anxiety disorders and their treatment

Diagnosis	*Symptoms*	*Treatment*
Anxiety states		
Panic disorder	Palpitation, fear	Propranolol (inderal), tricyclic antidepressants (TCA)
	Sweating, chest pain	Behavior modification, biofeedback
Generalized anxiety disorder	Anxiety	Propranolol, TCA, behavior modification, biofeedback
Obsessive compulsive disorder	Repeated thoughts or acts to ward off anxiety	TCA, monoamine oxidase inhibitor (MAO inhibitor), behavior therapy, individual psychotherapy
Posttraumatic stress disorders		
Acute	Psychic numbing, recurrent thoughts or "visions" of event	Group psychotherapy, individual psychotherapy
Chronic	Increased irritability	Group psychotherapy, individual psychotherapy
Phobic disorders		
Agoraphobia	Irrational fear of object, activity, or situation	TCA, propranolol, MAO inhibitor, behavior modification
Social phobia	Fear of specific social situation	Behavior modification, TCA
Simple phobia	Fear of object or situation	Behavior modification

signs, pupils, neck, skin, chest, heart, and abdomen. If doubt about a possible physical illness persists after hearing the history and examining the patient, appropriate further studies may include electrocardiograms (ECGs), arterial blood gas levels, electrolyte concentrations, blood urea nitrogen levels (BUN), glucose levels, complete blood counts, and possibly thyroid function tests. A toxicology screen may be warranted. If MVP is suspected, an echocardiogram may be indicated. When organic disorders seem unlikely, the physician can begin to evaluate the patient for one of the anxiety disorders.

Anxiety disorders are classified according to the DSM-III in one of the following three general categories:

1. Anxiety states
   a. Panic disorder
   b. Generalized anxiety disorder
   c. Obsessive compulsive disorder
2. Posttraumatic stress disorders
3. Phobic disorders

These categories have their own subdivisions. Some of the more common anxiety disorders and recommended treatment methods are presented in Table 9-3.

ANXIETY STATES

Panic disorder

The central features of panic disorder are recurring panic attacks, during which the patient experiences extreme and sometimes disabling symptoms of anxiety. These symptoms usually include palpitations, shortness of breath, dizziness, faintness, and trembling. The associated hyperventilation typically produces paresthesia (numbness and tingling or "pins and needles") in the hands, feet, and perioral region. Symptoms that could also be the result of a serious physical disorder include a sensation of choking, smothering, or chest pain.

The attacks usually last several minutes and rarely over an hour. They are typically spontaneous and may be associated with a phobic stimulus, (such as entering a crowded store or leaving home).

CASE EXAMPLE 2

A 32-year-old housewife was admitted to the emergency department complaining of severe anxiety. The physical examination was negative. She was jittery, had palpitations, and felt short of breath. She had mild perioral numbness and tingling. With calm questioning she revealed that her husband had left the day before on a business trip. She became intensely fearful while driving and developed her present symptoms.

The patient's severe anxiety is related to her separation from a figure on whom she is dependent. Reassuring her that no physical illness has been found in the examination helps diminish the symptoms. The physician can then point out that separations from loved ones are difficult for most people. The panic reaction is frightening but common and should be treated by a few visits to a psychiatrist/counselor. Medication is not necessary in the emergency department.

The anxiety associated with these symptoms can be monumental. The victims of panic attack report extreme apprehension, terror, and feelings of irrational fear. They may develop a sensation of unreality and experience fear that they are going crazy. Panic attacks may leave the patient with a sense of total exhaustion. This exhaustion was one of the predominant features of the "soldier's heart" or "Da Costa's syndrome," which left the soldier weak, virtually helpless (neurasthenic), and unable to fight.

At least three panic attacks must occur within a 3-month period to establish the diagnosis of panic disorder. A feeling of anticipatory anxiety may occur in association with recurrent panic attacks. The patient begins to fear the attack and becomes reluctant to be alone or in public places. When the fear of public places becomes the predominant symptom, the disorder is more appropriately diagnosed *agoraphobia*.

Panic disorders usually begin in the late teenage years or in the early twenties but may occasionally occur in the early thirties. It is unusual for the disorder to begin in later life. When the symptoms develop for the first time in older patients, the physician should search for an organic mental disorder or an underlying medical condition.

Approach to the patient with panic disorder. The panic may have subsided by the time the patient arrives in the emergency department. If not, the patient generally attracts the immediate attention of the emergency staff. Most experienced personnel correctly recognize a typical panic attack but remain alert for an underlying medical illness. The experienced clinician initiates a patient-assessment procedure that searches for a medical disorder. The patient's general appearance is noted, and vital signs are taken. The dyspneic condition of the patient is often stabilized with nasal oxygen at 2 liters per minute after an arterial blood gas level is obtained.

The physical examination of the patient with panic attack generally reveals a person with tachypnea and possibly mild tachycardia who otherwise appears well. The lungs are clear, and the heart sounds are normal. The association of MVP and panic attack has been documented. It is particularly useful to listen for the systolic murmur and midsystolic click of MVP during the cardiac examination.

Tachycardia greater than 120 beats per minute should prompt the emergency physician to obtain a cardiogram and look for paroxysmal supraventricular tachycardia or atrial fibrillation with rapid atrial response. Hypoglycemia could be a cause of anxiety and apprehension. When this is suspected in a diabetic, for instance, blood should be drawn to measure the glucose level. A Dextrostix bedside measurement of the blood glucose level provides an even more rapid screening test for hypoglycemia in this setting. Febrile illness may be a cause of tachycardia in some patients. Patients with hyperventilation, significant mouth breathing, and suspected fever may need a rectal temperature to be taken for an accurate measurement.

Hyperthyroidism, particularly thyroid storm, has several clinical features that are consistent with those of panic attack. There is typically tachycardia, palpitations, tachypnea, shortness of breath, anxiety, apprehension, and tension. These disorders may require immediate medical treatment and hospitalization. Since the results of thyroid function tests are rarely available immediately, the physician must rely on clinical signs and symptoms like exophthalmos, history of heat intolerance, and brisk deep tendon reflexes to make the diagnosis. Perhaps the best test is time, and thus a period of observation in the emergency department should decide the issue. Panic attack usually last minutes and rarely endures longer than an hour, whereas thyroid storm and other serious medical disorders persist, while the patient's condition remains the same or worsens with time.

Drug intoxication and withdrawal can produce the clinical symptoms and signs of panic attack. Caffeine or amphetamine intoxication can produce these features as can large doses of sympathomimetics like phenylpropanolamine (an ingredient in Coricidin, Ornade, and Dimetapp). Some sympathomimetics are packaged as "look alike" drugs (combinations of sympathomimetic agents packaged in capsules that look like amphetamines). Anticholinergic drugs (atropine or scopolamine) or effects from antihistamines or Jimson weed can produce the symptoms of a panic attack. Withdrawal from sedatives, particularly barbituates, precipitates a similar reaction.

Emergency treatment for panic disorder and panic attack

Hyperventilation. The time-honored treatment for hyperventilation is the rather inelegant but effective technique of covering the mouth and nose with a paper bag so that the patient rebreathes the expired air. This increases the alveolar and arterial Pa_{CO_2}. The increase in Pa_{CO_2} reverses the alkalosis caused by the hyperventilation and allows calcium to move back to the ionized state. These changes reverse the signs and symptoms of severe hyperventilation; tetany disappears, paresthesias diminish, shortness of breath diminishes, and anxiety gradually lessens. Sometimes patients are too anxious to accept the paper bag treatment and require mild sedation. Hypoxia should be ruled out, at least clinically, before asking the patient to breathe in and out of a paper bag.

Antianxiety medication. Antianxiety medication like diazepam (Valium) or chlordiazepoxide (Librium) has traditionally been used in emergency departments to treat panic attack. It does, in fact, allay anxiety and speed the patient's discharge. Though these medications are quite effective, they have at least two drawbacks. They may make the patient dependent on antianxiety agents, and they treat the symptom but not the source of the disorder. Alcohol and drug abuse are major complications of anxiety states like panic disorders. Physicians, friends, or family members often make these acute anxiety agents available to the patient in an effort to help. The patient typically experiences a rising level of anxiety, takes the medication, and experiences immediate relief. The patient may soon take the medication even when experiencing anticipatory anxiety. This anxiety-relief cycle reinforces itself, thus promoting eventual drug addiction or dependence. A similar mechanism promotes alcohol abuse in these patients.

Antianxiety agents may be used in the emergency department for the immediate treatment of the disorder simply because they are so effective for immediate management. The emergency physician should, however, attempt to explain to the patient and his family that the disorder requires psychiatric evaluation and probably further medical examinations. If possible, the patient should be instructed to avoid the antianxiety agents whenever possible. Ideally, the patient should not be sent home from the emergency department with minor tranquilizers (diazepam, chlordiazepoxide) because this discourages prompt follow-up with a psychiatrist.

A commonly used beta adrenergic blocking agent in clinical medicine is propranolol. The medication is remarkably effective in controlling the peripheral effects of the panic attack, including tachycardia, tremor, and palpitation. The patient experiences a reduction in anxiety when these symptoms abate. Propranolol is also the treatment of choice when disabling panic attacks are associated with MVP. The physician who hears the typical click-murmur of MVP may decide to refer the patient for further cardiac evaluation and may possibly treat him immediately with propranolol. The initial dosage of propranolol is 10 mg three or four times per day. The patient may be discharged with 3- or 4-days' supply of medication, but a medical or cardiac follow-up must be assured for him.

Tricyclic antidepressants. A tricyclic antidepressant like imipramine (Tofranil) may be useful for panic attack. Beginning at 75 mg per day, the dosage can be increased over 2 to 3 weeks to 150 to 200 mg per day. The patient should be warned about the side effects, like dry mouth and morning grogginess, to ensure compliance with the regimen. If the medication works at this level it may be continued for several months. At that point the dosage can be gradually decreased until the symptoms are controlled with the lowest possible dosage. Many emergency physicians prefer to let the referring physician or psychiatric consultant make the decision whether or not to use tricyclic agents.

Biofeedback and behavior modification. Biofeedback can be a very effective therapy in certain patients. By learning to control their alpha rhythm, these patients can often help themselves relax when experiencing the early stages of a panic attack. Behavior modification may also be a useful therapy, especially if a certain stimulus or type of behavior precipitates an attack. Self-hypnosis may be a helpful tool as well. Patients may be directed to practitioners or centers that specialize in these techniques.

Other therapies. MAO inhibitors like phenelzine (Nardil) may be helpful but should *not* be prescribed in the emergency department because of the extensive concomitant patient education about diet (e.g., low tyramine) that must accompany the patient's first prescription.

Generalized anxiety disorder

Patients with generalized anxiety disorder have persistent feelings of extreme anxiety and nervousness for at least 1 month's duration. This is between the discrete and brief episodes of overwhelming anxiety. The "free-floating" anxiety associated with this disorder typically does not cause major impairment in social or occupational functioning. Drug and alcohol abuse are frequently associated problems for the same reasons that they are for patients with panic disorder.

Although generalized symptoms of anxiety may vary from person to person, the DSM-III lists the following four major categories of symptoms in generalized anxiety disorder[3]:

1. Motor tension—shakiness, muscle tension, muscle twitching, jumpiness, jitteriness, and fidgeting
2. Autonomic hyperactivity—tachycardia, palpitations, sweating, flushed appearance, hyperventilation and frequent urination or diarrhea
3. Apprehensive expectations—generalized apprehension, worry rumination, and excessive concern about what will happen to himself (e.g., fear of fainting or losing control)
4. Vigilance and scanning—patient feels on edge or irritable, is unable to sleep, and may be easily distracted

Evaluation. The patient may initially select and emphasize a specific component of generalized anxiety when describing his complaint to the emergency staff. He may provide a chief complaint of dizziness, diarrhea, or abdominal pain, for instance. His overall jitteriness, restlessness, and increased motor activity may provide early clues to the diagnosis, which is established when the clinician confirms that the symptoms have been present for at least 1 month's duration or that another medical or psychiatric disorder is not responsible for the symptoms. Some authorities have claimed that the patient with generalized anxiety disorder has a less disturbed psychiatric history than the person with panic attack[4] and that the panic-attack victim has a higher degree of childhood separation or other early life disturbances.[5] Other authors have suggested that panic attack has a genetic basis, but families of these patients do not have a higher incidence of generalized anxiety disorder.[6]

Treatment. Propranolol or imipramine is probably the most appropriate medication for generalized anxiety disorder. The emergency physician may elect to refer these patients for further psychiatric assessment and management after reassuring them that a physical disorder is possible but not likely, based on the results of the history, physical examination, and relevant laboratory tests obtained in the emergency department. Antianxiety agents (minor tranquilizers) are avoided because of their high abuse potential in these patients. Antipsychotic medication is not indicated.

Crisis intervention may be helpful if there is an evident precipitating cause for the present anxiety. Crisis intervention techniques focus on a specific problem. The patient is interviewed briefly until the problem is identified, and then he is asked to develop alternative ways of solving the problem. Emotional support and reassurance that he will not get worse and indeed may get better over the next few weeks or months may be quite comforting to the patient and is helpful in treatment. The physician should encourage the patient to totally avoid the source of anxiety (if there is one) for 2 or 3 days and should help him accomplish this by work, exercise, family counseling, or whatever means seem appropriate. The technique emphasizes that the patient must begin to identify his problems and develop alternative behaviors, and this gives him a sense of mastery and discourages the belief that someone else will solve his problems.

Obsessive compulsive disorder

Obsessive compulsive disorder is a far less common cause of emergency complaints than panic attack or anxiety disorder. In its early stages, however, the disorder may cause the patient considerable anxiety and thus promote anxiety-related complaints.

Obsessions are recurrent thoughts, images, or impulses that seem to invade that patient's consciousness and cause great anxiety. The patient may suddenly have the impulse to hurt or kill someone or become agitated because he believes that germs are being passed by handshaking or contaminated food. He either tries to avoid activities that precipitate the anxiety (causing relief) or goes ahead and faces the situation (like shaking hands) and experiences increased anxiety.

Compulsions are mechanistic, almost ritualistic motor acts performed repetitively for some reason that presumably (according to the patient) relates to his safety or welfare. Common compulsions are checking the locks on the doors four or five times or checking the stove repeatedly to see that it is turned off. A compulsion may involve tapping the knee three times to prevent a certain obsessional thought. A common obsession that is frightening to a young mother is the impulse to kill her child. She may begin to avoid knives and other potential weapons and become frantic over this "unacceptable" thought. Repeated hand-washing may be another compulsion. The repetitious act is not a compulsion if it is necessary and causes little anxiety (such as the emergency physician washing his or her hands before examining each new patient).

Patients with this disorder are best referred for psychiatric evaluation and treatment that may involve behavior modification, tricyclic antidepressants, or psychotherapy. These patients need to be reassured that their symptoms are relatively common and treatable and that they are not "crazy" (something they invariably fear).

POSTTRAUMATIC STRESS DISORDER

Posttraumatic stress disorder may develop in anyone who has gone through a severely traumatic event like rape, assault, military combat, natural disasters, or physical torture. The typical psychological response to these events involves an early phase of "psychic numbing" that is characterized by emotional detachment from events and people. As the patient recovers from the numb sensation, he may then enter a long period characterized by anxiety, nightmares, and vivid sensations of reliving the experience ("flashbacks").

The patient with established posttraumatic stress disorder can be referred to the appropriate psychiatrist or facility (mental health center or Veterans Administration hospital). Allowing the patient to express his fear and describe the situation a few times may provide early relief of anxiety.

Emergency physicians also have an excellent opportunity to intervene when "victims of violence"[7] are first brought to the emergency department. Rape victims, for instance, can be counseled about predictable psychological reactions to the event, such as "numbing" and recurrent anxiety. It is generally helpful to arrange counseling for these patients as soon as possible and, if reasonable, to allow them to contact the emergency physician or nurse for counseling or support in the interim.

PHOBIC DISORDERS

Phobic disorders may be associated with panic attacks and therefore appear in the emergency department with the typical clinical portrait of panic attack. Routine questioning about the patient's attack and the source of anxiety may reveal the phobia. The emergency physician may encounter a phobic patient because he requests help dealing with the disorder, or it may be an associated diagnosis in a patient who requests emergency care for other problems.

Phobias are irrational, excessive fears of objects, situations, activities, people, or places. These fears are severe enough to interfere with or dominate the patient's life. The fear of the phobic stimulus is so severe that the patient goes to nearly any length to avoid it. There are three general classifications of phobia: agoraphobia, social phobia, and simple phobia.

Agoraphobia

Agoraphobia is the fear and avoidance of public places (derived from the Greek, *agora*—a place of assembly). Patients severely afflicted with this disorder virtually refuse to enter public places, especially away from home. The disorder may be so severe that the patient's activity becomes limited to a single area or room of the house. The patient may also complain of exhaustion, tremulousness, or the feeling that he is not himself. Agoraphobia is quite common, and in certain area lay groups have been organized to treat the symptoms. There is often a history of a recent severe loss, like the death of a child or parent, before the onset of the disorder, but a definite causal relationship has not been shown.

Social phobia

Social phobia differs from agoraphobia in that the patient's symptoms are related to other people. Various specific phobias relate to specific situations. The patient may be afraid to write checks in front of someone else, or he may fear vomiting in a dining room or restaurant. Other typical examples include people who are extremely fearful of performing in public or using public lavatories. Some of these fears are extreme; even the thought of participating in the feared endeavor causes a feeling of terror, sweating, and palpitations and is usually seen as unreasonable even by the patient. The patient goes to great lengths to avoid these situations and at times may come to the emergency department with the plea "you have to do something for my anxiety." It is crucial to take a full history at this point to rule out underlying medical causes for such feelings of anxiety. The patient may try to avoid feeling "silly" by not reporting his actual phobias and therefore only report his anxiety. Thus the patient with an anxiety disorder should be questioned routinely about phobias or specific fears.

Simple phobia

The simple phobia is an irrational and persistent fear with a compelling need to avoid certain objects or situations. The situation is one other than being alone or in public places. Simple phobias have traditionally been labeled with their Greek root to produce a lengthy name. This is not really helpful, however, since there is a phobia for any object or situation. Phobias can involve needles, physicians, pills, bridges, driving, heights, or flying. These patients have no other symptoms of generalized anxiety disorder, or panic attacks.

Most simple phobias that begin in childhood disappear without treatment. Some, however, persist into adulthood and rarely then remit without treatment. If the phobic object is rarely encountered in the environment, there is little impairment. However, if the phobia involves flying, for instance, it could be quite a handicap for a patient who is required to fly in the course of his occupation. Generally such a patient does not request treatment unless some unusual incident occurs, or his phobias begin to interfere with his work or social life. Therefore the case of a patient who has simple phobia and is brought to the emergency department usually involves a crisis in which he is confronted with his inability to carry through an important action (because of the phobia) and becomes desperate. At the time of crisis the patient may feel suicidal or extremely anxious and may request pharmacotherapy or referral for treatment.

Treatment

Treatment for the phobic disorders involves behavior modification therapy, antidepressants, and reassurance. Behavior modification therapy usually entails systematic desensitization. Imipramine and phenelzine have been used in this disorder but should probably not be initiated in the emergency department. Phenelzine, in particular, requires an extensive dietary education and medication review.

Reassurance may help the patient feel more comfortable in the emergency department. He should be made aware, however, that he need not suffer these symptoms indefinitely and should be encouraged to seek psychiatric help within the next few days. It is often difficult for the patient to keep the appointment because of the fear of leaving his home or environment. The person who brought the patient to the emergency department or a member of the family who can go along with him for the first meeting should be informed and recruited as an ally in getting the patient to the psychiatric appointment.

SUMMARY

Patients who come to an emergency department with the complaint of anxiety and its concomitant physical symptoms can easily be divided into specific subtypes. Differentiating these specific subtypes is helpful because the patient may be reassured that he has an illness that is common and treatable. The most difficult problem for the patient to manage is the fear that no treatment is available and that the disorder is so severe and pervasive it will permanently impair his ability to lead a normal life.

Important parts of emergency management, therefore are reassurance, education, support, and initiation of drug therapy if indicated. This scientific approach to these common problems gives rise to better medical care for the patient and a more systematic approach to a patient with such vague symptoms. Ideally this helps prevent immediate aggravation of the patient's fear and paves the way for formal psychiatric outpatient evaluation and treatment.

REFERENCES

1. Pariser, SF, et al. Diagnosis and management of anxiety symptoms and syndrome. In Davis, JM, and Greenblat, D (Eds.), *Pharmacology update: new and neglected areas*. New York: Grune & Stratton, 1979.
2. Pariser, SF, Pinta, ER, and Jones, BA. Mitral valve prolapse syndrome and anxiety neurosis/panic disorder. *American Journal of Psychiatry*, 1978, *135*, 246-247.
3. American Psychiatric Association. *Diagnostic and statistical manual of mental disorders* (3rd ed.). Washington, D.C.: The Association, 1980.
4. Raskin, J, et al. Panic and generalized anxiety disorders: developmental antecedents and precipitants. *Archives of General Psychiatry*, 1982, *39*(6), 687-689.
5. Klein, DF, and Davis, JM. *Diagnosis and drug treatment of psychiatric disorder. Baltimore:* The Williams & Wilkins Co., 1969.
6. Crowe, RR, et al. A family study of anxiety neurosis. *Archives of General Psychiatry*, 1981, *37*(2), 77-79.
7. Warner, CG, and Braen, GR. *Topics in emergency medicine: human violence* (Vol. 3, no. 4). Gaithersburg, Md.: Aspen Publications, Jan. 1982.

10 AFFECTIVE DISORDERS

Variations in mood, feeling, and emotion are integral, expected, and normally welcome components of human life. Happiness and sorrow are daily emotions for many people and cause no psychiatric impairment or pain. The extremes of these emotions, mania and depression, however, may be serious, intensely painful, and possibly life threatening. Depression and mania, serious disorders of mood and emotion, are illnesses that require thorough evaluation and treatment.

The term *affect* describes mood or "prolonged emotion that colors the whole psychic life."[1] *Affect* refers to the conscious subjective perception of emotion or feeling apart from the physical changes that accompany it. In this strict sense, tachycardia and flushing are physical changes that may accompany rage, for instance. The pure emotional response is the affect. As affective disorders are now defined, however, some of the associated physical manifestations for their diagnosis are extremely important.

Affective disorders are perhaps the most common class of psychiatric illness in emergency patients. At least one study has shown that affective disorders can be diagnosed in 23% of emergency patients.[2] Patients with these disorders often appear in the emergency department late at night as a suicide attempt or as having vague nonspecific complaints related to depression or mania. The two major affective disorders are major depressive episode (depression) and manic episode (mania).

DEPRESSIVE DISORDER

Major clinical depression, severe enough to require treatment, is an entity distinct from mild despondency or grief. Despondency is a normal response to a disturbing life situation or a medical problem. Grief or bereavement is a normal response to loss, especially of a loved one. Previous classifications of depression have used various categorizations like endogenous, exogenous, functional, and organic. At present, however, the depressive disorders are viewed as illnesses defined by their clinical characteristics and classified as either primary or secondary. *Primary depression* means that a depression appears before other significant medical or psychiatric illnesses and meets the criteria for major depression. *Secondary depression* develops after the onset of another serious medical or psychiatic illness and may be causally related to the primary condition.

MAJOR AFFECTIVE (MOOD) DISORDERS (DSM-III)

I. Major depression
  Primary (not due to another psychiatric or medical illness)
  Secondary (due to another psychiatric disorder, i.e., substance abuse, anxiety disorder, or a medical defect such as cancer, heart disease, or disfigurement)
II. Bipolar disorder
  Manic episode
  Depressive episode
  (or both)
III. Dysthymic disorder
  Less severe depression

Adapted from American Psychiatric Association. *Diagnostic and statistical manual of mental disorders* (3rd ed.). Washington, D.C.: The Association, 1980.

TABLE 10-1. Diagnostic features of major depressive episode originally developed by Washington University (Feighner criteria)

A. Dysphoric mood (sad, blue, down in the dumps)
B. Four of these eight symptoms every day for 2 weeks:

Category	Diagnostic features
1. Appetite	Increase or decrease
2. Sleep	Initial insomnia (inability to sleep for 1 to 2 hours) or early morning wakening (after 2 to 4 hours' sleep)
3. Activity	Loss of interest, decreased activity level
4. Interest	Reduced for usually pleasurable activities or hobbies
5. Energy	Tired, worn out or restless, tense
6. Guilt	Present over insignificant or incongruent things or events
7. Concentration	Decreased (cannot read or watch television for 1 hour at a time)
8. Suicide	Active suicidal thoughts or wishing he would not wake up

Adapted from American Psychiatric Association. *Diagnostic and statistical manual of mental disorders* (3rd. ed.). Washington, D.C.: The Association, 1980.

The diagnostic criteria for major depressive episode are listed in Table 10-1. These strict clinical criteria for the diagnosis of major depression enable the clinician to screen rapidly for the presence of depression with a relatively small number of questions and render an accurate diagnosis and treatment for this extremely common illness.

Dysphoric mood

The first criterion for a major depressive illness is a dysphoric mood. The term *dysphoric* refers to a state of being unwell or unhappy in contrast to *euphoria,* which refers to a feeling of being well or elated. The dysphoric mood is one of sadness. The patient feels blue, down in the dumps, hopeless, low, depressed, or irritable.

In depression the dysphoric mood predominates. The patient, for instance, feels sad continuously and typically thinks, speaks, and moves slowly (psychomotor retardation). The mood does not shift rapidly.

Individual symptoms

Strict criteria for the diagnosis of major depression have been developed by investigators at Washington University in St. Louis and are used in the DSM-III criteria for depression. They are extremely helpful for the emergency physician who wants to quickly screen patients for depression and yet maintain the tenor of the standard medical interview. Beginning with questions about sleep and appetite, the interviewer asks about loss of energy, loss of interest, and loss of ability to concentrate. If positive responses about these areas are obtained, the patient is actually depressed and questions about guilt, slowness of thought, slowness of action, and thoughts about death or suicide seem more appropriate for the interview and the patient's underlying condition.

The eight criteria for depression listed in Table 10-1 can be remembered under the following general headings: appetite, sleep, activity, interest, energy, guilt, concentration, and suicide. The diagnosis of major depression can be made if the depressed mood and four of the eight listed symptoms have been present every day for at least 2 weeks.

Psychotic symptoms

Affective disorders are one of the three major classes of psychiatric disorders (organic mental disorders, schizophrenia, and affective disorders) that can cause psychotic symptoms. The severely depressed patient may have mood-congruent delusions or hallucinations. The depressed patient may believe that he is dead, for instance, or being punished by "the voices" for a previous wrong. The grandiose delusions of the manic patient may result in his belief that he is a corporate president or a great prophet. The psychotic features of an organic or schizophrenic disorder may, in contrast, be incongruent with the mood. Here the content of the delusion or hallucination is not related to the patient's predominant mood.

When psychotic symptoms of affective illness are detected by the emergency physician, psychiatric consultation (and probably hospitalization) is indicated. The patient undoubtedly requires inpatient treatment with antidepressant medications and further evaluation.

Medical conditions causing depression

When the diagnosis of affective disorder is suspected, the clinician should complete the history and physical examination, looking especially for factors that can cause clinical depression. The major categories include medications, substance abuse, and neurological disorders.

Medication. Some medications are well-recognized causes of depression. The antihypertensives, reserpine and methyldopa (Aldomet), can cause a full-blown major depressive episode with both dysphoric and vegetative symptoms (sleep and appetite disturbance). Propranolol (Inderal) can cause a depressive syndrome. Oral contraceptives and corticosteroids can cause depression. Tranquilizers and hypnotics are depressants that can aggravate or create symptoms of depression. Barbiturates, diazepam (Valium), and chlordiazepoxide (Librium) are examples. Alcohol notoriously causes or worsens depression in a chronic abuser.

The examining physician should probably suspect nearly any drug the patient is taking chronically and at least consider withdrawing the medication for an observation period long enough to determine if the drug is responsible for the depression. Since this continuity of care is rarely feasible in emergency practice, this procedure must be carried out by the patient's own physician or an outpatient clinic.

Substance abuse. Substance abuse is clearly associated with affective disorders. Whether the alcoholic treats his underlying affective disorder with alcohol or develops depression following prolonged alcohol use is not really known. The association of alcoholism and affective disorder is frequently observed, however. For diagnostic and research purposes, the primary disorder is the one that appears first in time. The secondary disorder appears after the primary disorder is established.

Drugs like amphetamine and cocaine produce an early euphoria when initially taken but usually cause depression as the blood level and early peak effect diminish. As the amphetamine abuser begins to "crash," he experiences the urge to take more drugs, and the cycle may continue. Regularly used drugs like cocaine can induce a syndrome of dysphoria, anxiety, and weight loss that meets the criteria for a major depressive episode.

Neurological disorders. Chronic neurological disorders like multiple sclerosis can cause depressive symptoms as can certain traumatic neurological disorders like chronic subdural hematoma. When the dysphoric mood is accompanied by a new focal neurological deficit or symptom, neurological consultation and a computerized axial tomography (CAT) scan are clearly indicated.

Other medical disorders. Endocrine disorders like hypothyroidism and connective tissue diseases like lupus erythematosus may cause depressive symptoms. Chronic debilitating or painful diseases produce a quite understandable secondary depression. Chronic hospitalization may result in a secondary depression.

Initial complaints

Nonspecific symptoms. Emergency physicians who are prepared to zoom in quickly on a specific physical complaint like a sprained ankle or lacerated finger may back down immediately when they confront the patient who is "sick all over" or "weak and dizzy." In addition to completing a physical examination that includes postural vital signs and stool for occult blood, the emergency physician should routinely screen these patients for depression. The eight categories of symptoms, beginning with questions about sleep, appetite, and weight change, can be covered rapidly, even while the ex-

IN SAD CAGES

In	Interest
S	Sleep
A	Appetite
D	Depressed mood
C	Concentration
A	Activity
G	Guilt
E	Energy
S	Suicide

amination is being performed, if necessary. A mnemonic for remembering the symptoms of major depression is presented in the above box.

Patients with depression often seem to either feel that they must have a physical complaint or attribute their fatigue and listlessness to physical illness. The patient who insists that "it's not all in my head!" resists the suggestion that the symptoms may have a psychiatric cause (Fig. 10-1).

The best approach in this situation may be to complete the emergency history and physical examination and to assure the patient that no physical illness is present, based on the limited examination. He needs to be made aware, however, that a more complete medical evaluation and perhaps psychiatric testing are indicated. The patient can then be referred for appropriate medical and/or psychiatric follow-up care.

Chronic pain. Chronic pain syndromes, especially nonspecific facial pain, may be the initial complaints of the patient with a major depressive episode. In the case of facial pain, the emergency physician generally looks for disorders of the sinuses, ear and dental pathology, and tic douloureux. Along with this customary evaluation, screening questions for depression can generally be added. The ultimate treatment for the patient may include antidepressant medication that should, in time, alleviate the pain.

Anxiety. The patient with depression may complain about feeling agitated, nervous, or anxious, rather than being worn out or fatigued. He may appear irritable and look as if he suffers from anxiety disorder. The screening questions for depression should be asked of the patient, since the underlying disorders may be a major depressive episode.

Approach to the patient

Specific questions that can be asked in screening for depression include the following:

1. Has your appetite changed lately? Have you lost weight? How is your appetite in general?
2. Are you having trouble sleeping? If so, what kind of trouble?

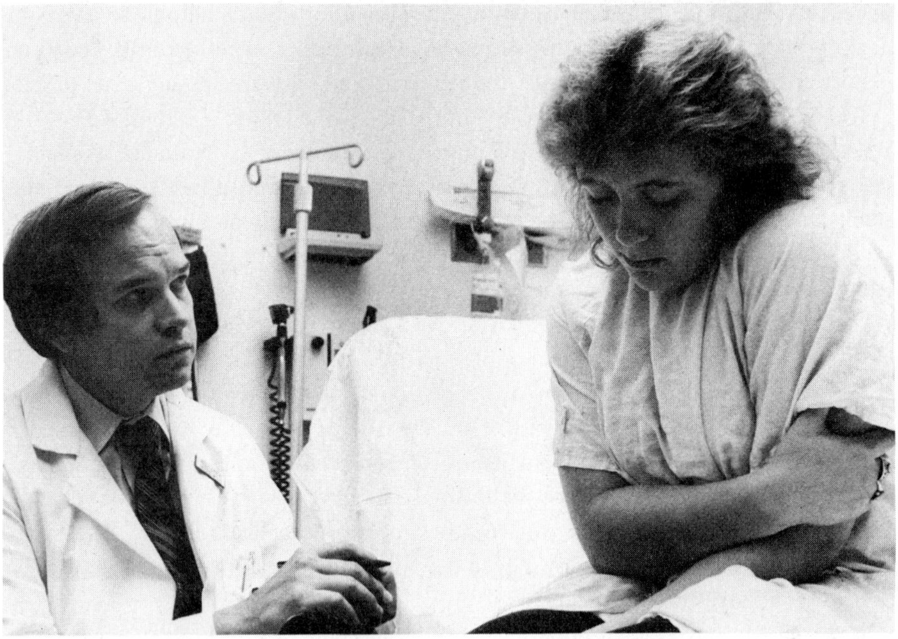

FIG. 10-1. Some patients who are severely depressed report vague physical symptoms as their main complaint. Screening for depression may be very rewarding in these patients. (Courtesy Lee Jansen, Columbus, Ohio.)

3. Are you as active as you used to be?
4. Has your interest in things like hobbies or your job changed recently?
5. Do you have much energy lately or do you feel tired most of the time?
6. Do you feel guilty about anything?
7. Can you concentrate as well as normal on things like television programs, the newspaper, or a book, or does your mind tend to wander to other thoughts?
8. Are you depressed, sad, or "down in the dumps"?
9. Have you ever thought of hurting yourself or of committing suicide?

Sometimes a patient gives a clear "yes" to four or five of these questions but refuses to acknowledge that he is depressed. He does not identify himself as depressed and may resist such a definition. It is helpful in this situation to discuss the typical cardinal symptoms of depression with the patient. The discussion may help him label his symptoms.

Sometimes a patient becomes tearful when asked questions about how he is feeling. This sometimes presents a somewhat awkward situation for the emergency physician, and a natural tendency is to change the subject or to leave the bedside. A more appropriate and therapeutic response, however, is to sit down beside the patient and wait for him to respond. The subsequent approach should be gentle and calm. The patient is thus encouraged to reveal inner feelings, fears, and guilt. Some helpful areas of subsequent questioning include how the patient has been feeling, whether he has been under pressure at work, how his marriage has been faring, and if there are any other problems.

If the patient does break down, burst into tears, and admit that there have been great difficulties, sympathetic listening and reassuring that there is treatment available for these feelings has quite a calming effect. The psychiatric consultant should be able to establish a specific therapeutic target for each particular symptom complex of the affective disorder. The consultant, for instance, can reassure the patient that sleeping patterns respond to therapy almost immediately.

Suicide

The major lethal complication of depression is suicide. When evaluating the depressed patient, suicide must be part of the inquiry. For the emergency physician, suicidal ideation and psychosis are major clinical indicators of the need for immediate psychiatric consultation and/or hospitalization. The physician must never be reluctant to mention suicide for fear of "putting the thought into someone's head." The truly depressed patient has at least acknowledged the possibility already and may need to search for help by telling someone.

If the patient has thought about suicide, the physician can ask about those thoughts and whether he has planned such an attempt. If the patient has, it is important to find out how close he came to ending his life and what means of suicide are currently available to him. The suicidal patient must be taken seriously and managed according to the principles outlined in Chapter 4.

Untreated depression

If depression goes unrecognized and untreated, it becomes a chronic condition associated with its own morbidity and potential mortality. In patients who manifest their depression by somatic complaints, the absence of effective treatment for their depression reinforces the somatic model. It encourages *doctor shopping;* the patient has definable symptoms, but no one can explain them. As the condition goes untreated, this pattern becomes a behaviorally learned response to symptoms of an otherwise treatable medical psychiatric illness.

Treatment

Related minor despondency or sadness should improve with brief psychotherapy, time, and needed changes in the external environment (e.g., removal of certain stresses at work or improvement in family relationships). The patient who meets the criteria for a major depressive episode, however, may need more intensive therapy with medication and psychotherapy.

Antidepressant medications are effective in the treatment of depression. The tricyclic antidepressants are probably the most widely used drugs for this purpose. Occasionally, monoamine oxidase inhibitors (MAO inhibitors), neuroleptic drugs, or lithium carbonate may be selected for treatment of a particular patient. Electroconvulsive therapy (ECT) is effective but is generally used as a second line of therapy only after drug treatment has failed. Psychotherapy, in conjunction with these medical treatments, greatly increases the effectiveness of the whole treatment regimen. These various treatment approaches are listed in the following outline:

A. Antidepressant medications
   1. Tricyclic antidepressants
      a. Imipramine (Tofranil)
      b. Amitriptyline (Elavil)
      c. Doxepin (Sinequan)
   2. MAO inhibitors
      a. Phenelzine (Nardil)
   3. Neuroleptic drugs (usually used only to control severe agitation or psychotic symptoms)
      a. Thiothixene (Navane)
      b. Haloperidol (Haldol)
      c. Thioridazine (Mellaril)
   4. Lithium

B. ECT

C. Psychotherapy

Antidepressant medication. There are some legitimate concerns about initiating antidepressant medication in the emergency department. One concern is that the patient could easily take a lethal overdose if enough medication is prescribed. The other concern is that the patient has not had the opportunity to develop a therapeutic alliance with a psychiatrist who can initiate and then follow the patient's progress.

On the other hand, the initiation of medication at the emergency visit allows the patient to begin treatment early and gives the referral psychiatrist the opportunity to evaluate how the patient responds to the medication. The best method of practice in a given instance should probably be determined by consultation with a psychiatrist about a general policy regarding such patients.

Tricyclic antidepressants. The tricyclic class of antidepressants includes imipramine, amitriptyline, doxepin, desipramine (Norpramin), and amoxapine (Asendin). The initial doses, early effects, side effects, and contraindications are perhaps the most important aspects of prescribing information for the emergency physician. As with many drugs, the physician should become familiar with the use of one or two of these drugs at initial doses.

Amitriptyline is more sedating than the other medications and may, therefore, be effectively used in patients with insomnia. The recommended initial dose is 50 mg at bedtime. The dose may be increased by 25 mg increments every 3 days (not to exceed 150 mg per day), or the 50 mg dose only can be taken each night. In either case the patient should be able to see a psychiatrist within 3 to 5 days. Since serious toxicity can occur with single doses over 1000 mg, only a 3- to 5-day supply of drugs at low dosages should be prescribed in case the patient suddenly takes an overdose of the medication in a suicide attempt.

Patients should be cautioned about the anticholinergic effect of the tricyclic antidepressants (dry mouth, constipation, blurred vision) and counseled that the effects should decrease in time, as the patient becomes accustomed to the medication. In older men, urinary retention may occur. When a depressed patient has been successfully treated in the past with a particular tricyclic agent, the same drug should be used again for the current depression.

Cardiovascular side effects are well-recognized complications of tricyclic antidepressant medication. Arrhythmias, conduction defects, or other signs of cardiovascular disease should contraindicate the initiation of tricyclic medication in the emergency department. Patients over the age of 45 should have a baseline cardiogram before initiating therapy. A cardiac abnormality noted in the history or on the electrocardiogram (ECG) would necessitate a delay in beginning therapy until further cardiac investigation had been completed. Some patients with cardiac disorders may have tricyclic antidepressant medication initiated, but they require close outpatient monitoring.

MAO inhibitors. MAO inhibitors such as phenelzine are mentioned here mainly to emphasize the point that they should *not be initiated* in the emergency department as treatment for depression. Patients taking MAO inhibitors must have a special diet free of tyramine, which causes a severe elevation of blood pressure in these patients. Other medications, particularly tricyclic antidepressants and meperidine, must also be avoided with these patients.

Because the patient must be reliable and educated extensively about diet and medication, the prescribing of these agents is best left to the psychiatrist who is familiar with the indications, contraindications, and precautions associated with their use.

Neuroleptic drugs. Neuroleptic agents are sometimes added to the tricyclic antidepressant regimen if the patient is severely agitated. Thiothixene or haloperidol in low dosages of 2 mg twice daily are appropriate for most patients, and these lower dosages should definitely be used for elderly patients. Thioridazine may be used in dosages of 25 to 50 mg twice daily. The addition of these agents to a tricyclic antidepressant outpatient regimen prescribed in the emergency department should be rare. For a full-blown depressive illness with agitation severe enough to require neuroleptic drugs, a psychiatric consultant should be notified and hospitalization considered.

Lithium. Lithium is most effective in the treatment of mania and bipolar affective disorders (both mania and depression). Because lithium is effective in treating both emotional extremes in bipolar disorders, it can be considered a mood stabilizer.

Although it is unusual that lithium therapy would be instituted in the emergency department, there are situations that require the emergency physician to decide to continue with previously established lithium therapy or to evaluate that patient for symptoms and signs that may be associated with lithium therapy.

Lithium is a salt that is almost entirely excreted by the kidney. Since lithium and sodium are reabsorbed competitively by the proximal tubule, lithium toxicity may develop in patients who use a diuretic, avoid the use of salt, perspire profusely in the summertime, or have been vomiting. Lithium dosages must be reduced or stopped in patients with renal failure.

The normal daily dosage of lithium is 300 mg three or four times a day. The desired blood level is 0.8 to 1.2 mEq/liter, but some patients require blood levels as high as 1.5 mEq/liter. Signs of toxicity develop above this dosage and include coarse tremor of the hands, nausea, vomiting, diarrhea, confusion, and lethargy in the early stages. Higher elevations of the lithium level may cause tetany, convulsions, fasciculations, and death. Lithium toxicity and its treatment are discussed in greater detail in Chapter 19.

ECT. ECT can be quite helpful in severe depression. There are strict criteria for the use of this therapy, however, and it is rarely the first line of treatment for depression. It is important to assure the patient that "shock treatment" is not the first choice and that other forms of therapy are available and attempted first. People who are depressed may have known others who have had shock treatment, and they may be quite fearful of it and, therefore, avoid appropriate treatment. Patients can be assured that ECT is not used unless absolutely necessary. It may provide hope for severely depressed patients, however, to know that ECT is effective for the treatment of severe depression.

Psychotherapy. Psychotherapy increases the effectiveness of somatic treatments for depression. The therapist provides the patient with the tools to fight against depression. The period of time required for the tricyclic antidepressant medication to alleviate depression is 4 to 6 weeks. This predictable course must be explained to the patient. The annoying side effects of the medication must also be explained and the patient reassured. These simple reassurances require the support of a therapist and regular meetings to assess problems and monitor the success of treatment.

Psychotherapy also offers some patients the opportunity to develop understanding of their vulnerability to depression either through an analysis of previous behavior and thought patterns or through genetic predisposition. An investigation of family dynamics and job and social activities can be carried out in psychotherapy and may be quite helpful in determining environmental changes that may help treat the depressive episode.

All of these features of treatment can be accomplished within the psychotherapeutic framework. A psychiatrist or therapist must spend enough time explaining the complicated issues involved in the treatment of depression. Therapeutic programs most commonly fail because patients drop out of treatment. They no longer receive psychotherapy or take their medication. Proper relationships between patient and physician, frequent explanations of therapies, and encouragement by the therapist help prevent these treatment failures.

MANIC EPISODE (MANIA)

Mania is a disorder of mood that runs a spectrum from mild grandiosity, distractibility, and difficulty sleeping to a completely psychotic state in which the patient acts "crazy" and may become unmanageable and require sedation and restraint.

When the acutely manic patient is encountered in the emergency department, one of two expressions of the illness may be evident. He may be euphoric, talkative, and energetic, or he can be irritable, belligerent, and argumentative. The latter appearance may be frightening, and security personnel may become involved in the patient's early management.

Sometimes mania is not suspected. The manic patient frequently drinks heavily, and it is presumed that he is simply intoxicated. He is treated largely by observation and discharged when relatively sober. The premature and inappropriate discharge of the patient can often be prevented by obtaining additional history from family and friends about his behavior.

At first glance, the manic with a euphoric, energetic appearance may seem somewhat charming. The patient typically seems gregarious, cheerful, and sociable. This sociability is unceasing, sometimes intrusive, and eventually annoying. Family and friends are able to relate that the behavior is not typical of the patient's normal personality.

Pressure of speech is one of the earliest indicators of mania. The patient just keeps talking; it is difficult to interrupt his steady stream of verbiage. The speech may be loud, rapid, and full of irrelevance, spontaneous creative thoughts, jokes, or puns.

Another hallmark of mania is grandiosity. The patient has an inflated self-esteem and sense of personal importance. He reveals that he alone can solve a particularly difficult national problem, for instance, and is in close personal contact with important government and business leaders. The manic patient may be psychotic. The hallucinations, delusions, and ideas of reference are mood congruent if they amplify the theme of self-importance. The patient, for instance, may have an auditory hallucination of God telling him that he has a special meaning to the world around him, or he may have the delusion that he is in command of a large multinational corporation or military effort.

The acute manic episode is characterized in part by a decreased need for sleep. The patient may stay up night after night and show no signs of fatigue. He may inundate himself with work or become involved in a project or creative effort that keeps him awake throughout the night. Regardless of talent (or the lack of it), a manic patient may undertake a huge creative project like writing a book or painting a portrait.

The most devastating aspect of an acute manic episode for the patient and his family is the tendency for him to become involved in dangerous, risky, or expensive ventures with little regard for the consequences. The manic patient may drive fast and wildly or become involved in sexual escapades with strangers. Spending sprees are common, and business judgment is typically poor.

The manic patient may buy a new car, an airplane, or real estate, or he may invest in some questionable business venture. These financial dealings may create an enormous family debt and impossible monetary burdens for several years. It is said that a marriage can survive only two or three manic episodes.

Talking to the family or friends of a patient who shows signs of mania allows the physician to define the time of onset of symptoms, their escalation, and the particular activities associated with the episode. For instance, the patient may deny that he has any problems, but when his wife is interviewed separately, she may tell stories of his inappropriate sexual advances toward other women, of spending money that he could not afford on extravagant items or travel, and of other signs of extremely poor judgment that could cripple the financial and social life of the patient and his family in the future. Questions that are particularly helpful in gaining information about the manic patient from someone who accompanies him to the emergency department include the following:

1. Has the patient been acting in an unusual way lately?
2. Has he recently spent money he did not have?
3. Has the patient been making plans that are inappropriate, such as renting a hall for a large meeting, making investments, or carrying out other business dealings that are inappropriate?
4. Has the patient been sleeping less recently?
5. Has the patient been acting inappropriately socially?

DIAGNOSTIC CRITERIA FOR A MANIC EPISODE

A. One or more distinct periods with a predominantly elevated, expansive, or irritable mood. The elevated or irritable mood must be a prominent part of the illness and relatively persistent, although it may alternate or intermingle with a depressive mood.

B. Duration of at least 1 week (or any duration if hospitalization is necessary), during which, for most of the time, at least three of the following symptoms have persisted (four if the mood is only irritable) and have been present to a significant degree:
   1. Increase in activity (either socially, occupationally, or sexually) or physical restlessness
   2. More talkative than usual or pressure to keep talking
   3. Flight of ideas or subjective experience that thoughts are racing
   4. Inflated self-esteem (grandiosity, which may be delusional)
   5. Decreased need for sleep
   6. Distractibility (i.e., attention is too easily drawn to unimportant or irrelevant external stimuli)
   7. Unrecognized excessive involvement in activities that have a high potential for painful consequences (e.g., buying sprees, sexual indiscretions, foolish business investments, reckless driving)

C. Neither of the following dominates the clinical picture when an affective syndrome (i.e., criteria A and B) is not present, that is, before it developed or after it has remitted:
   1. Preoccupation with a mood-incongruent delusion or hallucination
   2. Bizarre behavior

D. Not superimposed on either Schizophrenia, Schizophreniform Disorder, or Paranoid Disorder.

E. Not due to any Organic Mental Disorder, such as Substance Intoxication.

(NOTE: A hypomanic episode is a pathological disturbance similar to, but not as severe as, a manic episode.)

Adapted from American Psychiatric Association. *Diagnostic and statistical manual of mental disorders* (3rd ed.). Washington, D.C.: The Association, 1980.

Emergency evaluation

The floridly manic patient may draw so much attention in the emergency department that some form of immediate treatment or psychiatric evaluation is required. The differential diagnosis does, however, include organic disorders like amphetamine toxicity, steroid psychosis, and hyperthyroidism. The patient, therefore, should have a medical evaluation and examination. When a medical condition or drug toxicity causes the mania, the syndrome is called an *organic affective syndrome*.

The belligerent or assaultive patient may require initial restraint, and the security force is best called to the emergency department during the early evaluation. Several people should be present to subdue the patient, since he may become quite violent.

Treatment

Because the acute manic episode can be so destructive to the patient's career, family, and social life, prompt evaluation and treatment are required to prevent the horrifyingly disasterous consequences. The treatment should be aggressive and include hospitalization, following the initial evaluation in the emergency department.

Rapid tranquilization. Rapid tranquilization is most helpful for the patient who exhibits a full-blown manic episode with or without psychotic symptoms. Haloperidol is the agent of choice for rapid tranquilization. It is given in a dosage of 5 mg orally or intramuscularly every 30 minutes until the patient is calm or until a total dosage of 45 mg has been given.

Lithium. Lithium may also be added to this regimen later, but usually this is begun in the psychiatric unit after the patient has been transferred from the emergency department. Since the lithium level must be carefully monitored over the first several weeks, there is no hurry or need to begin lithium treatment in the emergency department.

Outpatient management

In a few cases the manic patient may be able to return home for outpatient management. A patient eligible for outpatient management should be well controlled with haloperidol, have an extremely secure social support system, not be dangerous or suicidal, and have a definite appointment with a psychiatrist within 24 to 48 hours. Sometimes a patient with a well-established diagnosis who has been noncompliant with his medication may be able to go home with an adjustment of his drug therapy or an addition of haloperidol to the regimen.

The first episode of mania, however, should be thoroughly evaluated on an inpatient basis for both medical and psychiatric causes. The ideal management of the patient includes a toxicology screen, medical evaluation, psychiatric consultation, and hospitalization to further evaluate the patient and begin lithium therapy.

BIPOLAR DISORDERS

Bipolar affective disorder (previously called manic-depressive illness) describes an ailment characterized by severe mood swings from a "high" or euphoria to a "low" or severe depression. These highs and lows are so extreme that the patient may appear psychotic. He usually has a period of depression lasting several days or weeks, followed by a manic phase lasting days or weeks. There may be a normal period between these extremes enduring from days to years. A patient may have more manic than depressed episodes, and it is rare to see these mood swings lasting only hours. If this history is given, the physician should suspect a drug effect or other illness (e.g., schizophrenic disorder).

Bipolar affective disorders are treated with lithium. Other drugs, as mentioned, may be helpful during the acute phase but are not used later. These drugs are the major tranquilizers such as haloperidol or chlorpromazine (Thorazine).

For the patient with depression as the predominate characteristic of his illness, concomitant use of tricyclic antidepressants is helpful. The patient may be maintained on lithium for his entire life. He should have periodic thyroid and renal evaluations.

Cyclothymic disorder

Cyclothymic disorder is a mild variety of bipolar affective disorder. The patient experiences mild "ups" and "downs" that cause some discomfort but no major impairment. This is a difficult diagnosis to make, included in this discussion more for completeness in presenting the DSM-III classification of affective disorders than for its applicability to general emergency practice.

DYSTHYMIC DISORDER

A garden variety depression without psychotic symptoms is called a *dysthymic disorder*. The term distinguishes it from the more severe major depressions. This disorder is common and often underlies vague somatic complaints. Dysthymic disorders respond to psychotherapy, and a trial of antidepressant medication is often indicated, whereas hospitalization is rarely needed. The emergency or family physician may explain that this is a common illness and should not be brushed off by the patient as "a weakness," which many depressed patients believe it is. It is eminently treatable in sometimes 6 to 10 visits to a psychiatrist or psychologist. Psychiatric evaluation is needed if medication is to be prescribed for the disorder. The emergency physician's concern, explanation, and professional referral result in far better compliance and, in the long run, better treatment of this common illness.

The important issue for the emergency physician is that the depression is identified. Whether this depression is labeled a major depressive episode with severe sadness, appetite and sleep disturbance, and loss of concentration or a dysthymic disorder with persistent sadness for no apparent reason is not important. The essential point is that depression is appropriately diagnosed.

SUMMARY

Affective disorders are the most common psychiatric illnesses seen in the emergency department. Along with organic mental disorders and schizophrenia, affective disorders can cause psychosis with hallucinations and delusions that are either mood congruent or incongruent. The affective disorders are extremely treatable once an accurate diagnosis is made. The emergency department management of these patients is of key importance in beginning excellent medical care. It is often the first contact the patient with mood disorder has with the medical profession. A good clear diagnostic evaluation, combined with reassurance and early psychiatric consultation, sets the stage for optimal management of the affective disorders.

REFERENCES

1. American Psychiatric Association. *Diagnostic and statistical manual of mental disorders* (3rd ed.). Washington, D.C.: The Association, 1980.
2. Summers, WK, Rund, DA, and Levin, M. Psychiatric illness in a general urban emergency room: daytime versus nighttime population. *Journal of Clinical Psychiatry,* Aug. 1979, *40*(8), 19-25.

11 SOMATOFORM DISORDERS

Somatoform disorders are psychiatric illnesses that have as their central feature physical symptoms for which there is no apparent organic basis. Further psychiatric evaluation generally provides evidence for the linkage of these symptoms with psychological factors. The somatoform disorders include conversion disorder, somatization disorder, psychogenic pain disorder, and hypochondriasis.

Previous classifications of somatoform disorders have emphasized terms like *psychosomatic* or *psychophysiological*. The symptoms and signs of somatoform disorders are not under the patient's voluntary control as they are in patients with factitious disorders. Rather they are thought to express unresolved psychological conflict, meet psychological needs, or reflect underlying psychiatric illness. Certain of these somatoform disorders, like conversion disorders, sometimes present the emergency physician with a difficult challenge—to prove that dramatic symptoms like paralysis, blindness, or inability to swallow are not the result of organic illness.

Other disorders (like somatization disorder) can be most frustrating when the patient rattles on about physical complaints and relates a totally positive review of systems. At night the hypochondriac may have what seems to be such a trivial complaint that no medical treatment is even needed. The recognition that these patients have somatoform disorders and do not require extensive evaluation can be of enormous help to the emergency physician besieged by such patients. The physician must, however, evaluate these patients with enough history and physical examination to rule out bodily disorders.

CONVERSION DISORDER

Clinical portrait

Conversion disorder is a condition in which the patient portrays an acute alteration in physical functioning that is an expression of psychological need, rather than a manifestation of medical illness. Common symptoms and signs of conversion disorder involve the voluntary motor system and sensory organs. Complaints of pain alone are not part of a conversion disorder but are considered part of a psychogenic pain disorder. The onset of symptoms and signs of conversion disorder is usually sudden. Fairly common conversion disorder syndromes initially suggest acute neurological disease. The patient may suddenly lose function of both legs and be unable to walk or appear to have lost a sense of balance acutely (astasia-abasia). Symptoms and signs suggesting sensory impairment include blindness, deafness, inability to smell, anesthesia, and paresthesia.

Often the description of loss of sensation to touch demonstrates the patient's lack of knowledge about neuroanatomy. The anesthesia is described as a loss of sensation over one entire side of the body. The dividing line is described as the midline of the body, often including the face, and all areas in the affected half are described as equally numb.

Similarly, the patient may report the entire hand as numb and describe a pattern of anesthesia that does not correspond to known dermatomes. When the onset is acute, a genuine neuropathy (producing glovelike paresthesia) is improbable. "Tunnel vision" is a fairly classic conversion symptom. The patient with tunnel vision typically perceives objects as being the same size, regardless of the distance from the eyes.

The patient with conversion disorder can produce dramatic clinical pictures. He may claim an inability to swallow or speak, for instance. This suggests pharyngeal or esophageal obstruction. Such a patient points to the neck, expectorates all saliva, refuses to talk, and may occasionally jump off the cart and begin to pace.

CASE EXAMPLE 1

A 21-year-old man was admitted to the emergency department with a chief complaint of inability to swallow or talk and chest pain. His accompanying family members related that he took no medication, had no allergies, and that the disorder had developed acutely. The patient's appearance was quite dramatic. He waved his arms, slowly pointed to his chest and throat, kept his mouth wide open, and intermittently expectorated his saliva into an emesis basin. The emergency staff feared a laryngeal or esophageal foreign body even though the actual respirations were quiet, breath sounds were equal bilaterally, and there was no cyanosis. Examination of the oropharynx and indirect laryngoscopy revealed no foreign body, epiglottitis, swelling, injury, or vocal cord paralysis. A chest x-ray film and a barium swallow were also normal.

A psychiatric consultant was asked to see the patient. The interview with the family revealed that the patient had mild mental retardation and was beginning to experience great difficulty at home where he had had several fights with his older sister. His mother and father had recently applied great pressure for him to seek work and help support the family. Following the psychiatric interview, the patient's symptoms subsided, and he was admitted to the psychiatric unit for further evaluation.

The portrait of possible acute airway obstruction generally arouses at least moderate anxiety among the staff as the emergency physician contemplates creation of an emergency airway. When laryngoscopy (direct, indirect, or fiberoptic) reveals no foreign body, the staff is generally relieved. When no organic lesion is found in a patient with conversion disorder, the physician may resent being "fooled." The patient may be ignored, casually discharged, or treated with hostility. Psychiatric consultation is clearly indicated for these severely impaired individuals.

The patient with conversion disorder may first appear as an individual experiencing a generalized seizure. Depending on the patient's medical sophistication, the genuineness of the seizures may be quite variable. The seizures may be extremely convincing or so obviously atypical that they seem almost ridiculous.

CASE EXAMPLE 2

A 28-year-old woman was admitted to the emergency department because of a generalized grand mal seizure. The emergency medical service (EMS) unit provided the history that she was found on the sidewalk of a busy street, "having convulsions and foaming at the mouth." The examination revealed an unarousable patient who had normal vital signs and no external signs of trauma. She became intermittently rigid and then developed diffuse muscular jerking. Her head was deviated to one side, and frothy saliva drooled from her mouth. She was initially treated with intravenous diazepam (Valium). The diazepam stopped the motor movements but left the patient unconscious. She was admitted to the neurology service where the medication was discontinued. Repeated electroencephalograms (EEGs) were normal. The patient subsequently had two normal EEGs during the apparent grand mal seizures. The remainder of the neurological evaluation, including a computerized tomography (CT) scan and lumbar puncture, was normal.

Because the seizures were felt to have no organic basis, psychiatric consultation was obtained. The psychiatric evaluation revealed that the patient, though unmarried, lived with a boyfriend whom she was desperately afraid of losing. He had remained close to her during her illness and had revealed no immediate intention of discontinuing the relationship. The patient was scheduled for psychiatric counseling. It was later learned that she soon discontinued her counseling sessions and was not seen again in the emergency department for her seizure episodes. Her symptoms had temporarily resolved her unconscious fears.

The symptoms and signs of physical illness are not under conscious voluntary control in conversion disorder. Despite the apparent magnitude of the deficit (e.g., inability to walk or speak), the patient may exhibit apparent emotional indifference (la belle indifference). The feature is classically associated with conversion disorder but is not of great diagnostic value, since it may not be present in the patient with this disorder and

DIAGNOSTIC CRITERIA FOR CONVERSION DISORDER

A. The predominant disturbance is a loss of or alteration in physical functioning suggesting a physical disorder.
B. Psychological factors are judged to be etiologically involved in the symptom, as evidenced by one of the following:
   1. There is a temporal relationship between an environmental stimulus that is apparently related to a psychological conflict or need and the initiation or exacerbation of the symptom
   2. The symptom enables the individual to avoid some activity that is noxious to him or her
   3. The symptom enables the individual to get support from the environment that otherwise might not be forthcoming
C. It has been determined that the symptom is *not* under voluntary control.
D. The symptom cannot, after appropriate investigation, be explained by a known physical disorder or pathophysiological mechanism.
E. The symptom is not limited to pain or to a disturbance in sexual functioning.
F. Not due to Somatization Disorder or Schizophrenia.

From American Psychiatric Association. *Diagnostic and statistical manual of mental disorders* (3rd ed.). Washington, D.C.: The Association, 1980.

can be seen in an individual with a genuine physical disorder. In contrast to the patient's unconcerned attitude about the deficit, the anxious family typically shows great concern over the sudden onset of disabling illness.

Psychological mechanisms

The conversion disorder is thought to achieve two psychological goals for the patient. It symbolically expresses a psychological conflict, and it partially solves the problem. The patient may be overcome with household chores and a new infant, for instance. She feels unable to handle the responsibilities and develops an acute loss of balance so severe that she cannot walk. A patient who is so angry that he wants to shoot his spouse may develop paralysis of the hand, or the patient who continually views traumatic events in the household may become "blind."

CASE EXAMPLE 3

A 22-year-old woman was admitted for inability to walk. She and the family related the history that she had rather suddenly lost her sense of balance, and her "legs were weak."

The examination revealed normal muscular tone, bulk, and strength. She had symmetrically normal deep tendon reflexes. When asked to walk, she exhibited a somewhat narrow-based gait with weight supported on the outside or lateral aspect of each foot. She weaved, waved her arms about, and swayed from side to side as if she could not keep her balance. Careful examination revealed, however, that she had incredibly good balance to keep from falling, while moving so far backward and forward and side to side.

A diagnosis of astasia-abasia (psychogenic ataxia) was made. Further history revealed that she had several small children at home and a new baby. Her husband had refused to help her with any of the housework until she lost her ability to walk. The patient was referred for immediate psychiatric consultation after the reason was calmly explained.

Physical illness

The inability to diagnose conversion disorder is probably not as important as mistaking real and treatable illnesses for conversion disorder. Lazare suggests, in his review of the literature regarding hospitalized patients with conversion disorder, that "from 13% to 30% will be patients with misdiagnosed organic illness."[1] Organic illness may be missed for several reasons; the illness may have a clinical cause that begins with vague, nonspecific, transient signs and symptoms. Myasthenia gravis, multiple sclerosis, and certain collagen-vascular diseases are examples. Another reason for missing organic illness is that true conversion disorder may coexist with medical illness. This situation is clearly difficult to detect in the emergency department.

It is in the best interest of the patient for the emergency physician to rule out organic illness in someone suspected of having conversion disorder. Several somewhat routine approaches guard against misdiagnosis in the emergency setting.

The first method is to obtain a clear history of the disorder, including any previous similar sudden massive motor or sensory deficits that subsided spontaneously and for which no medical cause was ever detected. Such a history supports the diagnosis of conversion disorder.

The second procedure is a physical examination that documents in detail the patient's deficit. The history and physical examination may suggest simple laboratory tests (e.g., a urinalysis, complete blood count, glucose level, or electrolyte concentration) that can be obtained easily in the emergency department.

A third mechanism for detecting physical illness is to ask for consultation, preferably with a specialist like a neurologist or the patient's family physician. Even consultation with a colleague in the emergency department may be extremely valuable. A second look by an independent examiner may be of great help in these cases. The patient may immediately appear well or ill to another physician who could support the suspicion that the illness might be functional rather than organic. A second opinion can usually confirm or refute the suspicion of the first physician rather quickly.

The final approach in guarding against misdiagnosis is to admit the patient to the hospital for medical and psychiatric evaluation. When admission is not possible, care should be taken to ensure proper subsequent outpatient evaluation.

Management of conversion disorder

The duration of symptoms in conversion disorder may be surprisingly brief. They may last only several hours and gradually resolve spontaneously. By contrast, some patients develop a personality adjustment associated with conversion disorder and remain incapacitated for many years.

When the diagnosis of conversion disorder is suspected, it is helpful to obtain a history of similar episodes or one of recent events or changes in the patient's life that could cause psychological trauma. The symbolic meaning of the conversion symptoms may be easily detected, as in the patient who witnesses a traumatic event and then rather suddenly develops total blindness.

Some excellent areas of questioning for the family of the patient include the following:

1. Has any family member or anyone the patient knows experienced the same or similar symptoms?
2. Did a significant life event occur at the time of the onset of symptoms?

When a family member has experienced the same symptoms or illness, the patient has a subconscious model to follow. The symptoms of such a disability are fairly easy for the patient to reproduce (unconsciously) in the conversion disorder.

Significant life events may involve a death in the family, death or sickness of a pet, family problems, children in trouble with the law, children having trouble with homework, parental fights, marital separation, loss of a boyfriend or girlfriend, or birth of a child. Trouble at work may constitute a traumatic event. Problems on the job, difficulties with the boss, or friction among co-workers are examples. More personal problems include sexual difficulties or the sudden discovery of a mate's infidelity.

If psychiatric consultation is immediately available, it can be offered to the patient. Often, however, the patient, and especially the family, is reluctant to accept the idea that the problem is "all in the head." It is best not to confront the patient with a firm statement that there is no physical illness. The emergency physician can never really be sure of this. The patient may indeed have a medical illness. The abrupt suggestion that the disorder is totally psychiatric may either convince the patient and family to seek care elsewhere or so discourage the patient that he does not keep the psychiatric outpatient appointment.

The best posture to take, perhaps, is one of concerned puzzlement; the symptoms do worry the physician, but their underlying cause has not yet been detected. The patient can be referred to a general physician and perhaps to a psychiatrist with the reassurance that psychiatric consultation helps the family "cover all the bases" in determining the cause of the disorder. The psychiatrist should be presented as a physician who deals with the interaction of the mind and body. This thorough approach ensures that no cause of the disorder is overlooked.

Insight-oriented psychotherapy is fairly unsuccessful in these patients because they actually have little of the psychological sophistication needed to understand the cause of their symptoms. This is one of the reasons that they respond to psychological trauma with conversion symptoms in the first place. These patients may be able to find solutions to the immediate problems, however, and gradually adjust their lives to reverse the changes that precipitated the conversion disorder. For instance, the patient may be able to move to a new department at work or resolve differences with other family members. The symptoms should abate as the patient makes these adjustments. Supportive psychotherapy with some direction giving is often the most helpful form of therapy. Medication should usually be avoided, since this reinforces the concept of an illness model.

SOMATIZATION DISORDER

The patient with somatization disorder can be quite frustrating to a busy emergency physician trying to evaluate all patients as quickly and efficiently as possible. Previously diagnosed as hysteria, or Briquet's syndrome, somatization disorder is a chronic condition, almost exclusively diagnosed in women, the predominant feature of which is the presentation of multiple somatic complaints for which no organic or physical cause can be discovered. The disorder begins before age 30 and takes a chronic fluctuating course. Typically the patient has sought medical attention for the symptoms, but previous evaluations have been either negative or have uncovered only incidental pathology. Occasionally patients with the disorder have undergone multiple surgical procedures for an explanation or a cure of the symptoms.

Common symptoms of patients with somatization disorder are various types of pain (abdominal pain, backache, or painful menstruation), vague pseudoneurological complaints (paresthesias, difficulty swallowing), and signs that suggest cardiovascular disease (chest pain, shortness of breath, palpitations, dizziness). Psychosexual dysfunction may be a prominent complaint; the patient may have little interest in sex and/or experiences pain during or after intercourse.

The presentation of the symptoms may be vague; the physician may have initial difficulty fitting the symptoms into one or several classifications of organic disease. The patient may present the clinical history in a dramatic or emotional way to emphasize the severity of the symptoms. A review of symptoms is usually totally positive. The patient responds affirmatively to the question, "Have you been in poor health most of your life?" or "Have you been sickly most of your life?" As the examiner proceeds through a review of symptoms, the patient does seem to have pain everywhere and active symptoms for most body systems. The symptoms must be serious enough to have caused the patient to change his life-style, take medication, or consult a physician. A partial listing of typical symptoms is presented here. If 14 of the symptoms are present (14 in women, 12 in men), the patient is under 30, and no physical cause is found, somatization disorder can be diagnosed.

A. Sickly his whole life
B. Pseudoneurological symptoms
    1. Loss of voice
    2. Inability to swallow
    3. Paralysis
    4. Numbness
    5. Double vision
    6. Blurred vision
    7. Urinary retention
C. Gastrointestinal symptoms
    1. Pain
    2. Vomiting
    3. Nausea
    4. Bleeding
D. Female reproductive symptoms
    1. Menstrual symptoms
    2. Excessive pain
    3. Bleeding or bloating
    4. Pregnancy symptoms (excessive vomiting)
E. Psychosexual symptoms
    1. Pain during intercourse
    2. Lack of satisfaction
F. Pain
    1. Back
    2. Joints
    3. Extremities
    4. Chest
G. Cardiopulmonary symptoms
    1. Shortness of breath
    2. Palpitations
    3. Dizziness

DIAGNOSTIC CRITERIA FOR SOMATIZATION DISORDER

A. A history of physical symptoms of several years' duration beginning before the age of 30.

B. Complaints of at least 14 symptoms for women and 12 for men, from the 37 symptoms listed below. To count a symptom as present the individual must report that the symptom caused him or her to take medicine (other than aspirin), alter his or her life pattern, or see a physician. The symptoms, in the judgment of the clinician, are not adequately explained by physical disorder or physical injury, and are not side effects of medication, drugs or alcohol. The clinician need not be convinced that the symptom was actually present (e.g., that the individual actually vomited throughout her entire pregnancy); report of the symptom by the individual is sufficient.

Sickly: Believes that he or she has been sickly for a good part of his or her life

Conversion or pseudoneurological symptoms: Difficulty swallowing, loss of voice, deafness, double vision, blurred vision, blindness, fainting or loss of consciousness, memory loss, seizures or convulsions, trouble walking, paralysis or muscle weakness, urinary retention, or difficulty urinating

Gastrointestinal symptoms: Abdominal pain, nausea, vomiting spells (other than during pregnancy), bloating (gassy), intolerance (e.g., gets sick) of a variety of foods, diarrhea

Female reproductive symptoms: Judged by the individual as occurring more frequently or severely than in most women—painful menstruation, menstrual irregularity, excessive bleeding, severe vomiting throughout pregnancy or causing hospitalization during pregnancy

Psychosexual symptoms: For the major part of the individual's life after opportunities for sexual activity—sexual indifference, lack of pleasure during intercourse, pain during intercourse

Pain: In back, joints, extremities, genital area (other than during intercourse), pain on urination, other pain (not including headaches)

Cardiopulmonary symptoms: Shortness of breath, palpitations, chest pain, dizziness

From American Psychiatric Association. *Diagnostic and statistical manual of mental disorders* (3rd ed.). Washington, D.C.: The Association, 1980.

The physical examination does not reveal pathology that explains the symptoms, but the patient usually claims to have tenderness to palpation if the primary complaint is one involving pain. Examination of the abdominal wall often reveals multiple surgical scars on the abdomen from previous exploratory operations and surgical procedures. All laboratory, electrocardiogram (ECG), and x-ray examinations are typically negative.

Management of somatization disorders

After taking a lengthy, inconclusive history, performing a physical examination, rechecking vital signs, and reviewing negative laboratory data (if ordered), the emergency physician is tempted to label the patient a *crock* and arrange a hasty discharge from the emergency department. This is a crucial period in the management of the patient, however, and a pause to review the case at this juncture should be rewarding.

The first consideration must be whether or not a physical disorder has been overlooked. Case example 4 illustrates that a medical diagnosis was mistakenly overlooked because the patient had a concurrent somatization disorder.

CASE EXAMPLE 4

A 35-year-old woman was admitted to the emergency department with vague abdominal pain. The patient had undergone numerous surgeries in the past, including an unrevealing exploratory laparotomy for chronic abdominal pain. She had a positive review of systems and answered affirmatively to questions about pain in virtually every area of her body and to the query of whether she had been "sickly all her life."

Her examination showed minimal diffuse abdominal tenderness but no guarding. She was discharged with a diagnosis of somatization disorder. Twenty-four hours later the patient returned with similar complaints. Her examination now revealed localized right lower quadrant tenderness and guarding. Her white count was 18,000. She underwent an appendectomy for a ruptured appendix.

The patient met the criteria for somatization disorder but had a concomitant physical defect responsible for her chief complaint. More careful attention to her physical symptoms and a more critical physical examination may have uncovered the correct diagnosis in the earlier stages of the disease.

A physical disorder may cause vague or confusing symptoms in its initial stages. Connective tissue diseases, certain neurological defects, and some endocrine disorders are examples. As in conversion disorder, the physician's best stance with the patient and the family is to share both concern and puzzlement. The opportunity to return to the emergency department for a worsening of symptoms must be emphasized. The patient should be referred for continuing medical evaluation as well as psychiatric evaluation, emphasizing the psychiatrist's role as a physician-specialist.

Having dealt with the possibility of organic disease, the emergency physician may have time to screen for other psychiatric disorders that can cause a similar clinical picture. Depression is one of the major differential diagnoses.[2] The patient can be asked about sleeping through the night, early morning awakening, or insomnia; change in appetite or weight; and a feeling of sadness or depression. Schizophrenia with multiple somatic delusions should be fairly easy to distinguish from somatization disorder. In schizophrenia the bizarre thought content, delusional nature of the complaints, loose associations, and data on previous psychiatric care should be evident in the history and examination. Various anxiety disorders, like panic attack, may produce symptoms referable to the cardiovascular system. The criteria for panic attack can be reviewed in these cases if the symptoms are strictly those considered for panic disorder (e.g., dyspnea, palpitation, choking, paresthesia, trembling).

Other psychiatric diagnoses that comprise the remainder of the differential distinction include conversion disorder, factitious conversion disorder, factitious disorder with physical symptoms (Munchausen's syndrome), psychogenic pain disorder, hypochondriasis, and malingering.

DIAGNOSTIC CRITERIA FOR PSYCHOGENIC PAIN DISORDER

A. Severe and prolonged pain is the predominant disturbance.
B. The pain presented as a symptom is inconsistent with the anatomical distribution of the nervous system; after extensive evaluation, no organic pathology or pathophysiological mechanism can be found to account for the pain; or, when there is some related organic pathology, the complaint of pain is grossly in excess of what would be expected from the physical findings.
C. Psychological factors are judged to be etiologically involved in the pain, as evidenced by at least one of the following:
   1. A temporal relationship between an environmental stimulus that is apparently related to a psychological conflict or need and the initiation or exacerbation of the pain
   2. The pain is enabling the individual to avoid some activity that is noxious to him or her
   3. The pain is enabling the individual to get support from the environment that otherwise might not be forthcoming
D. Not due to another mental disorder.

Adapted from American Psychiatric Association. *Diagnostic and statistical manual of mental disorders* (3rd ed.). Washington, D.C.: The Association, 1980.

PSYCHOGENIC PAIN DISORDER

Psychogenic pain disorder is similar to conversion disorder in the respect that no organic cause for the disorder can be found, and the symptom seems to be related to some psychological conflict or need. Pain is the predominant or only symptom in psychogenic pain disorder. The diagnosis of this disorder is difficult, if not impossible, to establish in the emergency department. Occasionally the description of the pain is so inconsistent with known organic mechanisms that the disorder can be suspected. Usually, however, more specialized diagnostic testing is required to exclude true physical pathology.

The main complications of the disorder are abuse and dependence on analgesics and multiple surgical procedures. Both complications are iatrogenic.

The differential diagnosis includes organic causes for the pain, depression, somatization disorder, and schizophrenia. Drug abusers who request drugs and feign various types of pain are classified as malingerers.

HYPOCHONDRIASIS

Hypochondriasis is fairly common in general medical and emergency practice. The hypochondriac believes he has a serious disease and becomes obsessively preoccupied with his health. Various minor signs or symptoms are unrealistically interpreted by the patient as indicators of serious disease. A small sore, muscle ache, sore throat, or minor cough may be seen by the patient as cause for alarm, despite reassurance by a physician.

DIAGNOSTIC CRITERIA FOR HYPOCHONDRIASIS

A. The predominant disturbance is an unrealistic interpretation of physical signs or sensations as abnormal, leading to preoccupation with the fear or belief of having a serious disease.
B. Thorough physical evaluation does not support the diagnosis of any bodily disorder that can account for the physical signs or sensations or for the individual's unrealistic interpretation of them.
C. The unrealistic fear or belief of having a disease persists despite medical reassurance and causes impairment in social or occupational functioning.
D. Not due to any other mental disorder such as Schizophrenia, Affective Disorder, or Somatization Disorder.

From American Psychiatric Association. *Diagnostic and statistical manual of mental disorders* (3rd ed.). Washington, D.C.: The Association, 1980.

When these patients arrive in the early predawn hours with a trivial complaint, they are rarely received with enthusiasm by the emergency staff. A quick examination and routine referral usually complete the interaction. Sometimes they are chastised for bothering the emergency staff with these minor complaints or for abusing the emergency department.

These patients are rarely satisfied by such treatment, even though the department may be so busy that this is all that is available to them. Sometimes these patients develop a relationship with a physician who seems to be more preoccupied with their health than the patients are themselves.[3] Such a physician can plan elaborate health regimens for the patient, including regular exercise and a healthful diet. The patient can be directed to keep a diary of daily symptoms that can be reviewed with the physician during each office visit. Such treatment reinforces the symptoms of hypochondriasis but may be the only realistic treatment available for the more severe cases.

Most of these patients are best handled professionally by an emergency physician who examines them, performs any necessary tests, and reassures them that a life-threatening illness has not been found but that further evaluations may be needed by their own physician.

OTHER PATIENTS WITH TRIVIAL COMPLAINTS

Three other classes of patients may have trivial complaints or lesions that ordinarily would not justify a visit to an emergency department. One category is the mentally retarded individual who is really not able to distinguish serious from nonserious conditions. Such an individual may have been instructed by a family member or friend to "get checked by a doctor." The patient with mental retardation has a history of school failure or institutionalization and has grossly impaired intellectual functioning when tested. These patients should respond cooperatively and gratefully when examined and assured that they have no serious illness.

Another class of patient is the adolescent or young adult who is preoccupied with developing sexuality and with the possibility of having venereal disease. A small penile abrasion or scrotal rash typically causes great alarm. The patient may try to seek care before transmitting the supposed infection to a sexual partner. He can be reassured on the basis of physical examination and perhaps by obtaining a urethral swab for gonorrhea and a serological test for syphilis. Further discussion about his sexuality may reveal activities and problems that he wants to discuss with a physician. Such a discussion in the emergency department can be quite therapeutic for the patient.

A third type of patient is one who does not have a disorder serious enough to be considered a psychiatric illness but who does have an acute situational problem that is worrisome. The following case example is illustrative of this third type of patient.

CASE EXAMPLE 5

A 52-year-old man entered a southwestern emergency department at 3:00 AM with the complaint of a small red papule on the lateral aspect of his lower leg. He had bumped against a cactus during the day and was afraid that he had been poisoned. The patient was reassured about the minor nature of the lesion and was asked about how things were going for him in general. With this opening he launched into a narrative about being recently separated from his wife and family. He complained of depression, loss of appetite, and insomnia. He had always depended on his wife for emotional and physical support but no longer had someone to meet these needs. The patient was given 5 minutes of brief psychotherapy, during which he was encouraged to focus on some of the real problems in his life and the potential solutions for them. He accepted psychiatric referral gratefully.

Patients who complain of seemingly insignificant medical ailments may, in fact, be seeking care for a variety of emotional problems. The patient described in the previous example was clearly depressed and had great needs for care and concern. He focused his anxiety on a trivial physical lesion and experienced a spiraling anxiety that propelled him to the emergency department. His arrival was an alternative to sitting down and thinking about his feelings, his problems, and their solution.

The patient with trivial complaints should be evaluated for depression with screening questions about appetite, sleep, and sadness and then asked about other tension-producing problems in his life. A mental status examination, checking for organic mental disorders and asking few questions about hallucinations, obsessions, or compulsions, provides a fairly good psychiatric screen. Some of these questions may seem inappropriate in the evaluation of a minor skin lesion, but to the patient with serious doubts about his emotional and mental health, it is reassuring to know that the physician is concerned about him, that all diagnostic bases are being covered, and that he can feel healthier by being able to answer "no" to most of these questions.

The management of the patient begins with the evaluation of the somatic complaint no matter how trivial, since he has focused his anxiety on the physical symptoms or lesion. Any treatment prescribed for the physical problem should make some sense and be as harmless as possible (e.g., an ice pack for a bruise or lozenges for minor throat irritation). These minor treatments help allay the patient's ailment and allow attention to be focused on the emotional problem.

Antianxiety agents are probably not indicated in this setting, especially if the patient is depressed. Certain patients respond to the suggestion that they should keep a diary in which the events of the day can be seen in relation to the appearance of symptoms. Some of these patients may need psychiatric referral, but many can be managed by brief psychotherapy and a referral to a psychologist, community mental health center, or clergyman.

SUMMARY

Patients with somatoform disorders or physical complaints linked to emotional problems can be diagnosed and managed effectively in the emergency department. Even though some of these patients are notoriously frustrating, a few extra minutes of time can mean the difference between skilled professional management and an abrupt ''brush off'' that terminates their care and perpetuates the symptoms.

REFERENCES

1. Lazare, A. Hysteria. In Hackett, TP, and Cassem, MH, *Massachusetts General Hospital handbook of general hospital psychiatry*. St. Louis: The C.V. Mosby Co., 1978.
2. Katon, W, Kleinman, A, and Rosen, G. Depression and somatization: a review. *American Journal of Medicine,* 1982, *72,* 127-134.
3. Fauman, B, and Fauman, M. *Emergency psychiatry,* Baltimore: The Williams & Wilkins Co., 1981.

12 SEXUAL PROBLEMS PRESENTED AS EMERGENCIES

Certain emergency patients present problems that involve sexual assault or abnormal sexual practices. The physician may, in fact, be quite surprised when confronted by a patient with a severe psychosexual disorder. While rape of all forms is considered a violent crime, the evaluation of these patients does involve a sexual history and pelvic examination. The topic is thus considered here along with the presentation of other sexual emergencies.

RAPE AND SEXUAL ASSAULT

Rape is a physical, psychological, and social attack on a person and is a common crime. It is the fastest rising violent crime in the United States. Rape increased 68% in reported incidence between the years 1968 and 1973.[1] Women's support groups have arisen to prevent its occurrence and assist the rape victim. Perhaps because these groups exist, the reporting of rape and prosecution of the rapist are becoming more frequent. In this chapter we consider rape as it applies to women and men and sexual abuse of children and adolescents. We divide these groups somewhat arbitrarily because their management differs in significant ways. Because the term *rape* is essentially a legal one (a crime with legal definitions for which guilt is determined by criminal prosecution and conviction), the term *sexual assault* or *alleged sexual assault* is probably more useful and appropriate in the clinical setting.

The female patient

The emergency department is the usual health care facility first used by rape victims. Fortunately most departments have protocols that guide the evaluation of these victims. Some of the better protocols are quite detailed,[2] as is the one presented in Fig. 12-1. Despite the availability of the protocol, some problems in rape management still exist. The psychiatric service of the hospital is usually consulted only if a management problem arises, and occasionally the medical and psychiatric follow-ups are inconsistent. Although these victims are not routinely evaluated or treated by a psychiatrist in the emergency department, many women show up months or years after the attack at adult psychiatry clinics with problems surrounding the rape.

One of the major difficulties that could possibly interfere with the appropriate management of women who have been sexually assaulted is the rather peculiar and quite outmoded belief that women somehow invite rape. This belief may even lead to a somewhat jocular or callous attitude toward the victim. If such is the case in the emergency department, community and institutional resources are not mobilized, which results in poor or fragmented medical, psychological, and social care. Because of this and the fact that women's groups have sometimes seen medicine as a male-dominated pathology-oriented institution, various women-supported rape counseling programs have developed. Good liaison between the emergency department and these groups can improve total care of the patient. These patients need both gynecological and psychological care. Legal documentation of the alleged rape is needed for criminal prosecution.

Sometimes prejudices get in the way of adequate medical care. The treatment model geared to most medical and surgical emergencies, however, may underestimate the emotional significance of rape to the victim. Anyone working in emergency service can

Text continued on p. 174.

AKRON GENERAL MEDICAL CENTER

ALLEGED ASSAULT/RAPE PROTOCOL

ACCOUNT NO.	EMD NO.
FULL NAME OF PATIENT	DATE

AUTHORIZATION FOR EXAMINATION AND FOR RELEASE OF INFORMATION

I hereby authorize physicians of AKRON GENERAL MEDICAL CENTER to:

- ☐ Perform a medical examination including pelvic (internal) examination
- ☐ Take necessary photographs by a competent hospital employed photographer, by examining physician, or by a police photographer
- ☐ Report to law enforcement authorities that an alleged assault/rape has been committed
- ☐ Record and maintain a file of the examination
- ☐ Collect and analyze necessary specimens in laboratories
- ☐ Administer treatment indicated

The procedures outlined above, all other procedures to be performed, and the purpose for performing such procedures have been clearly explained to the undersigned. The undersigned hereby authorizes their performance and the release of copies of all medical reports, including any laboratory reports, to the police department, the office of the District Attorney, or prosecutor having jurisdiction.

A minor may give his/her consent to all of the above. The hospital is required by law to give written notice to the parent, parents, or guardian of a minor that such an examination has taken place.

Patient: ______________________

Witnesses: ______________________ R.N. ______________________ M.D.

Date: ____________ Brought to EMD by Officer ______________________

of ______________________ Police Department. Badge No. ____________

If presented self and authorization to report has been granted, then the nurse in charge must notify the law enforcement authorities.

______________ Police Department notified at ____________ a.m. p.m. By ______________

Continued.

FIG. 12-1. Sample reporting form and protocol for management and documentation of alleged rape. (Courtesy Dr. Dan Schelble and the Akron General Medical Center.)

AKRON GENERAL MEDICAL CENTER

ALLEGED ASSAULT/RAPE PROTOCOL

ACCOUNT NO.	EMD NO.	
FULL NAME OF PATIENT		DATE

HISTORY: (Record in patients own words in so far as possible)

A. Date and Time of Incident ____________

B. Place of Incident ____________

C. Physical Abuse Other Than Sexual ____________

D. Describe All Types of Sexual Contact Whether Actual/Attempted.

1. Genital ____________
2. Oral ____________
3. Anal ____________

E. Time of Last:
1. Bath 2. Shower 3. Douche 4. Urination 5. Defecation

F. **GYNECOLOGIC HISTORY**

GRAVIDA ____________ PARA ____________ AB ____________

1. Date and Normalcy of LMP; If known to be Pregnant, how long?
____
2. Recent vaginal discharge/bleeding
____
3. Date and Time of last sexual experience prior to alleged rape. ____________
4. Date and Time of sexual experience(s) since alleged rape. ____________
5. Contraceptive practice (if any) ____________
6. Prior gynecologic surgery (especially hysterectomy, tubal ligation, PID, or venereal disease). ____________

G. History of Alcohol and/or Drugs Before or After Alleged Incident

PHYSICAL EXAMINATION:

Make generous use of color photographs to record positive, and significant negative, findings. This should be done, if available, by hospital biophotographer or police photographer.

A. General Appearance: Use of a Wood's Lamp - Filtered UV Light - to Detect Seminal Stains on Clothing or Skin may be helpful.

1. All areas for signs of trauma (scratches, hematomas, contusions, fingernails, or pulled hair). ____________
____
____
____
2. Torn clothing, blood stains, or seminal stains. ____________
____
____

Fig. 12-1, cont'd

AKRON GENERAL MEDICAL CENTER

ALLEGED ASSAULT/RAPE PROTOCOL

ACCOUNT NO.	EMD NO.
FULL NAME OF PATIENT	DATE

3. Unusual marks (e.g. rope, belt, etc.) ____________________

4. Evidence of alcohol/drugs (e.g. needle marks, breath order, etc.) ____________________

5. Emotional state ____________________

B. **GENITAL – RECTAL EXAM**

1. Evidence of trauma ____________________

2. Blood, moist or dried secretions – vulva, perineum, rectum, or thighs. ____________________

3. Hymen is:
   ______ present, intact, and free of evidence of trauma.
   ______ present, intact, and shows old scarring.
   ______ present and recently ruptured.
   ______ absent

4. Vaginal or Urethral discharge – quantity, color.

5. Vaginal mucosa (use **non lubricated**, water moistened speculum)
   a. Trauma – Hematomas, lacerations

   b. Secretions – quantity, color

Continued.

Fig. 12-1, cont'd

AKRON GENERAL MEDICAL CENTER

ALLEGED ASSAULT/RAPE PROTOCOL

ACCOUNT NO.	EMD NO.
FULL NAME OF PATIENT	DATE

6. Cervix, Uterus, and Adnexia ______________________________

7. Anus – appearance, evidence of trauma ______________________________

C. **LAB TESTS**

1. Wet Mount Results
   Sperm ☐ Present ☐ Absent
   If present ☐ Motile ☐ Immotile

2. Pregnancy Test
   ☐ Positive ☐ Negative

TREATMENT (Circle or write in which used)

A. Sedation ______________________________

B. Tetanus prophylaxis ______________________________

C. Venereal disease prevention
   1. Probenicid 1.0 gm P.O., together with 4.8 million units Procaine
   or Pen-G or Benzathine Pen G I.M.
   2. Probenicid 1.0 gm P.O. together with Ampicillin 3.5 gm P.O.
   or if sensitive to Pen. then,
   3. Spectinomycin (Trobicin) 4.0 gm I.M.
   or 4. Tetracycline 1.5 gm P.O. initially, followed by 500 mg P.O. QID for four days (total dose, 9.5 gm)
   or 5. For Pen allergic **pregnant** patients:
   Erythromycin base, Stearate, or Ethylsuccinate, 1.5 gm P.O., followed by 300 MG. P.O. QID for four days (total dose 9.5 gm)

   ALTERNATIVELY

   Ce-Fazolin 2.0 gm I.M. with Probenicid 1.0 gm P.O.

D. Prevention of possible pregnancy

   NOTE: Try to encourage patient to "Wait and See" regarding pregnancy. The Beta Subunit Test of HCG is a early (6 days), reliable test for pregnancy. If this test is positive, then patient should have a D & C. If, for whatever reason, this is unacceptable to the patient and she **demands** treatment for possible pregnancy, then use the following acceptable treatments. Do **not** use **DES** (see "Physician Advisory" HEW, October 4, 1978).

   1. Conjugated Equine Estrogen (Premarin) 2.5 mg P.O. QID for five days
   or 2. If doubt complience, then give Premarin 40 - 50 mg I.V. (single dose).
   or 3. If no menses within one week after end of above therapy, then consider D & C.

E. FOLLOW-UP INSTRUCTIONS
   To be seen in 3 - 5 days for follow-up care and counseling by:
   ☐ Patient's regular private physician ______________________________, M.D.
   ☐ Referral gynecologist from EMD call list ______________________________, M.D.
   ☐ AGMC Gynecologic Clinic

EMD Physician Signature ______________________________

Female Witness Signature ______________________________

Fig. 12-1, cont'd

AKRON GENERAL MEDICAL CENTER

ALLEGED ASSAULT/RAPE PROTOCOL

ACCOUNT NO.	EMD NO.	
FULL NAME OF PATIENT		DATE

****** ORIGINAL TO STAY WITH PATIENT'S CHART: DUPLICATE TO GO TO HOSPITAL LAB.**

	COMPLETED	TIME	INITIAL
MANDATORY SAMPLES (MAILED OUT)			
1. THREE VAGINAL SWABS (TC TUBE, DON'T BREAK)			
2. SALIVA SAMPLE (SPIT INTO EMPTY TUBE)			
3. BLOOD SAMPLES (TWO CLOT TUBES)			
VAGINAL POOL, UNDILUTED			
1. ACID PHOSPHATASE, ISOENZYMES			
2. PGM ISOENZYMES			
3. SECRETOR SPECIMEN			
VAGINAL SWAB DRYSMEAR			
PAP SMEAR FOR SPERM			
CERVICAL CULTURE			
ANAL SWAB, DRY SMEAR			
ANAL SWAB (TC TUBE, DON'T BREAK)			
ANAL CULTURE			
ORAL CULTURE			
ORAL SWAB			
BLOOD SAMPLE			
1. VDRL			
2. BLOOD TYPE			
3. ETOH (BIO SCIENCE BOX)			
4. DRUG SCREEN			
URINE SAMPLE STRAIGHT CATH			
1. ANALYSIS			
2. PREGNANCY TEST			
3. DRUG SCREEN			
OTHER			
1.			
2.			
3.			

EACH CONTAINER AND/OR ITEM MARKED WITH PATIENT'S NAME, DATE, TIME OF COLLECTION, SOURCE, EXAMINER'S NAME AND SEALED.

SIGNATURE (RECEIVED FROM)	DATE	TIME
SIGNATURE (RECEIVED BY)	DATE	TIME

Continued.

Fig. 12-1, cont'd

AKRON GENERAL MEDICAL CENTER

ALLEGED ASSAULT/RAPE PROTOCOL

ACCOUNT NO.	EMD NO.
FULL NAME OF PATIENT	DATE

ITEMS FOR SUBMISSION TO POLICE LAB.

	COMPLETED	TIME	INITIAL
FINGERNAIL SCRAPINGS			
SKIN STAIN SAMPLE			
PUBIC HAIR, MATTED			
PUBIC HAIR, COMBED			
CLOTHING IN SEALED BAG			
HOSPITAL BED LINENS, IN SEALED BAG			
OTHER			
1.			
2.			
3.			

EACH CONTAINER AND/OR ITEM MARKED WITH PATIENT'S NAME, DATE, TIME OF COLLECTION, SOURCE, EXAMINER'S NAME, AND SEALED.

SIGNATURE (RECEIVED FROM)		DATE	TIME
SIGNATURE (RECEIVED BY)	BADGE NO.	DATE	TIME

***** ORIGINAL TO STAY WITH PATIENT'S CHART: DUPLICATE TO GO TO POLICE LAB.**

Fig. 12-1, cont'd

become emotionally insulated to the significance of medical or psychological trauma in a patient.

Because of the well-publicized and now better understood meaning of rape, some medical centers and hospitals are developing a rape crisis intervention program. This program usually involves a team consisting of a patient advocate, an emergency department physician, and a hospital administrator. Each member of the team has distinct goals (Table 12-1).

One method of handling the female sexual assault victim is to assign an advocate to her immediately. This may be a nurse who has been trained in this area, a social worker, a crisis center team member, or a chaplain. The advocate stays with the patient while she is in the emergency department. This person can register the patient and explain the legal aspects and nature of the medical examination. The advocate may also tell the patient that the hospital must report the rape to the police.

TABLE 12-1. Treatment team concept for rape management in the emergency setting

Treatment team members	*Goals of members*
Physician	1. Assess and treat injuries 2. Gather evidence for court proceedings 3. Advise victim regarding venereal disease and pregnancy 4. Inform and support victim regarding referral for follow-up appointment
Patient advocate (nurse, social worker, volunteer, etc.)	1. Explain medical and legal procedures 2. Contact relatives and/or friends 3. Assess patient's view of the rape and convey to physician 4. Arrange follow-up appointment
Hospital administrator	1. Maintain good liaison with community groups 2. Document and keep material resulting from examination

The patient should be freely allowed to choose whether or not to prosecute the rapist. If the patient chooses not to prosecute, she should be warned that an examination at a later date cannot be done to obtain legal evidence for the rape prosecution. An examination and treatment, including the steps necessary to obtain legal evidence, should be completed if there is any question at all that the patient wishes to press charges.

The advocate can also contact relatives or friends at the patient's request. This advocate should be able to assess the patient's strengths and weaknesses in her handling of the rape and discuss these issues with the physician before the medical examination. The advocate may choose to arrange psychiatric consultation or support if deemed necessary. When the patient has finished the emergency department procedure for examination and treatment of rape, the advocate may give the patient several sources for help and counseling: the advocate's own name and number, the name and number of the rape crisis intervention center for long-term counseling, and perhaps the number of a psychiatric clinic. The availability of emergency psychiatric support should be discussed with the patient.

It is important, while this is going on, that no member of the team treating the victim makes a decision as to whether or not a rape occurred; this is a legal decision, not a medical one.

Management of the female victim. The problem of sexual assault is almost unique in the practice of emergency medicine. The physician knows immediately that evidence needs to be collected and that the patient has major psychological stress that requires proper management. The emergency physician thus has at least five goals in the assessment and treatment of a sexual assault victim. Although the initial priority in the management of *any* patient is the treatment of severe medical conditions or injuries, the first goal of the emergency physician in the management of the rape victim concerns the way the patient is handled from the first moment of contact. The method should be one that provides emotional support and empathy so that subsequent counseling and guidance can be provided.

The second goal is that the injuries are assessed and treated appropriately. The emergency physician must be sure that the patient does not have serious injuries, like stab wounds, that she cannot clearly describe because of serious emotional disturbances that may accompany sexual assault. This should be done in the gentlest possible way, and the patient should be well prepared for the pelvic and other physical examinations before they begin. The physician needs to make some contact with the patient emotionally, taking time to discuss her own feelings and the physical problems that she is now having. The physician should not discuss the incident of the rape in great detail unless the patient so wishes. In these cases the physician needs to recognize that in some ways he or she is symbolically recreating the act of sexual intrusion with the pelvic examination. It is important, therefore, to maintain a professional concern for the patient without appearing either too cool and disinterested or overly concerned or solicitous.

The physician's third goal is to gather all evidence necessary for anticipated court proceedings, and the fourth goal is to provide medical advice to the patient after the examination, regarding pregnancy or venereal disease.

The hospital administrator or a specifically designated nurse should have some plan to document and keep material resulting from the examination to ensure successful prosecution of the rapist. This person has an important role in maintaining liaison with community groups concerned about rape and related issues.

A woman who has been raped has experienced an intrusion into her physical and psychological identity. The victim may react to this in various ways. These reactions constitute a "rape trauma syndrome" (Table 12-2).

The "typical" rape trauma syndrome has two phases: an acute phase and a long-term phase. The acute phase is one characterized by disorganization, somatic symptoms, and various emotional reactions. The initial emotional impact of the rape may be so severe that the patient expresses disbelief or shock. As feelings return, some patients express their emotions openly as they cry, sob, pace, or display anger. Other victims react with a controlled style; their feelings are hidden, and they appear subdued, quiet, and composed. Several days or weeks later these patients may develop somatic symptoms like abdominal pain, headache, loss of appetite, or vaginal discharge or discomfort. Acute emotional reactions usually include embarrassment, fear, anger, and guilt. The long-term effects can include changes in life-style, sexual difficulties, nightmares, and various fears or phobias.

Occasionally a patient has experienced a previous rape. In general, this patient needs far more psychiatric care. Her reactions can include suicidal behavior, alcohol or drug abuse, and development of severe somatic symptoms.

The patient who refuses to reveal that she has been raped can develop a variety of new behavioral characteristics that include anxiety, irritability, phobic reactions, or loss of self-esteem.

TABLE 12-2. Rape trauma syndrome

Reactions	*Signs and symptoms*
Typical reaction	
Phase I: acute (disorganization)	Impact reaction—shock, disbelief, expressed emotion, controlled emotion Somatic reactions—physical injury, tension headaches, fatigue, sleep disturbance, abdominal pain, loss of appetite, vaginal complaints Emotional reactions—fear, humiliation, embarrassment, anger, guilt
Phase II: long-term (reorganization)	Relocation (change residence and obtain unlisted phone number), obtain support from out-of-town relatives, nightmares, multiple fears and phobias (e.g., indoors, outdoors, alone, crowds, strangers, sexual activity)
Compounded reaction	Severe psychological trauma, victim usually needs psychotherapy, possibility of suicidal behavior, alcoholism, drug use, severe somatic symptoms
Silent reaction	Persistent anxiety, marked irritability, change in sexual behavior, sudden onset of phobic reactions, sudden loss of self-esteem or development of guilt

From Burgess, AW, and Holmstrom, LL. Rape trauma syndrome. *American Journal of Psychiatry*, 1974, *131*(9), 981-986.

The early stages of the rape trauma syndrome are the best time for crisis intervention. The emergency physician is the most appropriate person to make this crisis intervention possible by either arranging social service or psychiatric consultation or by personally initiating the intervention.

The success of crisis intervention depends on the patient's ability to discuss her feelings. She must be encouraged to express them as openly as possible. The feelings may include both a sense of outrage and some component of self-blame. This early crisis intervention may be crucial in the patient's recovery. It is a time for the victim to mobilize strengths rather than to adapt to a lower level of psychological functioning.

Management of the spouse/boyfriend/relative. Boyfriends, husbands, and other relatives have a great deal of difficulty accepting the idea of sexual assault. These people need to be helped so that they can aid the victim. Therefore the physician and other emergency department personnel must see the assault victim as a member of a couple or family. There are four major methods in the management that are helpful to the victim. They are the following:

1. The mate or boyfriend should be able to express his own feelings.
2. The mate must be able to understand the meaning of the rape to the victim and not only to himself.

3. The family members or mate should anticipate psychological and physical sequelae from the rape.
4. The mate or family members may also need some support to get through the experience.

As the family members express feelings about the rape, several myths or beliefs may be discovered. They may feel that "nice women don't get raped." Family members or close friends may need some reiteration and reassurance about rape. In discussing the act of rape, the advocate or physician should concentrate on the violence of the crime, not the sexual meaning of it.

It is important to realize that the mate of the rape victim feels that his "possession" has been abused by another male. This arouses tremendous competitive and violent fantasies. These feelings need to be discussed in a protected environment, and, if possible, the mate should learn a way other than retribution to handle his feelings.

Some very obvious problems may arise following sexual assault. If sexuality is already a problem for a couple, it may become more so. If the husband has felt himself to be a poor protector in the past, he may now feel exaggerated feelings in this area. Counseling should encourage the couple to talk about these issues and build the closeness of a shared experience.

Follow-up of female sexual assault victims. Family members often patronize and overprotect the woman after sexual assault. This protectiveness may encourage regression and a sense of dependency in the victim. The family's tendency toward counterproductive behavior can be assessed in an interview in which the family is encouraged to talk openly about their feelings toward the victim. Even when such attitudes are not discovered, the family should be warned to begin treating the patient as a "normal" person as soon as possible.

In an open discussion with the patient's family, it may be helpful to discuss the rape trauma syndrome. The family can be told that the victim may make an outward readjustment following the sexual assault but may have nightmares, insomnia, somatic symptoms, and phobias. The victim may also have a good deal of depression with crying spells and feelings of guilt and self-blame. These can be predicted and reacted to by the family with support but not overprotection.

Such simple counseling in the emergency department helps educate the patient and allows early expression of fear and other emotions. The procedure is simple and can easily be taught to emergency department personnel. The early discussion provides a safety valve and sets the tone for further counseling. This procedure has tremendous potential for preventing or ameliorating psychiatric sequelae of rape.

After the patient has been physically examined, treated, and psychologically supported, she should be referred to a rape crisis intervention team for long-term follow-up. This may be within the hospital or in a community outpatient setting. Since a crisis intervention team should operate on a 24-hour-a-day basis, the patient should have a specific appointment time and location to which she can go within the next 72 hours.

The male patient

The rape of males has been little discussed in the literature. It is usually seen as a part of prison life and is, therefore, mostly covered in literature about prisoners. In prisons, rape has often been viewed as a vicarious sexual assault against women or a violent outgrowth of homosexual subcultures.

In a study at the University of New Mexico School of Medicine, an increase from 0% in 1975 to 10% in 1978 was seen in the reported incidence of male rape.[3] The male rape victims were compared to females, and several differences were found. The males were younger, usually had more than one assailant, were often beaten, and tended not to seek treatment for the sexual assault. They did seek treatment for nongenital trauma, however. In general these men tended to react to sexual assault in a more controlled way than women. They appeared quiet, embarrassed, withdrawn, and unconcerned. Such patients' apparent lack of emotional responsiveness may disguise real feelings and leads the emergency department team to inadvertently ignore their emotional needs.

The male victims often had a high incidence of instability in their home, social, and work life. They were likely to have been held captive for a longer period than female rape victims.

It has been estimated that 12% to 20% of women report rape. It is probable that a much smaller proportion of men report rape. This may be related to a fear of being labeled a homosexual or ridiculed in the emergency department.

Management of the male patient. The management of the male sexual assault victim is much the same as that of the female victim. The male feels helpless, damaged, and fearful of what others will think of him. He should be treated in a calm and accepting way. The physician can again concentrate on the violence of the act, rather than the sexual nature of it. The physician may also concentrate on the bodily damage while doing the examination. Joking or other light treatment of such an event is obviously inappropriate, and those kinds of glib comments that demean the patient or make negative social judgments may cause serious psychological harm and certainly may make the patient reluctant to seek medical attention for future problems.

Trying to minimize the number of staff involved in evaluating the patient is preferable. He probably thinks that he is a curiosity and that many people on the staff want to see him. Therefore any examination and discussion of the sexual assault should be done in complete privacy. Having an advocate go through the emergency department with him would be greatly helpful. It is always wise to remember that the male usually appears less concerned with the event than he actually feels. Therefore arranging for appropriate referral on discharge from the emergency department is important.

The management of the male rape victim includes a physical examination and medical advice about venereal disease. Predicting that sequelae such as nightmares, insomnia, excessive worry, or depression are common is helpful. The patient should be referred to a crisis intervention team, but he is probably less likely to follow up with this appointment than the female victim. Therefore it is even more important to spend extra time with this person and predict to him that he may have some difficulties adjusting to the event.

Child sexual abuse

The battered child syndrome was described by Kempe in 1962.[4] Since then, physicians in our society have become increasingly aware of the abuse of children by adults. Physical abuse has been emphasized, but emotional and sexual abuse is becoming more evident.

Adults who abuse children have become recognized as persons who were abused themselves during childhood. These people have been given a more compassionate view in recent years than adults who sexually abuse children. Everyone has had the experience of feeling like physically assaulting a child at one time or another, although most people do not do so. It is more difficult to identify with an adult who sexually abuses children. There is a universal taboo against incest, and this generalizes to all adult-child interactions. In one study (Hayman and Lanza)[5] a survey of 2190 women and child victims of sexual attack in Washington, D.C. between the years 1965 and 1969 revealed that the peak age of children being attacked was between 14 and 15. Forty-five percent of the victims were 12 to 19 years of age, and 13% were 0 to 9 years of age. Twenty-four children were admitted for severe injury (25%) and six of them ranged in age from 2 to 6 years. Eleven of these children required suturing in the emergency department. An occasional death has been reported as a result of sexual abuse of a child.

One of the difficulties of identifying sexual abuse in children is that physicians often do not report such suspected abuse, despite state laws that require it. In a canvas of physicians reported in the *Journal of the American Medical Association* (JAMA),[6] only 32% urged the family to report the incident of sexual abuse of a child. In this same group of physicians who did not report sexual abuse in children, two thirds thought that reporting such an incident would be harmful to the family or could be handled better privately. One third of these physicians were dissatisfied with the way social service agencies handled such cases.

In the emergency department a physician must have a high level of suspicion to pick up cases of sexual molestation in children. In general, four categories of these problems are seen in emergency practice. They include the following:

1. Genital complaints
2. History of encopresis, enuresis, difficulty in school
3. History of school phobias, sudden change in behavior
4. History of running away, unplanned pregnancy, fear of sex

Genital complaints like injury, irritation, or purulent discharge, which are not easily explained, should prompt further evaluation for sexual abuse. Childhood problems, such as difficulty with friends, difficulty in school, enuresis, or encopresis, may indicate sexual abuse and should at least be considered in the evaluation of these problems. Rather abrupt alterations in the behavior of a child should arouse suspicions of sexual

TABLE 12-3. Types of child molestation

Type	*Activity*	*Usual person involved*
Accidental	Fondling, exhibition of genitalia, one time only	Stranger
Participant	Intercourse or active sexual relationship lasting over long periods of time	Parent, relative, friend of the family

abuse. The sudden appearance of school phobia, extreme shyness, or a nasty disposition are other examples. Early adolescent problems like pregnancy, attempting to run away, drug abuse, or intense fear of sexual activity should arouse suspicions of sexual abuse.

The physician's failure to diagnose or ask about sexual abuse in a child probably stems from the fact that the thought of such abuse is rather repugnant to the physician who is probably uncomfortable asking the child about sexual problems. When the physician is hurried, it is difficult to establish a trusting conversational relationship with the child who may sense that the physician feels that sex or a sex-related topic is a taboo subject for conversation. This encourages the child to remain mute about such difficulties and initially deny these problems when asked.

If child abuse is suspected, certain types of evidence must be collected for the purposes of a legal prosecution and conviction. Careful documentation of these findings on the medical record facilitates subsequent legal review. The documentation should include the overall emotional and physical appearance of the child and any clearly obvious evidence of trauma. The patient or parent history and any discussion with the child about the injury or illness should be documented.

As in cases of rape, the examination should document all genital or other trauma. The child's clothing is generally saved in plastic bags with appropriate labels. Fingernail scrapings, photographs, or other data may be requested by police investigating the case.

Management of the sexually abused child. Two types of sexual abuse generally occur in children (Table 12-3). One type is considered "accidental" and involves the child who is typically approached by an exhibitionist or is fondled by a stranger one time only. The abuse may be rather nontraumatic or may be forceful or violent. Children abused in this way generally report it immediately. When the child is uninjured, the parent can discuss what happened and reassure the child. Unless there has been some physical assault on the child, there are no long-term sequelae from an exhibitionist or from a one-time fondling. When the child is injured, medical treatment may be required.

The second type of sexual abuse is "participant" or collaborative victimization. This type of molestation occurs when a usually well-acquainted friend or relative maintains a sexual relationship with a child over long periods of time.

Participant or collaborative types of child abuse are indicative of serious family pathology. Sexual relationships between brothers and sisters are the most common type of collaborative sexuality, but a sexual liaison between father and daughter is frequently reported. Usually the family appears perfectly normal but is actually quite chaotic.

Within these families the normal psychological roles of mother-daughter and father-son are generally obliterated. Often the mother appears to be more the "needy child." When a daughter-father relationship exists, the mother typically protests strongly that she did not know about the relationship, although at either a conscious or unconscious level, she almost invariably is aware. If a mother has a sexual relationship with a son, there is usually a psychotic problem present in one or both of them. The child must be looked on as a person seeking comfort, love, and warmth, whereas the adult must be viewed as someone exploiting this need.

The most obvious physician response to sexual abuse in a child is outrage. It is a natural reaction, but it gets in the way of medical care for the child and family. The physician and other staff members need to maintain a calm, thoughtful, and professional demeanor. All members of the family should be interviewed separately. The family must see the physician as a person who is a family helper and not as a policeman or fearful authority figure. Accurate records should be kept with complete notes concerning conversations with each person in the family.

Talking with the child. The art of talking with a child is a skill that can be learned fairly easily when simple principles are followed. One of the principles is that the adult must use simple words that the child understands. Another is to begin the conversation with nonthreatening things that the child knows well, like school or favorite sports, television shows, or toys.

Before interviewing the child, the physician should ask the parent about the child's words for various parts of the sexual anatomy. Using his own words for these areas helps avoid misunderstanding. The history of abuse is most easily obtained when the approach is calm, warm, and nonthreatening.

The child can be prepared for the examination in a simple, professional manner. The interview and examination demand strict privacy. The major goals of the evaluations are to determine if sexual abuse is present, and if so, which of the two forms, accidental or participant, has occurred. The following five areas of inquiry are most productive in determining which type of abuse has occurred:

1. Did the child know the adult?
2. Did the child tell an adult or parent immediately?
3. Did the child accept gifts from the adult?
4. Was the relationship prolonged?
5. Has the child been involved with more than one adult sexually?

In dealing with the parents of a child who has accidentally been exposed to an exhibitionist or a fondler, the physician should determine whether or not the parents can handle their own anxiety and anger. If they can handle their anxiety, they should be capable of supporting the child emotionally. If it appears that they are unable to deal with their anxiety, they may feel that the child is "forever damaged." Parents with these notions should be referred to a psychiatrist for further evaluation and treatment. If they appear capable of mobilizing their own protective and nurturing roles, they may need little future support. Parents need to be encouraged to talk about the event both between themselves and with their child. They should do so in a calm, thoughtful manner, even using humor if it is appropriate. The enormity or intensity of the event should be minimized, and bringing it up in the future (for several weeks) when appropriate might be helpful, particularly if the child shows any interest in talking about his feelings.

In participant molestation the family should be considered pathological, no matter how it appears. In this case all parties of the family need a referral for psychiatric intervention and further evaluation. If it is not done, the sexual relationship will probably continue and the child may become a child abuser when he grows up. All cases of child abuse should be reported to the authorities, and the family should be prepared for this.

Preventive measures should be taken for venereal disease, pregnancy, and tetanus. Appropriate pediatric or psychiatric referral should be made if it is deemed necessary. The emergency evaluation of child abuse sets the tone for the family's future handling of the event. The evaluation must, therefore, be calm and professional.

Sexual abuse of an adolescent

In a study of adolescent sexual abuse at Boston City Hospital, three types of abuse were identified:[7] sex stress situation, incest, and rape (Table 12-4).

Sex stress situation. The first type of adolescent sexual abuse is the sex stress situation. Adolescents who are having a sexual relationship of one kind or another become concerned about it. The girl may come to the emergency department to find out whether or not she is pregnant. She may be very concerned about this but not able to admit that she was a consenting partner in the sexual relationship. She may even plead that she has been raped to avoid admitting her complicity.

This same sex stress situation may occur when an authority figure or parent discovers two adolescents engaged in sexual activity. The parent or police officer may create an uproar and bring the two adolescents to the emergency department. The management of the sex stress situation requires the emergency personnel to try to reduce the anxiety of all parties. The prevailing anger must be defused. Defusing is best accomplished by holding separate interviews with the parents and the adolescents.

Unless it is deemed absolutely necessary (e.g., claim of rape), the gynecological examination should be deferred for a subsequent appointment. The emotional condition of all parties involved constitutes the most important consideration in the early stages

TABLE 12-4. Types of sexual abuse of an adolescent

Type	*Activity*
Sex stress situation	"Found out" or concerned about consenting sexual activity
Incest	Sexual abuse by family member
Rape	Violent physical attack

(Adapted from McCausland, MP. Sexual development and sexual abuse: emergencies in adolescents. *Pediatric Clinics of North America,* Nov. 1979, *26*(4), 895-901.)

of management. If one of the parties appears ignorant about sexuality, he or she can be referred for guidance about sexual matters. For some patients the best referral may be to their own minister, rabbi, priest, teacher, family physician, or community health service.

Incest. Incest involves sexual activities between family members. An adolescent may engage in sexual activity with a parent or sibling for various reasons. The adolescent may have been pressured to enter into sexual activity and may fear rejection, punishment, or blame for discussing the sexual liaison. The symptoms and signs of incest are similar to those of other forms of child abuse. The adolescent may undergo sudden behavior changes, become pregnant, or contract veneral disease. Alternatively, the patient may come to the emergency department with vague somatic complaints like abdominal pain or headache. The adolescent's school performance or personal relationships with peers may deteriorate suddenly, or the victim may run away from home or begin abusing drugs or alcohol. These elements of history should arouse a suspicion of sexual abuse. The elicitation of further sexual history requires a small amount of time to establish some rapport.

If incest is discovered, the situation must be reported to the local children's services agency, and the family needs counseling. The adolescent must also be protected from retribution and ongoing sexual abuse. Therefore the adolescent should be removed from the home. If necessary, the patient can be admitted to the hospital and subsequently transferred to a temporary foster home.

Rape. As discussed previously, a prompt referral to a rape crisis team is most valuable. Adolescents are deeply anxious about sexuality, and rape intensifies all of these normal conflicts. The adolescent male or female who has been raped requires understanding and particularly sensitive handling.

SEXUAL CONCERNS OVER SEEMINGLY INNOCUOUS PROBLEMS

Often patients come to the emergency department with seemingly inconsequential questions. This frequently occurs late at night when there is the tendency to focus on things that may, in the light of day, seem less important. A number of concerns occur to people, and many of them are sexual. Most emergency department physicians have had a case of a young man who has a bump on his penis and is in a panic about it. It turns out to be a normal vein or skin tag. Other examples include minor pains in the genital area, frequently after masturbation or intercourse. Concerns about masturbating (or not masturbating), petting, getting pregnant in a bath tub, contracting venereal disease from a toilet seat, or other sexual problems may seem amusing to the emergency staff but are not to the patient.

In dealing with these seemingly trivial concerns, the most important issue is to listen carefully. The patient may be embarrassed and need encouragement to express the full extent of his anxiety. He should be heard in a calm, thoughtful way. The physician who listens thoroughly to the concern can then respond. A careful physical examination should be done to avoid missing real pathological conditions and to convince the patient that the physician has not overlooked an important clue. The examination should be done deliberately and thoroughly. Any minor abnormal findings should be minimized or not even mentioned at all. Informing the patient of even a normal variance may arouse panic.

Unless the complaint seems bizarre or psychotic, the patient can be educated. This is most easily done by providing a simple explanation for the phenomenon and repeating it several times in different ways. The patient can be raised to a level of commonality by explaining that the concern about a possibly abnormal finding is quite common. The patient can thus be reassured that he is normal and that no untoward results should occur. If neither reassurance nor brief education (perhaps with appropriate drawings or photographs) seems to relax the patient, referral sources should be suggested. A student health service, local phychiatrist, psychologist, community mental health center, and the patient's own family physician are appropriate referrals.

Occasionally nonadolescents suddenly develop fears or phobias about sexual matters. A middle-aged man may suddenly be unable to urinate in a public toilet, for example. The situation may require one or two sessions of psychiatric treatment, involving brief psychotherapy and perhaps a minor tranquilizer. The important feature of emergency treatment is the physician's genuine concern. Some patients have actually killed themselves over seemingly inconsequential worries about the important matter of sexuality. When the patient feels the physician is lending a sympathetic and professional ear, the anxiety can be shared and then reduced.

IMPOTENCE OR OTHER SEXUAL DYSFUNCTION

A man or woman arriving at the emergency department with the chief complaint of impotence or other sexual dysfunction is probably in a state of acute anxiety. A careful assessment is necessary and includes a history of drug use, a thorough physical examination of the genitalia, and a full sexual history. This reassures the patient that nothing is being overlooked and often determines the problem. If no precipitating factor is obvious, the patient needs to be reassured that this is a common problem and that there is specific and rapid treatment for it. Any educational issues, such as discussion of anatomy or the impact of fatigue and alcohol on sexual performance, should be presented to reduce the patient's anxiety. The patient may be sent home with the reassurance that if this continues after a couple of restful days, he or she should be referred to someone adept at sex therapy, like a private psychiatrist, psychologist, or community mental health center.

GENITAL FOREIGN BODIES

Emergency department physicians occasionally encounter foreign bodies in the rectum, vagina, urethra, or bladder. The patient may be acutely embarrassed and often blame an unusual or unbelievable mechanism for the insertion of the foreign body. When a pencil is lodged in the bladder, for instance, the patient may say she "accidently" sat on it. Occasionally the complaint is so vague that the discovery of the foreign body may be almost by chance. The patient may complain, for instance, of inability to urinate or defecate or of bloody urethral discharge. After a thorough physical examination, the patient should be gently asked about his or her sexual history, and the topic of the present situation can be introduced in the following way: "All of us at one time or another want to experiment sexually. It looks as though you may have been doing this. Would you like to tell me about it?" If the patient does not respond to this approach, the physician should not press the question immediately. The physician may merely seem to accept what the patient says and provide reassuring information about any anatomical injury or lack of injury that has occurred. Reassuring the patient that the behavior is not crazy is important. Following extraction of the foreign body, the patient may benefit from being given a referral source to further explain any other issues about sex. A brief screen for psychosis should determine whether or not the patient needs immediate psychiatric evaluation.

Quite often a sexual partner accompanies the patient to the emergency department. When such a person is present, each may be interviewed separately. At the end of these interviews both patient and partner can be brought together for a few minutes of general discussion. The discussion helps ease tension and aids in preventing any distortion of things that have been discussed separately.

PSYCHOSEXUAL DISORDERS

Patients with psychosexual disorders may be encountered in the emergency department with complaints relating to their disorder or to nonrelated problems. Sometimes their appearance is so flamboyant or bizarre that they immediately attract the amused attention of the entire staff. As with patients who have other psychiatric disorders, the approach to these individuals must be professional and nonjudgmental. As mentioned previously, some of these patients interpret the staff's private ridicule as extremely threatening. They may leave without treatment, become violent, or become extremely withdrawn.

The psychosexual disorders include gender identity disorders, paraphilias, and psychosexual dysfunction. The most common gender disorder is transsexualism.

Transsexualism

Few events cause greater surprise to emergency physicians than the experience of examining a patient thought to be one sex and discovering the genitals of another. Transsexuals feel a persistent desire to change their anatomical sex. They adopt names and dress appropriately for the opposite sex and occasionally request sex change surgery. Sometimes these patients have had one operation and await surgery for the remainder of the change. The anatomical male, for instance, may have received mammary prostheses, but the penis and the testes remain. Transsexuals generally find the genitals of their anatomical sex repugnant and wish to be rid of them.

Transsexuals are not psychotic. The presence of psychosis suggests a different diagnosis (schizophrenia, affective disorder, or organic mental disorder). Transsexuals sometimes have personality disorder and/or depressive episodes that can lead to a suicide attempt. The official diagnosis of transsexualism requires that the disorder be present for at least 2 years.

The most appropriate response to these patients is to deal objectively with their chief complaint and treat them as the sex with which they identify. Patients requesting psychiatric help regarding their transsexualism can be referred to a psychiatric consultant or to a center specializing in these problems.

Paraphilias

Paraphilias are characterized by sexual arousal in response to objects or situations that do not normally cause such arousal. This abnormal arousal pattern may interfere with normal sexual relationships and in some cases result in assault, battery, indecent exposure, or some other crime. Examples of paraphilia are fetishism, transvestism, exhibitionism, zoophilia, voyeurism, pedophilia, sexual masochism, and sexual sadism.

Fetishism. The central characteristic of fetishism is that nonliving objects cause sexual excitement and arousal; a typical example is sexual arousal (in the male) associated with a woman's shoe. The objects causing sexual arousal are not ones like a vibrator, specifically designed for such stimulation.

Transvestism. The transvestite male achieves sexual gratification and relief of anxiety by dressing as a female. The male is heterosexual and considers himself basically male. This is an important distinguishing feature from transsexualism in which the male patient considers himself female and wishes to be rid of his male genitals.

Exhibitionism. Exhibitionists are males who experience sexual excitement from exposing their genitals to unsuspecting children or adult women. Sexual excitement seems to be associated with causing shock or surprise. There is no associated rape attempt. Since this behavior is clearly abnormal, repugnant, and frightening, the patient may be apprehended by the police and brought to the emergency department for treatment of an injury or evaluation before incarceration. When apprehended, these patients are best treated for associated injury or illness and returned to the authorities.

Zoophilia. Zoophilia is the use of animals as a preferred method of achieving sexual excitement.

Voyeurism. Voyeurism involves deriving sexual excitement and gratification from viewing naked bodies or the sexual acts of others. The arousal is especially high when the viewing is done secretly.

Pedophilia. Pedophilia can be an act or fantasy of sexual activity with children. When the sexual activity occurs, it is considered sexual abuse of a child and must be reported as discussed previously.

Sexual masochism. Sexual masochism is defined as a preferred or exclusive mode of producing sexual excitement by being made to suffer. This may occur by being beaten, bound, or tortured. The disorder also includes the individual who has intentionally participated in an activity in which he was physically harmed or threatened to produce sexual excitement.

Individuals with this disorder may mutilate themselves repeatedly over the years. To be considered under this diagnosis the individual must have engaged in serious masochistic acts and must prefer such acts to other sexual activities as a means of achieving sexual pleasure. The proper approach to such patients is to adopt a nonjudgmental attitude and to refer them for psychiatric evaluation or follow-up.

Sexual sadism. Sexual sadism involves the "infliction of psychological suffering in another person in order to achieve sexual excitement," according to the definition provided in the DSM-III. The diagnosis may be made if any of the following three criteria apply:

1. On a nonconsenting partner the individual has repeatedly and intentionally inflicted psychological or physical suffering to achieve sexual excitement.
2. With a consenting partner a repeatedly preferred or exclusive mode of achieving sexual excitement combines humiliation with simulated or mildly injurious bodily suffering.
3. On a consenting partner bodily injury that is extensive, permanent, or possibly fatal is inflicted to achieve sexual excitement.[8]

The sadist may commit rape, although this is not usually the case. All rapists are not sadists. The diagnosis of sexual sadism should be suspected when the patient or his partner shows signs or symptoms attributable to being bound, hanged, or in other ways acting out unusual sexual fantasies. If sexual sadism is suspected, particularly if there is any genital trauma or other bodily harm, the patient should be questioned about his sexual history after a rapport is established. The possibility of engaging in unusual sexual activities can be mentioned in a nonthreatening way by saying something like the following: "Many people experiment with sex. Have you been involved in any unusual sexual activity lately?" Establishment of this diagnosis can be important. Patients involved in sadomasochistic sexual behavior may inflict permanent injury or kill someone.

Because of the dangers to the patient and others involved in sadistic sexual activity, early referral to a psychiatrist or perhaps obtaining immediate psychiatric consultation most effectively keeps the patient and others from possible harm. A nonjudgmental and nonthreatening attitude toward these patients is most likely to elicit their cooperation.

EGO DYSTONIC HOMOSEXUALITY

Homosexuality per se is not considered a mental disorder. When the patient sustains an overt pattern of homosexual activity yet still expresses the desire to maintain heterosexual relationships in spite of homosexual preferences, and when this conflict causes the patient persistent emotional pain or disability, he can be diagnosed as having ego dystonic homosexuality. Many patients with this disorder eventually give up the effort to maintain heterosexual relationships and accept themselves as homosexuals. A strong homosexual subculture supports this tendency. Such patients can be referred for psychiatric counseling if they need help in dealing with their situation.

HOMOSEXUAL PANIC

Homosexual panic may manifest when a patient enters the emergency department in a state of acute anxiety. The patient is usually male but may be female. A typical history is one of experiencing acute anxiety when suddenly coming into close contact with people of the same sex. A student, for instance, may have recently moved into a dormitory or rooming house. The patient may or may not admit his fear of homosexual thoughts or feelings. When the patient does not admit such fears, the complaints range from vague generalized anxiety to absolute panic. If the patient does not broach the fear of homosexuality, the physician should not mention it.

The most effective temporary therapy involves moving the patient out of close contact with members of the same sex. This advice does not need to be explained in any great depth. There is no point in mobilizing or uncapping a deep concern about homosexuality in a busy emergency department. This can be done more effectively and gently over a period of time in psychiatric counseling.

If the patient does bring up homosexual thoughts and feelings that are frightening to him, the physician should respond in a calm, professional, nonjudgmental manner, which allows the patient to continue to express his feelings. He can even be assured that this is a relatively common problem, that adequate treatment is available, and that his concerns should certainly be explored further with a therapist. The patient should not be mistakenly reassured that he is not a homosexual. He needs to accept his own feelings of ambivalence in this situation. Allowing him to have such feelings without commenting on them is the most important response the physician can make.

SUMMARY

Emergency department personnel can be trained easily to respond to patients with sexual difficulties in a calm way. Training may involve some desensitization and education for the staff about sexuality and its attendant difficulties. Since the emergency department personnel are often the first to be contacted with such difficulties, their response to them may set the tone for future therapeutic intervention and provide early stabilization to prevent painful or dangerous consequences.

REFERENCES

1. McCombie, SL, et al. Development of a medical center rape crisis intervention program. *American Journal of Psychiatry,* April 1976, *133*(4), 418-421.
2. Schelble, DT, and Bradford, JC. An 18-month evaluation of the Akron General Medical Center assault/rape protocol. *Annals of Emergency Medicine,* Jan. 1982, *11*(1), 9-17.
3. Kaufman, A, et al. Male rape victims: noninstitutionalized assault. *American Journal of Psychiatry* Feb. 1980, *137*(2), 221-223.
4. Kempe, CH, et al. The battered child syndrome. *Journal of the American Medical Association,* 1962, *181,* 17-24.
5. Hayman, CR, and Lanza, C. Sexual assault on women and girls. *American Journal of Obstetrics and Gynecology,* 1971, *109,* 480-486.
6. James, J, Womack, WM, and Strauss, F. Physician reporting of sexual abuse of children. *Journal of the American Medical Association,* Sept. 1978, *240*(11), 1145-1146.
7. McCausland, MP. Sexual development and sexual abuse: emergencies in adolescents. *Pediatric Clinics of North America,* Nov. 1979, *26*(4), 895-901.
8. American Psychiatric Association. *Diagnostic and statistical manual of mental disorders* (3rd ed.). Washington, D.C.: The Association, 1980.

13 FACTITIOUS DISORDERS, MALINGERING, AND OTHER UNUSUAL AILMENTS

With the exception of malingering, most of the disorders considered in this chapter are unusual but important in emergency practice. One vital distinction about most of these disorders needs to be made at the outset. Patients with factitious disorders are controlling their symptoms but are expressing severe emotional conflict with them. This distinction needs to be made, since referral for appropriate psychiatric treatment and support can sometimes lead to dramatic improvement. Malingerers are fairly common in emergency practice but are rarely referred (or rarely comply with the referral) to psychiatrists. They feign illness consciously and purposefully to obtain some obvious gain. Thus the emergency physician is often the primary medical contact with malingerers who want drugs, an excuse for not working, or disability compensation. The initial symptoms and suggested disposition of disorders presented in this chapter are listed in Table 13-1.

FACTITIOUS DISORDERS

Factitious disorders include the chronic factitious disorder with physical symptoms (Munchausen's syndrome), the chronic factitious disorder with mental symptoms (Ganser's syndrome), and malingering. Factitious disorders are "characterized by physical or psychological symptoms that are produced by the individual and are under the individual's control. The sense of voluntary control is subjective, and can only be inferred by an outside observer."[1] *Factitious* means artificial, contrived, unnatural, or false. Therefore the patient with a factitious disorder is consciously simulating or causing symptoms and signs of a physical or psychiatric ailment. The reasons for such symptoms are not immediately apparent to an observer.

Malingering is a condition also characterized by the creation of artificial symptoms or signs. However in the case of malingering, the goal of the mock illness seems quite apparent; a drug user wants an injection of a narcotic; a prisoner wants a few days in the infirmary; an employee wants several days off work. Other common conditions include patients who are seeking disability or trying to evade the police. In emergency

TABLE 13-1. Diagnostic categories of factitious disorders and their disposition

Diagnosis	*Initial Symptoms*	*Disposition of patient*
Chronic factitious disorder with physical symptoms (Munchausen's syndrome)	Simulation of physical symptoms, lying, demands for painful or dangerous procedures, shifting complaints, evidence of prior treatment or surgery, vague and elaborate medical history, medically sophisticated	Psychiatric consultation, minimal procedures
Chronic factitious disorder with psychological symptoms (Ganser's syndrome)	"Approximate" answers, amnesia, usually prisoner or patient facing loss of autonomy (chronic illness, etc.)	Psychotherapy, amobarbital interview
Malingering	Lying, vague history, goal for symptoms, symptoms present only when observed	Confront gently, encourage alternate behavior
Voodoo	Possession state (usually based on religious or cultural beliefs)	Admit to medical or psychiatric hospital for support, encourage family involvement
Tourette's disease	Motor or verbal tic often with coprolalia	Haloperidol (Haldol) and psychotherapy as outpatient
Capgras' syndrome	Patient believes one or more people around him are imposters	Refer for outpatient psychiatric treatment
Folie à deux (shared paranoid disorder)	Psychotic symptoms (usually paranoid delusions) shared by two or more people close to each other	Hospitalize and separate
Cotard's syndrome	Nihilistic delusions (body is empty of organs)	Admit to psychiatric hospital
Autoscopic hallucinations	Patient fleetingly sees own face or body as if in mirror	Treat organic cause, no treatment otherwise
Amok	Wild rage (Malaya)	Restrain, admit
Latah	Mimic words or actions (Malaya)	Admit, psychotherapy
Koro	Penis shrinking (South China, Malaya)	Psychotherapy, evaluation for brain tumor

practice malingering is far more common than factitious disorders, and it is more understandable from a psychological standpoint. The nature, cause, and treatment of factitious disorders are still frought with uncertainty.

Chronic factitious disorders with physical symptoms

Chronic factitious disorders with physical symptoms are perhaps better known as the *Munchausen's syndrome*. Baron von Munchausen was a character who wandered about telling fantastic fabricated anecdotes. The syndrome has been called many other names, including *hospital addiction syndrome* and *hospital hobo syndrome*. This syndrome was first described by Asher in 1951.[2]

Patients with this disorder fabricate the symptoms and signs of a physical illness and present them to physicians in such a believable way that they are able to gain repeated hospital admissions and surgeries.

The hallmark of this disorder is that hospitalization or surgery produces no obvious gain for these patients. This is, therefore, completely different from malingering. Patients with this disorder crave hospitalization for its own sake and are willing to endure the discomfort of painful medical and surgical procedures to gain admission. The psychological gains of hospitalization may include a sense of caring or nurturing and the drama of being a patient.

Some of these patients may seem to crave abdominal surgery. They describe severe abdominal pain and mimic tenderness in that area with guarding and distention. Because they have done this successfully in the past, multiple abdominal scars are usually discovered during the physical examination. The intersection of multiple linear scars produces the "road map" or "gridiron" abdomen commonly described in these patients.

Other patterns of alleged physical illness are seen. Some patients, for instance, have complaints related to hemorrhage. These patients simulate bleeding from various orifices by inserting sharp objects into the area and lacerating the tissue or by swallowing human or animal blood and then appearing to have hematemesis. Patients have been known to insert pins or sharp objects in their urethra to simulate hematuria. They may do the same in other orifices, including the nasal passages, where they inject sharp objects and produce bleeding that can be interpreted as a bloody nose or as hematemesis or hemoptysis. They may also prick their fingers and add blood to urine samples.

A neurological type of syndrome has been described in which patients complain of headaches, seizures, or sensory loss. Some have undergone craniotomy for these factitious symptoms. Some patients emulate cardiovascular diseases with chest pain, shortness of breath, or syncope. Other patients have simulated chest disease like tuberculosis or chronic lung conditions. Dermatoses have also been caused by injecting substances into the skin or by repeated dermal self/excoriation, which is denied. Some highly sophisticated patients (from a medical standpoint) have injected infectious or toxic substances into their veins to produce high fevers. Some patients take oral medications to produce a factitious disorder. An example of such a symptom, which is not rare, is a patient who takes various types of anticoagulants, bruises himself, and comes to the emergency department with a bleeding disorder.

These patients typically wander from one hospital to another and travel widely within the country and abroad seeking hospital admission. Because they may become well known as "phonies" or "fakers" at each hospital they enter, they obtain surgery or admission at many different hospitals. They are often vague and nonspecific about previous hospitalizations and surgeries. They never have any of their medical records with them, and they may have had many aliases.

Another intriguing symptom of this disorder is the patients' dramatic and extremely convincing lying. They tell incredible tales of previous illnesses, complications, and surgeries. They do this in an entertaining and fantastic way, and thus the symptom has been called *pseudologia fantastica*.

Individuals with this disorder also have great familiarity with medical terms and, therefore, may be intimidating. They know medical idioms and hospital procedures and may annoy the physician or nursing staff with the use of medical terminology or with their demanding questions regarding hospital procedures. They often have a background in the medical field and frequently have occupations such as orderlies, nurses, or physicians, or they may be related to a physician or nurse.

These patients are difficult to understand, since they are so willing to submit to painful procedures. This also differentiates them from malingerers who obviously do not want to undergo painful or offensive procedures. These patients are very lonely and have few if any family or friends. They are rarely visited while in the hospital or emergency department. They often have shifting complaints, and over 50% of them have a history of drug abuse, usually analgesics.

If these patients are admitted to a medical or surgical service, they usually become increasingly hostile and belligerent. They anger the staff, make increasing demands, and are generally considered "obnoxious patients." Often before there is a definitive discovery of this syndrome, patients sign out against medical advice. They then begin their trek to a new medical facility.

The evident etiology for this illness often relates to patients' backgrounds, when they were rejected, lonely, or unhappy as children. They receive intense gratification by becoming a patient, often in a dramatic way, in a hospital setting where physicians, nurses, and other staff members care for them. They may also have unconscious wishes to be punished, thus explaining their seeming indifference to painful or dangerous procedures.

Management. The first objective in managing these patients is to distinguish real from factitious pathology. The physician should suspect a factitious disorder, however, when the presentation of symptoms is dramatic and vague and there is evidence of numerous previous surgeries or other medical procedures. The combination of symptoms of medical sophistication, indifference to dangerous procedures (even a demand for them), shifting complaints, evidence of previous treatments, presumptive evidence of drug abuse, and no supporting family or friends should point quickly to this disorder.

These patients are notoriously difficult to treat with psychotherapy or psychoactive medications. Psychiatric consultation is advised, however, if only to make the diagnosis and attempt to engage the patient in a treatment program. The most effective role the psychiatrist can play in the patient's treatment is to organize other physicians in the community to continuously refer this patient back to a psychiatrist whenever they see him. This prevents "doctor hopping," multiple prescriptions, numerous potentially dangerous procedures, and confusion and divisiveness within the medical community. If the patient is always met with referral back to a treating psychiatrist, he is more likely to receive appropriate treatment eventually. The treatment of choice is psychotherapy combined with appropriate major tranquilizers or antidepressants.

The disorder that has been described is intriguing, puzzling, and often results in rejection by physicians. Nonetheless, this disorder incapacitates the patient. Social, family, and employment performance are all seriously impaired. Criminal activity, prison sentences, psychiatric hospitalization, and continued progress toward self-destruction are the milestones that mark the lifetime road of these patients. Therefore a plan of action should be developed by a team of physicians and emergency department staff so that a therapeutic referral can be made when these patients appear.

Factitious disorders with psychological symptoms

Also known as Ganser's syndrome, factitious disorders with psychological symptoms seem to be observed most often in prisoners. The central feature of these disorders is the simulation of psychiatric illness for no apparent gain except that of assuming the patient role. These patients typically give answers that are approximate. That is, the patient, when asked what 3 + 3 is, usually responds with "7" or an approximation of the correct answer. The theory behind this unusual symptom is that the patient is under a great deal of stress, is mimicking mental illness at an unconscious level, and, therefore, is not malingering.

The patient may show symptoms and signs that suggest both organic mental disorder and functional psychosis. These symptoms include memory loss, impaired ability to calculate, hallucinations, and delusions. It is clear that the individual understands what is asked of him and is aware of the sense of the questions. The approximate answer, however, makes the patient appear psychiatrically impaired. It becomes apparent that the patient is presenting symptoms based on his own impression of what psychiatric illness should be. The patient is usually below average in intellectual ability or comes from a severely disadvantaged cultural or educational background.

These symptoms often occur in patients who are in a difficult situation. The most common appearance occurs in patients who are in jail or in some way feeling a loss of autonomy. This may occur in patients with chronic medical problems who are facing increasing physical impairment.

Management. These patients usually recover within days or weeks. The treatment can be carried out in the emergency department to speed the recovery and might include an intravenous amobarbital injection with a therapeutic interview. This can be accomplished by the emergency department staff or by a consulting psychiatrist. These patients often benefit from psychiatric or medical hospitalization where they can be treated in a protective and secure environment. When discharged, they should have definite psychiatric referral for follow-up, which has been found to be beneficial.

Whether or not the emergency physician recognizes this particular syndrome is probably not critical to the patient's emergency management. The fundamental rules of eliminating organic mental illness in the emergency department and referring appropriate patients with functional psychiatric illness to a psychiatrist continue to hold true in the management of these patients.

MALINGERING

Malingering is a particularly common problem in emergency medicine. The malingerer is distinguished from the patient with factitious disorders by the observation that the malingerer has the chance of fairly obvious gain if taken seriously.

CASE EXAMPLE 1

A 24-year-old man complained of pain caused by a kidney stone. The patient claimed that he had experienced ureteral stones off and on for several years and that renal stones ''ran in the family.'' He complained of excruciating back, flank, and inguinal pain, and he requested narcotics for relief. The patient was asked to produce a urine sample. When he thought he was unobserved, he picked a blood-soaked alcohol swab from the wastebasket and squeezed a few drops of blood into the urine specimen. The urinalysis demonstrated hemoglobin and red cells. The patient continued to writhe about begging for narcotics. An intravenous pyelogram was suggested, but he refused the procedure, claiming that he was ''allergic to the dye.''

When the patient was confronted with the observation that he had falsified his urinalysis, he denied it and became angry, saying that doctors ''never help anyone who really needs it.'' He refused psychiatric consultation and stormed out of the department.

CASE EXAMPLE 2

A 38-year-old city worker came to the emergency department with the complaint that he had strained his back while loading heavy boxes onto a truck. His physical examination revealed only slightly limited range of back motion, minimal paraspinous spasm, and a normal neurological examination. The patient readily accepted an excuse from work for 1 week and promised to use a heating pad and take aspirin for the pain. He was referred to an orthopedic surgeon for further evaluation.

Both of these cases represent extremely common situations in emergency medicine. One patient requests narcotics for feigned pain; the other requests compensated time off work (paid sick leave) and possibly a future disability status. The goals of the malingerer in each case are fairly obvious and represent external gain, rather than the solution or fulfillment of an intrapsychic conflict or need.

The malingerer is generally reluctant to accept extensive, possibly painful, physical testing or surgery. The patient may undergo minimal pain, however, if the goal seems fairly sure of being met.

The diagnosis of malingering can only be confirmed by the patient's own confession. He would have to state that the symptoms were faked to get drugs or to be excused from work. Such a confession is not likely to come from the patient.

The malingerer may give an inconsistent or unlikely history. The location, radiation, and nature of pain complaints, for instance, may be atypical enough to arouse suspicion. Even more suspicious, perhaps, is the patient's description of previous medical treatments and hospitalizations. The malingerer is characteristically vague about these details and may list his previous physician as being out of state, out of practice, or no longer alive. He may enlist the assistance of one or several accomplices.

CASE EXAMPLE 3

A 26-year-old man claimed to have a history of severe lumbosacral disc disease, treated effectively by an out-of-state physician with relatively high doses of hydromorphone (Dilaudid). The patient requested "just 1 or 2 days worth of medication" until he could return to his home state to see his physician. The emergency physician asked for the name and city of the patient's alleged physician. The information operator for the city given reported that the physician in question was a veterinarian. The emergency physician later received a call supposedly from the physician in question who recommended narcotics for his patient. Further questioning about the pathophysiology of the disease and the details of previous diagnostic tests revealed that the alleged physician was an imposter. When confronted with the information obtained from the operator, the bogus physician promptly hung up the telephone. The patient had also disappeared by this time.

Medical personnel in military and prison environments have encountered malingerers throughout the ages, probably more than other physicians. In a military setting, one of the major objectives of the malingerer is to escape unpleasant work or front-line combat or to attempt to be discharged from the service. Care must be taken to differentiate the malingerer from the patient suffering from a posttraumatic stress syndrome, conversion disorder, or severe depression who focuses on physical symptoms.

The objective of the prisoner is often hard to discern. It may be that he wants a few days in the infirmary or hospital; he may want to obtain drugs, or he may be trying to substantiate a claim for a later suit against the prison or its officials. He may be seeking placement in a hospital setting from which he feels escape would be more likely.

The emergency department may be fertile ground for a malingerer. The interactions are expected to be episodic; the patient has a reasonable hope of seeing a different physician on each visit (in teaching hospitals he expects to see a different house officer on each occasion). The necessity of the emergency staff to keep patients moving creates pressure to give in to the demand for drugs or time away from work. This results in the discharge of a highly satisfied patient but one who has abused the medical system.

UNUSUAL DISORDERS PRODUCING PECULIAR SYMPTOMS

Voodoo

Voodoo and other "possession states" are often a result of cultural and religious beliefs. This is sometimes called *root work* in the North American black ghetto. Patients with such beliefs may develop symptoms that seem to the emergency department to be organic or psychological. Patients may appear to have seizures after being whipped to a frenzy in a meeting with a "witch doctor." These patients should not be dismissed easily. They may believe that they are going to die; there have been documented cases in which patients become withdrawn, stop eating and drinking, and go on to die, despite their apparently satisfactory physical health.

Patients suffering from such possession states should probably be admitted to a medical or psychiatric ward and observed for a few days. If they believe that they will die on a certain date, it is wise to hospitalize them before this date and nurture them through it. The cause of death in some of these patients is speculative but has been related to increased vagal tone (causing cardiovascular depression), increased epinephrine (producing arrhythmias), dehydration, and malnutrition. A differential diagnosis should include an examination for evidence of psychosis or an organic cause for such mental symptoms.

Tourette's disease

Tourette's disease was first described in 1885 by Gilles de la Tourette. The disease usually begins in childhood between the ages of 3 and 12 years. The patient has multiple or single motor tics. He may shrug his shoulders, stick out his tongue, grimace in some other way, or appear to be doing a brief dance step. These motions usually require some coordination. They may be associated in over 50% of the cases with coprolalia or sudden and loud utterances of obscene or vulgar language. The patient is embarrassed, sometimes desperately so, about his symptom. He may also at times repeat what the examiner or other persons say (echolalia). The patient may sometimes bark like a dog.

The etiology of this disorder is unclear but probably organic. It occurs three times as often in men as in women. The disorder causes intense psychological suffering in the patient and often results in complete social isolation. He is sometimes overly protected by his family and may not be brought to a physician's attention until the disease has completely incapacitated him. This illness should be thought of when the patient has any unusual motor tic or sudden and apparently inappropriate use of obscene or foul language. A level of suspicion should be maintained regarding children who suffer any motor or verbal tic. These patients often find ways of concealing their tics by incorporating them into other elaborate gestures.

The drug treatment of choice for Tourette's disease is haloperidol in varying dosages. The medication is best administered in conjunction with a program of psychotherapy to help the patient readjust to his improved medical condition and discuss his feelings about his illness. Haloperidol can be used in dosages from 5 to 200 mg per day for this condition and needs to be titrated over a period of weeks or months. Patients are dramatically helped in a large percentage of cases with this medication.

The important differential diagnoses in the symptom with such a motor or verbal tic are cerebral-vascular accident, postencephalitic disorder, Huntington's chorea, Wilson's disease, or Sydenham's chorea. Usually, however, in these illnesses coprolalia, the sudden use of loud and inappropriately foul language, does not occur. Once these illnesses have been ruled out, referral to a psychiatrist or neurologist for appropriate follow-up care is important. Generally patients are relieved to find that the illness is fairly common and treatable, often with dramatically good results.

Capgras' syndrome

The Capgras' syndrome is uncommon and has a fascinating symptom. The patient with this syndrome believes that other people in his environment are not who they claim to be but instead are doubles or imposters. This patient shows no intellectual impairment and is oriented. He usually believes that his spouse, family member, friend, or neighbor has been replaced by a double or impostor. He may believe this about one or several people.

This complaint is usually a symptom and not a syndrome. That is, it generally occurs as a symptom of another psychosis. If the patient is examined carefully and repeatedly over a period of time, he usually ends up with a primary diagnosis of a bipolar affective disorder (manic-depressive illness) or a schizophrenic disorder. Therefore referral for appropriate psychiatric follow-up would be important.

Folie à deux syndrome

Folie à deux is an unusual syndrome that occasionally is seen in an emergency department and is otherwise known as a shared paranoid disorder. Patients with this symptom complex show psychotic signs that are shared by one or more people living with the patient. Therefore two or three people may have the same auditory or visual hallucination or believe the same delusional system, such as having taken a trip on a spaceship together, their house being watched by the Central Intelligence Agency or some other group, or any other elaborate paranoid system.

The interesting thing about this syndrome is that one of the two or more patients has a psychosis, and the other is in such need of that relationship that he shares the psychosis. The treatment is to admit these patients to a psychiatric unit, separating the psychotic from the nonpsychotic patient who is usually the more passive one. Generally the more passive and nonpsychotic patient recovers within a few days or weeks. The psychotic patient is treated in a traditional manner with appropriate medications and supportive therapy.

Cotard's syndrome

Cotard's syndrome involves symptoms that are considered nihilistic delusions. The patient believes that not only does he have no energy and feels fatigued, but he has no heart or internal organs, and he may believe that time has stopped. Because the patient frequently has these delusional symptoms, it is common for him to be brought first to the emergency department. Such unusual and bizarre symptoms require a differential diagnosis separating these patients from those with schizophrenic disorder or severe psychotic depression. The patient should be referred for appropriate psychiatric treatment and follow-up care. This syndrome may also occur in early presenile and senile dementias. These symptoms may be seen in patients with delirium or acute organic brain syndrome. Therefore it is important to rule out an underlying central nervous system disorder as a cause of these symptoms.

Autoscopic hallucinations

Autoscopic hallucinations are unusual symptoms that involve the patient's face or whole body appearing in front of him as though he were looking in the mirror. These hallucinations may last from seconds to minutes and usually mimic the patient's own movements. These symptoms are generally brief, are fleeting, and should be differentiated from symptoms of schizophrenia. A differential diagnosis is easily accomplished by a mental status examination, ruling out schizophrenia. The patient who has a vivid imagination but no other psychiatric disorder often has such symptoms and can be reassured and sent home. No other psychiatric or follow-up treatment is necessary unless the symptoms change or progress.

Amok, Koro, Latah

There are some dramatic psychiatric symptoms in pure cultures. Amok occurs primarily in Malaya. This syndrome appears when the patient has an outburst or goes into a wild rage, often harming or killing others around him in a rampage through his village. Usually this patient is psychotic and must be physically restrained. Latah also occurs in Malaya and involves the patient mimicking the words or actions of others around him. He responds to psychotherapy and tranquilizers.

Koro occurs in South China and Malaya. The patient fears that his penis will shrink into his body, and at that point he will die. He may have bound his penis with cord or ribbon and thus must be differentiated from the patient with sexual fetishes or deviations.

Another differential diagnosis that becomes important in this syndrome is to rule out amphetamine abuse or a brain tumor, which can sometimes cause such symptoms. Therefore a workup for a central nervous system disease with such bizarre symptoms would be helpful.

SUMMARY

The factitious disorders (Munchausen's and Ganser's syndromes) are puzzling to most physicians. Common sense dictates that most people want to enjoy good health, and it seems perverse that some feign illness to enter the hospital. When genuine illness is ruled out, the management of the factitious disorders is best left to the psychiatrist, even though the results of such treatment may be less than optimal.

The malingerer, by contrast, feigns illness for goals that are usually quite evident. The emergency physician can only refer these patients for further evaluation and be as sparing as possible in prescribing narcotics or offering work excuses.

REFERENCES

1. American Psychiatric Association. *Diagnostic and statistical manual of mental disorders* (3rd ed.). Washington, D.C.: The Association, 1980.
2. Asher, R.. Munchausen's syndrome. *Lancet,* 1951, *1,* 339.

14 PERSONALITY DISORDERS

Personality is the sum of behavioral traits, attitudes, habits, and characteristics that determines the way the patient interacts with other people and the environment. These traits usually endure throughout the person's lifetime. When the personality interferes with the patient's social or economic functioning or causes the patient persistent discomfort, a personality disorder is probably present. Minor variations of personality are normal characteristics that make each individual unique and distinguish one person from another.

All emergency physicians encounter patients with personality disorder. As the interaction with the patient proceeds, an early clue surfaces when the physician begins to feel intuitively that there is something not quite right about the patient's personality. A vague dislike of the person may evolve as the examination proceeds; the physician may become unusually involved in the patient's story or emotionally aroused to a vivacious, attractive, yet seemingly helpless patient. Such intuitive, nonverbal, "gut" reactions are generally quite valid; the physician has probably never seen the patient before and thus has had no opportunity to have formed a previous opinion about the patient. Rather the physician reacts de novo to the person's characteristics, way of thinking, and behavior patterns.

Personality disorders are important to the emergency physician because patients with these disorders appear rather frequently in that department. Some reports have estimated that personality disorders are present in 11% of the general population. Personality disorders are perhaps more commonly diagnosed in certain populations that find their medical care in emergency departments, such as lower socioeconomic groups, institutionalized persons, and prison inmates.

Two particular hazards of emergency evaluation of personality disorders deserve early emphasis: diagnosis of personality disorders is difficult in the compressed, tense atmosphere of an emergency assessment, and patients with previously diagnosed personality disorders may develop new causes of abnormal behavior (i.e., organic mental disorders caused by hypoglycemia, drug abuse, or encephalopathy) that may be overlooked because a personality disturbance has been previously diagnosed.

The emergency department is an environment where the need for a rapid diagnosis and assessment nearly always precludes prolonged interviews or formal psychological testing. The physician who develops a general idea of the patient's personality type may

TABLE 14-1. Clusters of behavioral characteristics that suggest various groups of personality disorder diagnoses

Behavior	*Personality disorder group*
Eccentric, odd, isolated, withdrawn, suspicious, inhibited, no friends, overly sensitive	Paranoid Schizoid Schizotypal
Emotional, dramatic, angry, seductive, impulsive	Antisocial Histrionic Borderline Narcissistic
Anxious, fearful, "nervous," cautious	Dependent Avoidant Compulsive Passive-aggressive

suspect one of various disorders based on some obvious behavioral characteristics, as shown in Table 14-1. It is often difficult, however, to precisely diagnose specific personality disorders. The patient may immediately seem unusually odd, inappropriately dramatic, or intensely anxious, for instance. Fortunately it is rarely, if ever, necessary for the emergency physician to make such an exact diagnosis of personality disorders to proceed with emergency management of the patient.

The second pitfall, missing a serious medical condition or acute psychosis superimposed on a previous personality disorder, is a more important concern for the emergency physician. As stressed repeatedly, organic mental disorders or acute psychoses require careful evaluation and treatment. A review of previous emergency department and/or psychiatric records helps the physician sort out the patient's chronic baseline mental status and personality from superimposed acute organic or functional illness. When psychotic features (delusions, hallucinations, ideas of reference, loose association, autism) are discovered in the patient, hospitalization provides the time required for a full evaluation.

It is usually only necessary to recognize this patient in the emergency department and interact with him accordingly. Unless the patient with a personality disorder experiences extreme psychological pain, he usually does not request psychiatric help. He is typically unaware of the problems caused by his behavior and is rather comfortable with his own personality. Psychotherapy, therefore, is usually of little help (unless the patient seeks it), and antipsychotic or antianxiety agents have no place in his management.

The physician and emergency staff, however, should be much more comfortable dealing with the patient once the specific type of disorder is determined. As a general rule, it should be sufficient to manage the patient's medical problem and merely make a mental note of the personality disorder.

TYPES OF PERSONALITY DISORDERS

Various specific personality disorders exist, and beginning with the more common types of disorders seen in emergency patients, the following list is presented:

Antisocial
Borderline
Histrionic
Compulsive
Passive-aggressive
Dependent
Avoidant
Schizoid
Schizotypal
Paranoid
Narcissistic

Antisocial personality disorder

In at least one study antisocial personality was the most common personality disorder seen in emergency patients in an inner-city hospital.[1] The disorder was found more often in the nighttime patient population than in those requesting care during the day. When evaluated according to strict research criteria, 17% of nighttime patients (midnight to 8 o'clock AM) had a diagnosis of antisocial personality, whereas 4% of daytime patients met the criteria for the diagnosis.

The diagnosis requires that the patient be at least 18 years of age and that the antisocial behavior developed *before age 15*. Antisocial acts or behavior for the under-15-year age group include truancy, expulsion or suspension from school, delinquency, running away from home, persistent lying, repeated casual sexual intercourse, repeated drunkenness, repeated substance abuse, theft, vandalism, poor school grades, initiation of fights, and general disregard for home and school rules.[2] Other childhood symptoms can include sexual deviation, recklessness, lack of guilt, enuresis, slovenly appearance, impulsivity, bad companions, and general incorrigibility.[3] The three most common symptoms before age 15, easily queried as a screening device, include truancy, fire setting, and shoplifting.

After the age of 15, antisocial persons typically have just as much trouble with authority as they did during childhood and adolescence. Adults with this disorder have poor work records; they are frequently late or absent, have a record of numerous firings, and have wandered from job to job. If they have a military service record, they may have suffered disciplinary actions, been absent without leave, spent time in a military prison, or been dishonorably discharged.

It is likely that these persons may spend time in prison. Their offenses can include theft, prostitution, drug dealing or use, assault, and battery. A hallmark is that these patients rarely experience guilt or remorse for their crimes.

Antisocial patients' marital and family lives are bound to be stormy. The families

DIAGNOSTIC CRITERIA FOR ANTISOCIAL PERSONALITY DISORDER

A. Current age at least 18.
B. Onset before age 15 as indicated by a history of three or more of the following before that age:
   1. Truancy (positive if it amounted to at least 5 days per year for at least 2 years, not including the last year of school)
   2. Expulsion or suspension from school for misbehavior
   3. Delinquency (arrested or referred to juvenile court because of behavior)
   4. Running away from home overnight at least twice while living in parental or parental surrogate home
   5. Persistent lying
   6. Repeated sexual intercourse in a casual relationship
   7. Repeated drunkenness or substance abuse
   8. Thefts
   9. Vandalism
   10. School grades markedly below expectations in relation to estimated or known IQ (may have resulted in repeating a year)
   11. Chronic violations of rules at home and/or at school (other than truancy)
   12. Initiation of fights
C. At least four of the following manifestations of the disorder since age 18:
   1. Inability to sustain consistent work behavior, as indicated by any of the following: *(a)* too frequent job changes (e.g., three or more jobs in 5 years not accounted for by nature of job or economic or seasonal fluctuation), *(b)* significant unemployment (e.g., 6 months or more in 5 years when expected to work), *(c)* serious absenteeism from work (e.g., average 3 days or more of lateness or absence per month, *(d)* walking off several jobs without other jobs in site (Note: similar behavior in an academic setting during the last few years of school may substitute for this criterion in individuals who by reason of their age or circumstances have not had an opportunity to demonstrate occupational adjustment)
   2. Lack of ability to function as a responsible parent as evidenced by one or more of the following: *(a)* child's malnutrition, *(b)* child's illness resulting from lack of minimal hygiene standards, *(c)* failure to obtain medical care for a repeated defaulting on debts, failure to provide child support, seriously ill child, *(d)* child's dependence on neighbors or nonresident relatives for food or shelter, *(e)* failure to arrange for a caretaker for a child under six when parent is away from home, *(f)* repeated squandering, on personal items, of money required for household necessities
   3. Failure to accept social norms with respect to lawful behavior, as indicated by any of the following: repeated thefts, illegal occupation (pimping, prostitution, fencing, selling drugs), multiple arrests, a felony conviction
   4. Inability to maintain enduring attachment to a sexual partner as indicated by two or more divorces and/or separations (whether legally married or not), desertion of spouse, promiscuity (ten or more sexual partners within 1 year)

Continued.

DIAGNOSTIC CRITERIA FOR ANTISOCIAL PERSONALITY DISORDER—cont'd

5. Irritability and aggressiveness as indicated by repeated physical fights or assault (not required by one's job or to defend someone or oneself), including spouse or child beating
6. Failure to honor financial obligations, as indicated by failure to support other dependents on a regular basis
7. Failure to plan ahead, or impulsivity, as indicated by traveling from place to place without a prearranged job or clear goal for the period of travel or clear idea about when the travel would terminate, or lack of a fixed address for a month or more
8. Disregard for the truth as indicated by repeated lying, use of aliases, "conning" others for personal profit
9. Recklessness, as indicated by driving while intoxicated or recurrent speeding

D. A pattern of continuous antisocial behavior in which the rights of others are violated, with no intervening period of at least 5 years without antisocial behavior between age 15 and the present time (except when the individual was bedridden or confined in a hospital or penal institution).

E. Antisocial behavior is not due to either Severe Mental Retardation, Schizophrenia, or manic episodes.

From American Psychiatric Association. *Diagnostic and statistical manual of mental disorders* (3rd ed.). Washington, D.C.: The Association, 1980, p. 320-321.

of these persons are torn apart by frequent domestic fights, separation and divorce, and general family neglect. Children of these individuals are likely to receive poor medical care and nutrition. They experience repeated episodes of desertion by the parent. The personality disorder may be more frequent among patients whose biological fathers had antisocial personality disorder and in those raised in an environment of an antisocial personality.

These patients lack the ability to form meaningful interpersonal relationships. Sexual promiscuity and casual relations create insurmountable problems in their marriages. A past spouse may have deserted, and two or more divorces or separations form part of the diagnostic criteria for the diagnosis. These patients typically cannot manage their finances competently. Their poor work records inevitably place them in financial "hot water." They have unpaid debts, broken financial obligations, or economic dependency on someone else.

Alcohol and substance abuse are common concomitant disorders with antisocial personality. The patient typically uses drugs or alcohol to excess as part of his overall reckless and impulsive behavior. The patient enters the emergency environment for a variety of reasons linked to his antisocial behavior. Such behavior includes public intoxication, bar fights, struggles with police after an arrest, or feigning illness to obtain drugs.

CASE EXAMPLE 1

A 28-year-old divorced unemployed man was brought to the emergency department after fighting the police in a local bar. The arresting officers brought him in for a medical evaluation of injuries before taking him to jail. The intoxicated patient had sustained multiple contusions over the face and body and had a 3 cm laceration of the parietal scalp. The remainder of the examination was unremarkable. The patient alternatively rambled on about police brutality and then taunted the arresting officers with verbal abuse.

Initially the patient refused a suture repair of the scalp wound. Eventually, however, he became more calm and agreed to sutures. While the wound was being sutured, the physician tried to question him about his employment. At first the patient seemed to welcome the chance to talk about himself and related a story of a few short-lived jobs over the past several years with long intervals of unemployment. He said he made his money by playing pool and from his "old lady" who had a steady job. He then became quiet, grabbed the sterile drapes, and attempted to get off the cart. The repair was hastily completed, while the police held him down. The patient was sent off to jail, and the staff seemed quite relieved to have him leave the department.

The case illustrates several points. One is that the patient is likely to be brought in by a law enforcement official, family member, or friend, rather than coming in alone. Another important point is that it is often extremely difficult to distinguish alcohol abuse from antisocial personality, and both disorders are often present simultaneously, as they were in the patient just discussed. A final point is that making the diagnosis of antisocial personality is generally not a primary goal of the evaluation because psychiatric treatment is of so little value in these cases.

Similar patients are undoubtedly discharged regularly from the emergency department. Patients may be brought in by friends, family, or police for the evaluation and repair of traumatic injuries. Some of these patients merely want drugs and typically feign an illness that produces a great deal of pain for which there are few objective physical signs and for which immediate surgery is not generally required. Ureterolithiasis (kidney stones) in men and migraine headaches in women seem to be the most common complaints. In these cases patients who meet the criteria for antisocial personality carry the additional diagnosis of malingering. The physician should be reluctant to prescribe outpatient narcotics for these patients. A general emergency department guideline about not prescribing any outpatient narcotics unless there is objective evidence of disease and an absolute departmental rule that no more than a 48-hour supply of narcotics may be prescribed at one time help limit the yield of narcotic medications patients obtain with these ploys.

Most antisocial personalities do not benefit from psychiatric treatment. This simple observation is perhaps the most useful information the emergency physician can have. Patients with antisocial personality, almost by definition, see no wrong in what they do and have established a lifelong pattern of behavior that is almost impossible to change. They are comfortable with their personality; it defines them as a person. The physician need not feel guilty, therefore, about sending such a patient out with the police or back to his usual environment without psychiatric intervention. The most the emergency physician could be expected to do is recommend psychiatric counseling to the patient for some of the problems he seems to be having.

The important differential diagnosis for these patients includes organic mental disorder, acute mania, drug or alcohol abuse, and schizophrenia. A chronic organic mental disorder can manifest as poor judgment and impulse control. A mental status examination, vital sign determination, and brief physical evaluation, along with the history of the ailment, should allow the physician to distinguish between the two disorders. Acute mania produces the impulsive activity, sexual promiscuity, and irritability characteristic of antisocial personality. The early history (before 15 years of age) of antisocial behavior signifies a personality disorder; the onset in adult life and the presence of psychosis, if any, indicate that mania is the correct diagnosis.

Substance abuse is perhaps the most common concomitant diagnosis in these cases. When alcohol or drug abuse develops earlier in the patient's life than antisocial behavior, it can be considered the primary diagnosis, whereas antisocial behavior is considered secondary. Schizophrenia can result in antisocial behavior. The presence of a psychotic episode, complete with delusions and hallucinations, a previous mental hospitalization, or earlier response to antipsychotic medications points toward schizophrenia as the primary diagnosis.

Borderline personality disorder

Borderline personality disorder is presented here so that the emergency physician may become familiar with the term, but not so that the condition can be diagnosed in the emergency department. The term *borderline* reflects early thinking that these patients tread along the border of schizophrenia. The predominant feature of borderline personality includes impulsivity, unstable interpersonal relationships, inappropriate intense anger, identity disturbance, frequent dramatic mood shifts, self-damaging acts, and chronic feelings of emptiness or boredom.

Borderline personalities have been described as follows:

> ". . .today's borderlines are still known by their impulsivity, drastic swings from love to hate and irrationality bordering on madness. . . Borderlines are extremists who split the world into exaggerated dichotomies of good and evil, black and white. Infants emotionally, they cannot tolerate ambiguity; nothing is neutral, everything is personal. A middle ground does not exist. These are patients who by biologic flaw or by developmental bad luck have never reconciled the positive and negative extremes of mental life. Not merely neurotic yet not quite psychotic, but somewhere on the border the borderlines lie."[4]

The emotional instability of the borderline personality may be the first clue the emergency physician notices. The patient may suddenly display anger of unusual inten-

FEATURES OF BORDERLINE PERSONALITY DISORDER

- *Impulsivity or unpredictability* in at least two areas that are self-destructive, such as money, sex, gambling, drugs, shoplifting, overeating, or physical self-damage
- A pattern of *unstable and intense interpersonal relations,* fraught with rapid shifts in attitude, idealization, devaluation, or manipulative exploitation of others
- Inappropriate, frequently uncontrolled, or extremely *intense anger*
- *Disturbed identity,* manifested by uncertainty about personal image, gender identity, goals, values, or loyalties, or even by transient confusion in the fundamental sense of the self
- *Unstable mood,* with marked shifts from a normal to a depressed, anxious, or irritable mood, usually lasting for a few hours and only rarely for more than a few days
- *Intolerance to being alone,* with frantic efforts to avoid being alone or severe depression and emptiness when alone
- *Physical self-damage,* such as suicidal gestures, self-mutilation, recurrent accidents, or fighting
- Chronic feelings of *emptiness or boredom*

From Groves, J.E. Current concepts in psychiatry: borderline personality disorder. *New England Journal of Medicine,* July 1981, *305*(5) 259-262. By permission.

sity about a seemingly innocuous statement or trivial incident. Additional history may reveal that these outbursts are frequent and may have been responsible for the destruction of the patient's family life or for unstable social relationships.

Self-destructive acts may be another feature of the disorder that brings the patient to the physician's attention. The patient may make suicidal gestures or mutilate himself (the "slasher"). Sometimes the patient creates an accident causing self-damage. Appropriate treatment for such an individual entails medical management of the injury and perhaps psychiatric referral.

We say "perhaps" because treatment for the disorder is so unsatisfactory. Borderline personality does not respond to any specific medication, and psychotherapy requires great effort, time, and persistence. At present psychiatric treatment helps maintain the patient, rather than attempting to produce a dramatic change in behavior.

Like other patients with personality disorders, the first clue to the borderline personality disorder for the busy emergency physician may be that the patient rapidly generates fairly intense emotion (usually anger) within the physician. Because the patient is so emotionally labile and manipulative, the physician may begin to dislike him, even while performing a simple procedure like suturing a wrist slash. This early clue may be ignored as the physician proceeds with the repair, or it can be followed with a series of questions to the patient and family about his emotional history and personality. For the experienced physician who easily sutures a laceration, even such brief probes may be enough to suggest a disorder like borderline personality.

The physician or staff need not necessarily "like" all emergency patients, or feel guilt when warm empathic feelings do not appear. Rather than feel intense urges or guilt, however, the physician and staff must realize that the patient with borderline or antisocial personality has a physical or emotional complaint like other people and may also have a personality disorder so severe that practically *no one* likes him. Usually the most important aspect or case for any patient is not how the staff feels about him but how the patient *perceives* they feel.[5] The physician or nurse who feels aversion to the patient should begin channeling professional energies into setting limits on the patient's behavior or focusing on a personality disorder that may have features amenable to treatment.

Histrionic personality disorder

The histrionic personality is probably familiar to emergency physicians. The patient is typically a dramatic, intense, vain, and often seductive woman. In men the syndrome has been most often diagnosed in homosexuals. When the emergency physician is male and the patient female, the first intuition to the disorder may be one of sexual attraction to a colorful, attractive, yet helpless person. An alternate clue surfaces when the physician begins to feel annoyed or angered by the patient's incessant demands for attention or continuing reassurance.

These patients are typically lively and theatrical. They crave notice and call medical attention to themselves because they portray themselves as "helpless victims." They frequently complain of poor health with nonspecific problems like weakness, dizziness, or headache. Sometimes the role-playing is so overt that they seem to be a caricature of a textbook hysteric. Their gestures are flamboyant; they talk incessantly, flutter their eyelids, and make suggestive overtures to the physician.

The male counterpart of the disorder seems to be diagnosed most frequently in homosexuals or in promiscuous males who develop shallow, superficial sexual relationships with men or women.

The diagnosis rests on two fundamental characteristics: (1) behavior that is overly dramatic and intensely expressed and (2) chronic disturbances in interpersonal relationships. The dramatic behavior includes angry, irrational outbursts, restlessness, craving for excitement, flamboyant dress in the latest fad fashions, overreaction to minor events, and incessant drawing of attention to oneself. The disturbances in interpersonal relationships create a weak marriage; thus the patient is typically unmarried or has been divorced at least once. The interpersonal relationships are perceived by others as superficial, shallow, and lacking genuine feeling or commitment because the patient is so vain and self-centered; others tend to be treated off-handedly or inconsiderately. These patients are vain, demanding, and manipulative, yet portray themselves as dependent and helpless.

The management of these patients as well as other individuals with nonspecific com-

DIAGNOSTIC CRITERIA FOR HISTRIONIC PERSONALITY DISORDER

The following are characteristic of the individual's current and long-term functioning, are not limited to episodes of illness, and cause either significant impairment in social or occupational functioning or subjective distress.

A. Behavior that is overly dramatic, reactive, and intensely expressed, as indicated by at least three of the following:
   1. Self-dramatization, e.g., exaggerated expression of emotions
   2. Incessant drawing of attention to oneself
   3. Craving for activity and excitement
   4. Overreaction to minor events
   5. Irrational, angry outbursts or tantrums

B. Characteristic disturbances in interpersonal relationships as indicated by at least two of the following:
   1. Perceived by others as shallow and lacking genuineness, even if superficially warm and charming
   2. Egocentric, self-indulgent, and inconsiderate of others
   3. Vain and demanding
   4. Dependent, helpless, constantly seeking reassurance
   5. Prone to manipulative suicidal threats, gestures, or attempts

From American Psychiatric Association. *Diagnostic and statistical manual of mental disorders* (3rd ed.). Washington, D.C.: The Association, 1980, p. 315.

plaints that seem to be psychiatric or supratentorial in origin is to proceed in the early stages as if the complaint is actually organic. A description of the complaint, brief medical history, pertinent physical examination, and referral or medical follow-up may be all that is required. Psychiatric referral is generally necessary if the patient asks for psychiatric help or appears so impaired that the disorder obviously interferes greatly with daily functioning. As with other personality disorders, these patients are more or less comfortable with their personality and, therefore, fairly resistant to change.

When psychiatric treatment is indicated, psychotherapy takes alternate routes depending on the severity of the symptoms and the insight of the patient. The healthier patient may respond well to insight-oriented psychotherapy and group therapy (including family therapy), whereas the more primitive hysteric responds better to goal-limited supportive psychotherapy.[6] The major mistake made with the very difficult patient is that medical personnel make the diagnosis of "hysteric" and dismiss him. The patient needs a careful workup. If this is negative, gentle explanations linking stress to physical symptoms (muscle spasm, etc.) may open the door to pulling together emotional pain and physical symptoms. Referral to a psychiatrist may be broached then, or later, when the patient reappears.

Compulsive personality disorder

Compulsive personality disorder creates an individual whose world is small, cold, and frustrating. These individuals tend to be perfectionists; they are preoccupied with small tasks that must be completed exactly. Their relationships are unemotional and, they tend to be formal, stiff, self-righteous, and demanding that others conform to their ways. Perhaps because it is difficult to achieve perfection and complete control over the actions of someone else, these patients eventually become anxious or depressed and seek professional attention.

Patients with compulsive personality disorders can be referred to a psychiatrist, but the benefit of psychotherapy may be quite small; the therapist who tries to change old, ingrained, comfortable habits that partially define the person, generates a high level of patient anxiety and typically meets considerable resistance to change.

Patients with a compulsive personality disorder often come to the emergency department or to physicians' offices with trivial complaints. They are extremely concerned about a bump on the penis or a normal bone protrusion of the foot or hip. They seem quite anxious and tense and continue to ask minute questions, seeking detailed underlying anatomical reasons for their problems. This form of questioning may persist even after a reasonable explanation has been given.

When the patient persists in complaining, despite normal reassurance, and if he continues to exhibit the characteristics just mentioned, the physician may want to switch the line of approach. At this point it may be helpful to ask the patient whether or not he has been under stress recently. Asking about his marriage, his job, or recent changes in his life may provide a helpful hint that he is feeling stressed. He may respond with his compulsive focusing on medical complaints. Linking the fact that he is presently under stress with his extreme concern about his physical condition may be helpful to the patient. This may cause an alleviation of his symptom and begin to open the door to talking about psychological issues rather than medical ones.

Passive-aggressive personality disorder

The passive-aggressive personality disorder is characterized by the patient's passive resistance to compliance with demands made in his business, social, and personal life. The emergency physician may encounter a patient with this disorder who is not at all compliant with his medical regimen. The patient with renal failure who ignores a prescribed diet, the hypertensive individual who does not take the prescribed medication, or the diabetic who does not take insulin properly may appear in the emergency department with exacerbation of his disease. Although passive-aggressive personality certainly cannot be diagnosed in all noncompliant patients (since at least one third of all patients are noncompliant), it may be a cause in some cases.

The hallmark of the passive-aggressive personality disorder is a "pouting" resistance. The patient tends to make everyone else feel responsible for his problems. He may portray himself as a martyr. He may be quite whiney and demanding and yet not responsive to others' helpful suggestions. Since this dominant theme of resistance to the requests or helpful advice of others is all pervasive, the patient suffers significant impairment in functioning in his business and family life. He is quite resistant to being referred to a psychiatrist or mental health facility, and the results of psychiatric treatment are poor.

The best way of communicating with these patients is to respond to their questions or demands with simple and straightforward answers. Repeating these answers, despite various forms of questions, is helpful. This does not allow the patient to distort or twist the meaning of any advice given and tends to cut down on the number of transactions that can occur between the physician and patient.

Dependent personality disorder

The dependent personality has the following three characteristics:

1. He lets someone else assume responsibility for major portions of his life (e.g., where to live, what kind of job to have, who his friends are).
2. He subordinates his own needs to those of the supporting person (e.g., a spouse may tolerate major forms of abuse to remain married).
3. He lacks self-confidence.

Some of these characteristics are seen in many individuals. The condition becomes a personality disorder only when it causes the patient enough pain to want to change or when the condition interferes in a major way with the patient's functioning.

The emergency physician may encounter female patients who are victims of repeated physical abuse by a husband or boyfriend. Sometimes these patients return several times with the same black eyes, contusions, abrasions, and even facial fractures. Unless they are making a supreme effort to preserve a family life for their children, they may be suffering from dependent personality disorder.

When these patients lose the individual or group on whom they are dependent, they become severely depressed. In these cases symptoms of depression or a suicide attempt may bring them to the emergency physician's attention. The differential diagnosis includes mental retardation or an organic mental disorder that makes them seem dependent.

Psychiatric therapy is as difficult for this disorder as it is for the other personality disorders. It involves individual therapy, support for a change in the patient's life-style, and group therapy.

Avoidant personality disorder

The individual with avoidant personality fears rejection so greatly that he is unwilling to enter into a relationship unless there is an almost absolute guarantee of security. Unlike the cold schizoid who remains withdrawn and aloof or the eccentric schizotypal patient who shuns the rest of the world, the avoidant personality seeks affection and acceptance but has such low self-esteem that he is afraid to trust others with his feelings.

In the emergency setting the avoidant personality remains wary of the physician and staff. In most cases only a superficial relationship develops and the patient does not ask for help with the personality disorder. Psychiatric therapy is rarely helpful. The avoidant does not trust the psychiatrist with his thoughts or feelings and retreats back to his lonely, private shell.

Schizoid personality disorder

Like the avoidant personality, the schizoid patient lacks the ability to form warm, trusting social relationships. The schizoid individual generally prefers to be alone. He is typically reserved, withdrawn, reclusive, cool, and aloof and appears humorless or dull.

The schizoid personality functions poorly in occupational settings that require public contact and human interaction. He may function quite well, however, in settings where human interaction is rare. The patient with this disorder is perceived as a loner; the male rarely marries, and the female may accept courtship and marriage passively.

The terms *schizoid, schizotypal,* and *schizophrenia* may cause confusion. The schizotypal personality disorder is not as well organized and may produce symptoms similar to schizophrenia. A schizoid personality disorder is indicative of a better organized personality structure with no psychotic symptoms and is not related to schizophrenia. These differences are outlined in Table 14-2.

Schizotypal personality disorder

The schizotypal diagnosis comes closer to that for schizophrenia than the schizoid personality. The two essential features of the diagnosis are disorders of perception-cognition (patient can predict the future, and others can read his thoughts, "magical" thinking) and odd personality (eccentric, suspicious, aloof).

TABLE 14-2. Schizoid and schizotypal personality disorders*

Schizoid	*Schizotypal*
Emotional coolness	Magical thinking
Aloofness	Clairvoyance
Absence of warm tender feelings for others	"Sixth" sense
Indifference to praise or criticism from others	Ideas of reference
Few close friendships (no more than one or two, including family members)	Social isolation
	Recurrent illusions
No eccentricity of speech or behavior	Odd speech
No psychosis	Inadequate rapport as a result of inappropriate affect
No hallucinations	Suspiciousness
	Paranoid ideation
	Undue social anxiety
	No hallucinations

Adapted from American Psychiatric Association. *Diagnostic and statistical manual of mental disorders* (3rd ed.). Washington, D.C.: The Association, 1980, pp. 311-313.

*Schizotypal personality is more bizarre and closer to the diagnosis of schizophrenia.

The emergency physician may have great difficulty distinguishing schizotypal personality from schizophrenia. When hallucinations are detected, the examiner can be fairly confident of the diagnosis of schizophrenia.

Patients with schizoid and schizotypal personality are generally resistant to both psychotherapy and medication. When doubt exists about the differentiation from schizophrenia, psychiatric referral or consultation is indicated.

The emergency physician may encounter patients who seem uncommonly aloof, odd, or eccentric, yet do not appear psychotic or meet diagnostic criteria for schizophrenia. These patients may be schizoid or schizotypal. They probably allow their medical condition or injury to be treated and then are admitted or discharged without fanfare. Since they respond poorly to treatment, it is not necessary to make a precise diagnosis of these disorders in the emergency department.

Paranoid personality disorder

The characteristics of paranoid personality include generalized suspiciousness and mistrust of others. The patient is hypersensitive to criticism and rather cold emotionally. Some of the symptoms are similar to those of the patient with paranoid schizophrenia, but hallucinations and bizarre delusions are absent. The paranoid person expects trickery or harm at every turn and remains wary of others. He typically avoids blame, continually questions the loyalty of others, exaggerates trivial difficulties, and lacks a sense of humor or tender feelings.

The patient is generally so suspicious that he rarely requests psychiatric help. When this disorder is suspected, charts should be carefully documented. The patient may sue the institution or physician, particularly if he feels he has been slighted. Therefore, whenever treating such a patient, careful documentation should be kept, and the physician should always maintain a neutral emotional attitude toward the individual. This tends to dampen any distortion that the patient may develop about the physician's attitude toward him.

Narcissistic personality disorder

In Greek mythology Narcissus rejected Echo's offers of love. Zeus punished Narcissus by making him fall in love with his own image in a pool of water. When he moved to touch or embrace his loved one, the disturbance of the water caused the image to disappear. He slowly pined away, unable to possess his beloved, and became the flower that now bears his name.

The patient with narcissistic personality disorder exhibits an exaggerated sense of self-importance. The person is preoccupied with unlimited success and shows great anger and resentment about criticism.

The patient's interpersonal relationships are impaired by the lack of empathy for others and the tendency to manipulate them for his own selfish needs. This patient may also, to bolster his own sense of importance, bring litigation against physicians or institutions that he feels may not have met his grandiose expectations. The patient should be treated with reasonable respect, and a careful record of his treatment should be kept. He can become quite infuriating, but the treating staff and physicians must maintain a neutrality.

SUMMARY

The first clue to a patient's personality disorder may be the feeling that the physician experiences when first contacting the patient. Though some personality disorders may be quite evident, others are difficult to diagnose in the emergency department. Personality disorders are notoriously difficult to treat because the patient is generally quite comfortable with his personality and is reluctant to change. The personality disorders per se rarely require emergency treatment.

Nevertheless it is important to recognize someone who has a personality disorder, even if the exact diagnosis is unclear. This allows the treating physician and staff to focus on the patient's medical problem, appropriately evaluate it, and make recommendations. Overt anger, hostility, or another strongly expressed emotion rarely has a place in the treatment of the patient. The physician can use emotions to generate a hypothesis about the patient's personality disorder and then channel residual feelings of anger into a constructive course for the patient. The physician who avoids entering into the patient's manipulations and abrasive interpersonal style makes the emergency department more effective in the treatment of these patients as well as others. The avoidance of becoming embroiled in power struggles with the patient cannot be over-emphasized. The patient's best interests are served when the staff remains professional, nonjudgmental, and supportive.

REFERENCES

1. Summers, WK, Rund, DA, and Levin, M. Psychiatric illness in a general urban emergency room: daytime versus nighttime population. *Journal of Clinical Psychiatry,* Aug. 1979, *40*(8), 340-343.
2. American Psychiatric Association. *Diagnostic and statistical manual of mental disorders* (3rd ed.). Washington, D.C.: The Association, 1980.
3. Robins, LN. *Deviant children grown-up: a sociological and psychiatric study of sociopathic personality,* Baltimore: The Williams & Wilkins Co., 1966.
4. Groves, JE. Current concepts in psychiatry: borderline personality disorder. *New England Journal of Medicine,* July 1981, *305* 259-262.
5. Groves, JE. Taking care of the hateful patient. *New England Journal of Medicine,* 1978 *298*(16), 883-887.
6. Tupin, JP. Histrionic personality. In Lion, JR (Ed.), *Personality disorders: diagnosis and management (2nd ed.).* Baltimore: The Williams & Wilkins Co., 1981.

15 THE PATIENT WHO "SIGNS OUT" OR REFUSES TREATMENT

One of our fundamental legal and moral principles is that a conscious, competent adult or emancipated minor has the right to determine what someone else may do to his body. This general principle applies to the patient and health professionals. An individual may at any time during the hospital evaluation refuse to consent or withdraw previously given consent to undergo medical evaluation and treatment. When the patient's consent is refused or withdrawn, the physician and the hospital are obligated to release the patient from the emergency department. For their own legal protection the physician and the hospital generally ask the patient to sign a form that declares that he has been advised by the physician that further medical treatment is required, that his leaving may be dangerous to his health, and that he is, therefore, leaving against medical advice. A competent, conscious adult can legally refuse treatment (Fig. 15-1) and should sign an against medical advice form to help protect the physician and hospital from subsequent liability (Fig. 15-2).

The "catch" in the system of letting any patient refuse treatment is that he may be neither conscious nor competent to make a decision about the need for medical treatment. He may be mentally incapacitated by various kinds of organic or functional mental impairment. Typical causes for this kind of mental impairment are alcohol intoxication or withdrawal, drug intoxication, and functional psychosis. Other forms of mental disorder may also cause impairment of this competency or judgment.

In most states physicians have the legal right to hold such a patient if they feel that his release would place either the individual or someone else in imminently grave danger.

Each of the existing procedures to deal with the patient who refuses treatment (having him sign an against medical advice form or holding the dangerous or incompetent patient against his will) has major disadvantages. Each involves risk for the patient and physician. The patient may be harmed by the lack of proper medical treatment, and the physician faces the two-edged dilemma of being liable legally for allowing the incompetent patient to leave or for holding a patient against his will.

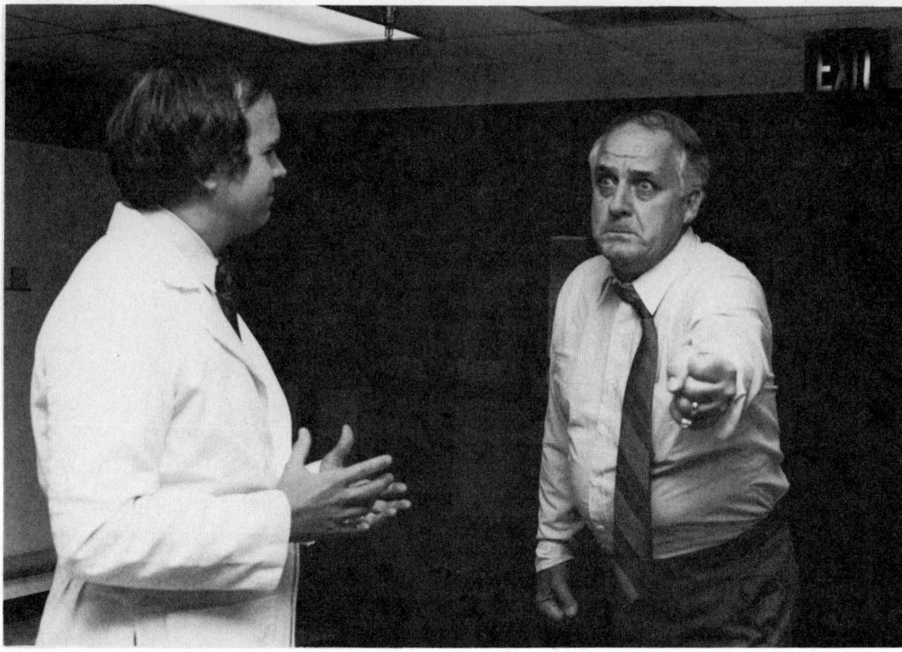

Fig. 15-1. Competent, conscious adult has right to refuse evaluation and treatment in emergency department. (Courtesy Lee Jansen, Columbus, Ohio.)

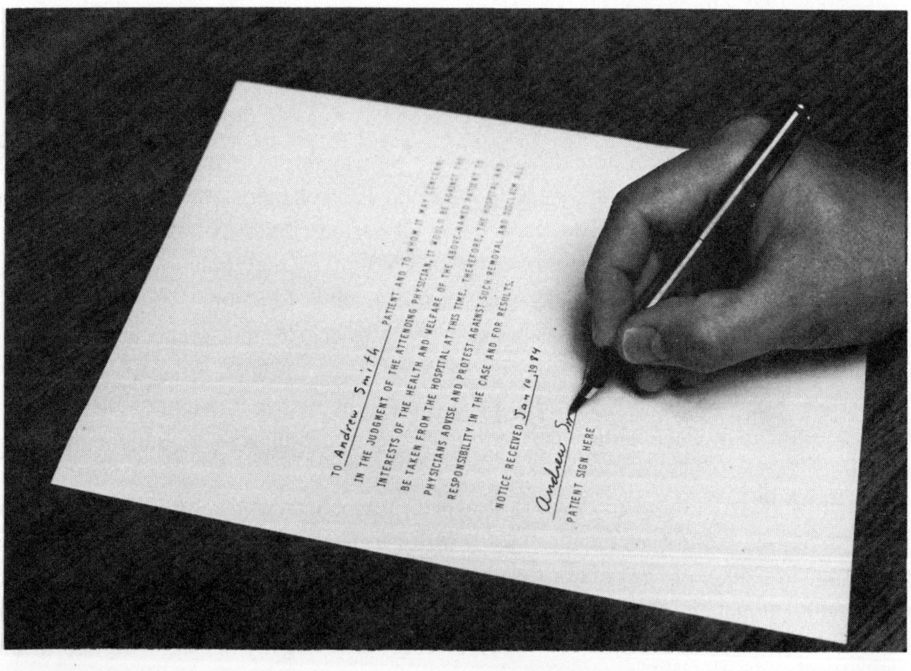
TO Andrew Smith PATIENT AND TO WHOM IT MAY CONCERN:
IN THE JUDGMENT OF THE ATTENDING PHYSICIAN, IT WOULD BE AGAINST THE
INTERESTS OF THE HEALTH AND WELFARE OF THE ABOVE-NAMED PATIENT TO
BE TAKEN FROM THE HOSPITAL AT THIS TIME. THEREFORE, THE HOSPITAL AND
PHYSICIANS ADVISE AND PROTEST AGAINST SUCH REMOVAL AND
RESPONSIBILITY IN THE CASE AND FOR RESULTS.
NOTICE RECEIVED Jan 10, 1984
PATIENT SIGN HERE

Fig. 15-2. When patient refuses treatment, against medical advice form is signed to release hospital and physician from liability. (Courtesy Lee Jansen.)

CATEGORIES OF PATIENTS WHO REFUSE TREATMENT

Not all patients who refuse treatment are the same. Some of these patients can be skillfully managed in such a way that they finally accept proper medical treatment. The purpose of this chapter is to present various types of patients who are likely to refuse medical treatment and the recommended approach to their management. The overall goal is the patient's well-being.

In general there are seven categories of patients who refuse treatment. These categories include patients with the following characteristics: delirium or dementia, anxiety, suicidal ideation, major psychiatric illness, noncompliance, anger, or rational refusal of treatment for personal reasons. These categories, their signs and symptoms, and their suggested treatments are outlined in Table 15-1.

Delirium or dementia

The patient with a generalized clouding of consciousness caused by an organic mental disorder may be confused and frightened by the rather complex events involved in his medical care. He tends to be uncooperative because his cerebral function is impaired. He is unable to orient himself and he has difficulty interpreting each new stimulus. This inability to understand the situation makes the patient irritable, angry, and uncomfortable. The only way to reduce these feelings and escape the uncomfortable situation may seem to be to leave the hospital.

The patient with such an organic mental disorder may have been brought to the hospital for treatment of a medical emergency like myocardial infarction, cerebrovas-

TABLE 15-1. Categories of patients who refuse help (or sign out) and recommended treatment

Category	*Signs and symptoms*	*Treatment*
Delirium or dementia	Confused, disoriented, paranoid	Haloperidol (Haldol) intramuscularly
Anxious patient	Frightened, denying	Ask about "hidden" agenda, chlordiazepoxide (Librium) or diazepam (Valium) intramuscularly
Suicidal patient	Refusing life-saving medical regimen	Institute prearranged commitment procedure
Major psychiatric illness	Psychotic	Admit to psychiatric unit
Noncompliant patient	Ignoring medication, depressed, dependent	Reassure, involve in treatment plan
Angry patient	Hostile, questioning regimen	Listen, compromise
Competent conscious individual who wishes no medical treatment	Alert, intact mental status, rational explanation of refusal	Politely allow patient to leave hospital against medical advice

cular accident, or major motor signs. The cerebral effects of the medical condition (hypoxia, ischemia, or postictal state) can lead to mental confusion. Similar effects may be seen in the patient with hypoglycemia or head injury.

The clinical evidence of organic mental disorder may be subtle. In patients with minimal impairment, the history provided by family or close friends is invaluable. Since they have a close day-to-day association with the patient, they are able to detect and report rather subtle changes in personality and mental function.

Occasionally the confusion and changed behavior only becomes noticeable when the patient is brought to the emergency department and confronted with many new tasks that require orienting skills. The patient may develop paranoid delusions to help explain a complex and confusing environment where other people stick needles in his arms, strap electrodes on his chest, and examine him with lights, reflex hammers, and x-ray beams (Fig. 15-3).

When the activities of the emergency staff are viewed from this confused, paranoid perspective, it is easy to see why the patient soon feels that nothing but evil and personal injury can come from this continued hospital evaluation. The patient then tries to pull out the intravenous line and leave the hospital.

Management. The management of the patient with delirium or dementia, who wishes to sign out and leave the department, consists of the following basic approaches:

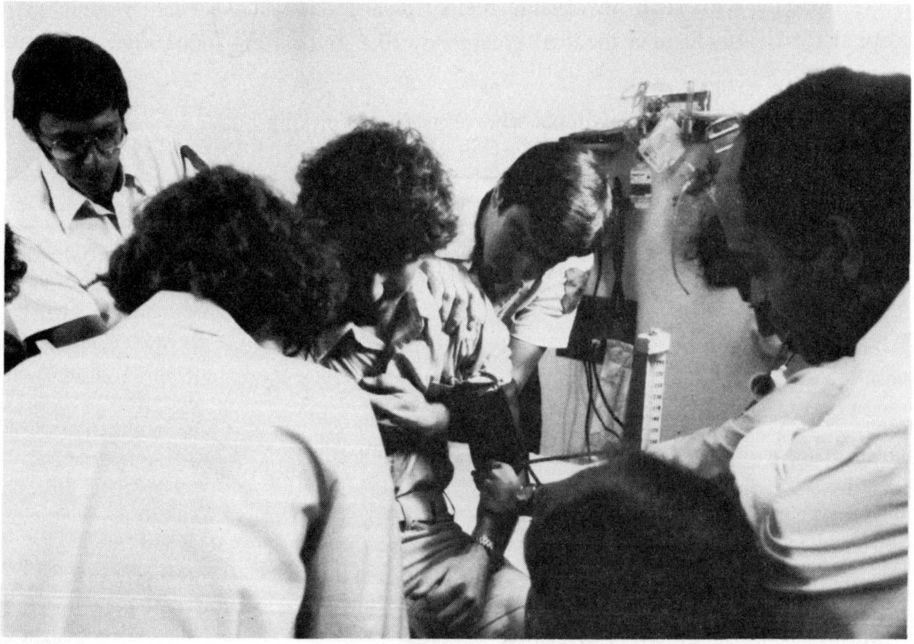

FIG. 15-3. Patient with organic mental disorder may deteriorate significantly in confusing environment where multiple persons interact with patient, and variety of procedures are done simultaneously.

treatment of the responsible medical condition, removal of ambiguous stimuli from the environment, and antipsychotic medication.

Treatment of the medical condition. The underlying cause of the impaired mentation should be corrected when possible. Hypoxia, ischemia, hypoglycemia, and infection are conditions that can usually be reversed by appropriate intervention.

CASE EXAMPLE 1

A 38-year-old man was brought to the emergency department because he had assaulted his wife and son. The patient appeared belligerent and claimed that he wasn't himself and wanted to leave. He repeatedly attempted to leave the department and was finally locked in a small detention room until a physician was available to evaluate him. When examined, his temperature was 103°F and he was diaphoretic. His wife provided the history that he had been hit in the nose 3 days previously and had experienced some intermittent clear nasal drainage. A lumbar puncture confirmed the clinical suspicion of bacterial meningitis, and the patient was admitted for treatment.

Wernicke's encephalopathy resulting from thiamine deficiency may be seen in an alcoholic patient and can be precipitated by the administration of glucose. Wernicke's encephalopathy may be diagnosed when the patient exhibits ocular paresis, ataxia, and mental confusion. Thiamine given intramuscularly in dosages of 50 to 100 mg rapidly reverses the condition.

Organic mental syndromes resulting from drug or alcohol intoxication or withdrawal are perhaps the most common conditions associated with refusal of treatment in everyday practice. Management of the patient requires a clinical judgment about the seriousness of the medical condition and the risk (to the patient) of allowing him to sign out. If an intoxicated patient has been in an automobile accident, for instance, and sustained a cervical fracture, he should not be allowed to refuse treatment and walk away. The patient has a clear risk of sustaining permanent damage to himself but cannot appreciate the seriousness of the situation because he is intoxicated. Such a patient must be restrained, forcibly if necessary, and secured to a backboard with adequate cervical protection until a neurosurgeon assumes care.

By contrast, the population of alcoholics with trivial or chronic complaints in some emergency departments is so high that the staff almost breathes a sigh of relief when the patient even hints about signing out. Against medical advice forms appear instantly, and the patient is assisted to the door. When such a patient leaves before medical evaluation (at least a history and physical examination), the staff assumes some risk that the patient may have a serious, acute condition like pneumonia or subdural hematoma that requires urgent medical care.

The intoxicated patient who wishes to sign out should be allowed to do so if he has no "life or limb" threat and is mentally competent as determined by the clinical judgment of the physician, the history, his vital signs, and as much of a physical examination as possible (including his general appearance and gait), documented clearly in the patient's record. A blood ethanol level may be unreliable for making the judgment about competence, since many chronic alcoholics are tolerant to the effects of high alcohol levels, including those higher than levels that "legally" signify intoxication. Documentation of a high blood alcohol level in the record, therefore, could cause subsequent problems for the physician when questions are raised about the patient's capability to function when leaving the hospital. The documented clinical observation of the physician *without* a recorded blood alcohol level may be more accurate in predicting capability and may be a safer course in terms of subsequent questions of professional liability.

If there is serious suspicion that leaving the hospital against medical advice will result in serious harm to the patient or someone else, he must be physically restrained, if necessary, and treated appropriately.

CASE EXAMPLE 2

A 50-year-old man who claimed to be an attorney was involved in an automobile accident and brought to the emergency department. The patient's behavior and breath odor suggested alcohol intoxication. The patient complained of neck pain. He was cooperative until two radiographs of the cervical spine were taken. He then tried to get out of bed, remove his cervical collar, and leave the hospital. The x-ray films revealed a superior facet fracture of the sixth cervical vertebrae. The patient's wife, the hospital attorney, and the administrator on call were notified, and the patient was physically restrained, despite threats of criminal charges if he were not allowed to leave. When the patient became sober, he apologized for his actions and thanked the staff for taking care of him.

Environment. Delirium tends to become worse when few stimuli are presented or when the stimulation is ambiguous. When there is very little noise, few visual cues, and dim lighting, the patient has little with which to orient himself.

The patient has similar difficulty dealing with the activity and speech of several people at once in the apparent confusion of an emergency department. At the very least such a patient becomes irritable and demanding. As the patient becomes increasingly anxious and confused, he may become somewhat paranoid in an attempt to explain the confusion of the world around him.

The management of the patient involves manipulation of his environment and the adoption of a clear unambiguous approach that reassures him. If the patient's room is alive with the bustle of nurses, orderlies, students, attendants, and family, it is best to ask everyone to leave the room. This diminishes the patient's fear of attack. The physician should then sit down in a nonthreatening posture, adopt a calm and comforting demeanor, use firm but warm reassurance, and explain to the patient that the hallucinations or delusions are normal under these conditions and that the medical problem can be treated successfully. Rather than argue about misinterpretation of reality, the clinician should constantly refer back to the original medical problem and its treatment. If the patient is confused and delusional, the clinician may elect to join him in his delusion, if necessary. If the individual believes that someone is following him, he could be told that he is not alone and that the physician is watching for anyone trying to attack the patient.

It is important to remember that the patient who is confused and fearful needs clear unambiguous limits. These limits are set by the responsible physician who maintains an authoritative approach. After the patient has responded to the treatment, it is important to describe what happened to him, explain the cause of his "crazy behavior," and tell him that this is entirely normal. The patient can be reassured that the confusion is not a sign of underlying insanity or craziness.

Medication. When the source of confusion in the combative patient cannot be easily reversed with treatment of the underlying cause (e.g., hypoglycemia, hypoxia, hypotension), haloperidol may be helpful. Usually an initial dose of 5 to 10 mg is given intramuscularly or orally. An additional 5 mg dose of haloperidol can be given in 30 minutes if the behavior persists. When the medication is continued for several days, it is usually given as follows: one half of the total dosage required to cause mild sedation is administered every 12 hours for 24 to 48 hours. Haloperidol has few cardiovascular side effects and does not cause significant respiratory depression. It should prevent a return to the delusional or combative behavior of the confused patient who requires medical-psychiatric care.

Anxiety

Nearly everyone experiences some anxiety when admitted to an emergency department. There is often separation from the family, loss of some control over what is happening to the body, fear that a serious medical-surgical condition is present, a fear of pain, and generalized anxiety associated with removing one's clothes and donning a hospital gown. In some patients the anxiety becomes so great that the desire to get out of bed, get dressed, and go home is overwhelming. Some of these stresses, the emotions they arouse, and the resulting behavior are portrayed in Fig. 15-3.

CASE EXAMPLE 3

A 38-year-old man entered the emergency department with a complaint of severe chest pain. He was diaphoretic and anxious. Occasionally he would press his fist to his chest and lean over as if in excruciating pain. After an initial examination, the patient noted that he felt better. His chest pain was diminished, and he planned to leave the department. He got off the cart, pulled off his monitor leads, and began getting dressed, stating that he would return if he had any recurrence of chest pain, but he did not want to waste everybody's time with further testing or hospitalization.

This type of patient certainly generates a sense of frustration in a busy emergency staff. The most understandable response could be to say "Go ahead and leave . . . we have to take care of other patients who are *really* sick."

It is helpful to understand the patient's anxiety and feeling of stress that form the reaction to leave the hospital. It is also beneficial to realize that the patient who responds this way is often quite simple or primitive in his view of things. He may have grown up in a rural or socially deprived area and functioned all his life in rather simple, unchanging roles. His reaction to stress is not modified by complex social experiences that allow him to tolerate the frustrations and uncertainties of hospitalization.

The patient in the emergency department must sense multiple stresses—a threat to his own integrity, the chance of dying, the loss of control over his body, a separation from loved ones, a loss of health, or perhaps a loss of manhood. Viewed from this perspective, one can understand the patient's attempt to leave. He wishes to deny his illness as a part of his response to a fear of dying. The patient reasons that if he does not have a heart attack, he will be allowed to leave the emergency department, and this denial of illness, manifested by leaving the hospital, relieves the patient's anxiety.

The patient also wants to return home to those he trusts and who he feels will take care of him. They have a greater investment in him than the hospital staff, according to his view, and will do a better job in caring for him. He wants to be united with those who nurture him.

The emergency staff's understanding of the forces causing the anxious patient to refuse care is really the key to rational management. Some patients have a "hidden agenda." They want something from their emergency visit but do not communicate their expectations spontaneously. Generally these patients are embarrassed to discuss their hidden agenda for fear that they will be ridiculed. An example of the hidden agenda is the patient who believes that he has cancer and enters the emergency department with a variety of seemingly unrelated complaints but no mention of a fear of cancer. Such a patient may have heard about a family member who had similar symptoms and then learned about the presence of his malignancy. Other patients may fear that their heavy alcohol or drug abuse will be discovered, yet hope it will be to obtain treatment.

The discovery by the emergency staff of the hidden agenda should lead to increased patient cooperation. This discovery requires subtle questioning and a sensitivity to clues the patient provides about the real reason for his visit. This type of patient needs to be reassured that the staff is concerned about him as a person, not a disease. The physician must ask him what he thinks is wrong with his health. It is important to find out his worst fears. This approach is often enough to calm the patient and permit the taking of a meaningful history. The patient should not be falsely reassured but calmly convinced that as full an evaluation as possible will be done.

Patients who fear separation from their family or loved ones must be reassured that they will be able to visit for a time in the emergency department at the conclusion of the examination. Some patients request the presence of a family member or friend, and it is usually quite acceptable to have the requested person present for at least some portion of the patient interview. Having such a person present should lessen anxiety resulting from the separation.

The patient who fears loss of control over his life and body responds most favorably to an approach that is direct, yet respectful of his wishes. The patient who fears loss of control may have worked for many years to prove his independence and importance to himself and others. When he is being placed in a completely dependent position with powerful figures ordering him about, he becomes frightened and wishes to leave. The physician managing this type of patient must clarify diagnostic reasoning and explain any procedures that are planned. Each procedure should be explained in sufficient detail so that the patient comprehends what will happen and why it is necessary. It is most helpful to ask the patient's explicit permission to allow these procedures. In so doing the physician becomes a powerful ally, working for the patient. The nurses should be instructed to explain the procedures again before they are performed. The patient should be allowed to walk in the hall and participate in his care as much as possible. This decreases his sense of loss of control.

If these procedures are ineffective and the anxious patient still considers leaving the department, the physician should at least consider offering an antianxiety agent like diazepam or chlordiazepoxide. As the patient's anxiety is lessened, his cooperation should increase.

The patient with steadily rising anxiety may begin to have delusions and misinterpretations of his surroundings. The individual in this more serious category probably requires an antipsychotic agent like haloperidol. If this is effective and the patient is to be discharged, he may be given a 24- or 48-hour supply of the medication for temporary use until follow-up care is available.

The suicidal patient

Three large classes of patients who refuse treatment can be considered within this broad category. They are the patient who makes a suicide gesture for secondary gain, the truly suicidal patient, and the patient with chronic illness who is withdrawing from treatment for deliberate reasons.

The patient who makes a nonlethal suicide attempt and achieves some secondary gain, such as attention and concern from his family, may wish to leave the emergency department for one of two reasons: either the goal of the attempt has been achieved, or the patient wants to continue to be considered a risk for suicide. The patient who makes these minor attempts (low risk and high likelihood of rescue) probably has a personality disorder that makes him rather resistant to psychiatric treatment.

If the patient in this category is medically stable (i.e., normal vital signs, awake, alert,nontoxic blood drug levels) and professes to be no longer suicidal, he can generally be discharged from the emergency department. The patient who continues to profess suicidal intent requires psychiatric evaluation and a medical "hold" for 1 to 3 days for further evaluation.

The suicidal patient who survives a serious attempt or relates to the emergency physician the desire to commit suicide falls into a second category of patients who may refuse treatment.

CASE EXAMPLE 4

A 52-year-old man was found unconscious in his bedroom by his daughter who became suspicious about possible suicide when no one answered the phone for several hours one evening. The patient was a widower who lived alone. He had seemed depressed for several months and had mentioned suicide to his daughter on more than one occasion. An empty bottle of diazepam was found near the patient's bedside. Shortly after arrival in the emergency department, the patient became more responsive. Over the next 6 hours he gradually regained consciousness. Soon after awakening, he attempted to remove his intravenous (IV) tubing and get out of the examining bed. He claimed that he saw no use in living anymore and that he ''just wanted out.''

The patient illustrates a serious suicide risk. Further questioning would undoubtedly reveal that he is profoundly depressed. This category of patient most definitely requires mandatory hospitalization and psychiatric treatment. The emergency physician must point to the suicide attempt and continued suicidal ideation as justification for placing the patient under a temporary legal hold because he represents a grave danger to himself. Such a patient may be restrained by whatever means are necessary, including physical restraint by security officers or placement on a locked psychiatric unit.

The third category includes the patient with chronic illness who withdraws from treatment for deliberate reasons. The key to evaluating this patient is the word *deliberate*. Suicide is at some level an angry interpersonal statement. The typical patient who is suicidal exudes a feeling of anger, appears to be pouting perhaps, and offers passive resistance to any procedures requested by the hospital staff.

On the other hand, the patient who has made a deliberate decision to withdraw from treatment has probably reviewed his life and discussed with his family and medical staff the implications of stopping treatment. Such a patient has an accepting, peaceful feeling about his decision. He undoubtedly demonstrates this feeling in interactions with the staff. The patient is neither angry nor depressed. He has reviewed his options and, faced with chronic illness, is ready to die. A patient like this is highly unusual. The acceptance of death should be a product of a several-month period of discussion with a psychiatrist and attending physician. Such a patient should be discharged but only after consultation with the attending physician and family. If the feeling is positive and life centered, the choice to withdraw from medical treatment is often rational, competent, and deliberate. If the feeling is hostile, angry, and death centered, the choice to refuse treatment is suicidal and irrational.

Far more likely in clinical practice is the chronically ill patient with major depression. A patient with chronic renal failure and a superimposed medical illness may suddenly refuse his dialysis treatment. The physician should suspect a major clinical depression and ask about sleep disturbance, appetite loss, crying spells, and feelings of sadness or irritability. Since depression is one of the most common illnesses seen in the emergency department, it should always be considered when a chronically ill patient refuses treatment. The patient should eventually respond positively to a discussion of depression as a medical illness, with the attendant description of adequate treatment. If depression is suspected, the patient should be considered for hospitalization, psychotherapy, and treatment with tricyclic antidepressants.

The exact procedure to be followed for holding a patient against his will because of risk to himself or others varies from state to state. The safest course to follow involves a team like the following: (1) the hospital administrator of the department, (2) a psychiatrist to determine whether or not the patient is impaired (by reason of mental illness) in his ability to refuse medical treatment, and (3) the patient's attending physician to document the fact that refusal of treatment creates an imminent risk of death to the patient.

Advanced planning for such commitments requires a specific written plan for handling these cases; an in-service program or seminar for the entire emergency department staff to review the procedures should prove helpful and eliminate prolonged and painful delays. Planning and consultation beforehand with hospital attorneys, psychiatrists familiar with these problems, and judges who handle such commitments permit smooth emergency commitment to a psychiatric or medical service with minimal fear of subsequent legal reprisal.

The patient with a major psychiatric illness

A patient who refuses or sabotages treatment to an alarming extent may be psychotic.

CASE EXAMPLE 5

A 24-year-old intoxicated man sustained multiple fractures of limbs and face in an automobile accident. On arrival to the emergency department, he was active and talkative. He attempted to get up from the examining table and walk around. He seemed euphoric and attempted to flirt with several of the nurses and joke with the physicians. The patient appeared to have little concern for his serious injuries. As he became more grandiose and talkative, acute mania was suspected. An interview with his family revealed a history of bipolar affective disorder. During his manic phase the patient customarily drank excessively and had been involved in a previous accident under similar circumstances.

CASE EXAMPLE 6

A 19-year-old man had accepted chemotherapy for acute leukemia. He was brought to the emergency department because he refused further treatment. A short interview revealed rambling, paranoia, and delusional thought and speech. He felt that people were walking in and out of the television set at home. The patient could hold together briefly with social chitchat but became more irrational as the conversation continued. A diagnosis of paranoid schizophrenia was made after several days of inpatient observation on a psychiatric service.

Both of these patients must be evaluated for medical causes of abnormal behavior and thought, such as head injury, hypoxia, hypoglycemia, and shock in the former and toxic psychosis, encephalitis, or meningitis in the latter.

The addition of a mental status examination, including drawing a clockface as discussed in Chapter 3, should help distinguish organic from functional psychosis. It is also helpful to take a few minutes to listen to the patient. This allows him to "fall apart" as he becomes less coherent.

The psychotic patient needs firm yet gentle reassurance that people often become confused under these circumstances. When a patient has a serious medical and psychiatric illness, a close liaison between the staffs of these two departments offers the best overall therapy to the patient.

The noncompliant patient

Noncompliance or refusal to adhere to the prescribed medical regimen is a major problem in medical practice. It is possible that as many as two thirds of the patients either take their medications sporadically or not at all. Some patients who are generally noncompliant may refuse emergency medical treatment altogether. At least four types of patients may become noncompliant. If the syndrome is identified, the proper treatment mode can be selected. Some guidelines for the management of noncompliance include the following:

1. Assure congruence between patient expectations and treatment plan.
2. Encourage truthfulness (openness) in the patient.
3. Ask the patient for other ideas he may have.
4. Compromise with the patient.

Depression. The most common psychiatric cause of noncompliance is depression. The depressed patient is in effect saying, "I'll show you; I'll kill myself" by refusing to comply with medical treatment. Clinical clues to the depression are crying spells, early morning awakening, decreased appetite, and increased irritability. The depressed patient may actually look sad to the examiner. When the diagnosis of depression is made, the treatment emphasis must be toward alleviating the condition first and then concentrating on the medical illness with the patient's cooperation. Once the patient can discuss his feeling of depression, he usually complies at least minimally with treatment.

Characterological problems. Certain patients feel the need to be in control. They may picture themselves involved in a power struggle with the medical profession and sense a need to defeat the physician. These patients need to be made to feel that they are part of their own treatment. They do best when invited to join in the planning of their own treatment. Questions that generally elicit greater patient cooperation include the following:

"When would you like to take your medication?

"Does the number of pills you have to take bother you?"

"Do you think this is a good plan, and is it working for you?"

Patient suspicion. Some patients are so suspicious of others' intentions that they are noncompliant with their medical treatment. These persons tend to blame others, including their physician, for their problems, and to appear rigid, arrogant, and intent on having the upper hand. The proper approach to such a person is one that maintains a neutral friendliness. The physician cannot and should not try to get close to this type of patient but needs to keep a neutral distance. Patient instruction should be carefully explained, and a clearly written record of the encounter, including the patient's instructions, must be documented in the chart. The patient should be instructed to return to the emergency department for a follow-up visit if he is unable to contact his physician.

Dependency. Dependent patients often become noncompliant. These people tend to resent their own dependency. They typically ask for increasing medical supervision and may repeatedly come to the emergency department for a minor change in medication. Therefore they trigger the staff's irritation and their own rejection. When unchecked, this creates a spiral of increased clinging, followed by staff rejection, and then by the patients' self-sabotage of their own medical treatment programs. Whatever medical problems they had initially are certainly not well served by this behavior. Because these dependent patients see successful treatment of their illness as resulting in the physician's abandonment, they cannot afford to get well because they fear the physician will leave them. When severely dependent patients are identified, they need to be reassured that the physician will follow them closely "in sickness and in health." They must be openly reassured that they will not be abandoned.

Adolescent patients

Adolescent patients generally test everyone's limits. The whole fabric of an adolescent's life is involved in testing authority, rules, and regulations. The adolescent symbolically asks persons on whom he is dependent the following question repeatedly: "Do you love me? If so, prove it!" The adolescent patient is best handled with an approach that demonstrates both concern and patience. Most important is that the adolescent must be shown a reasonable degree of acceptance and given a fair amount of freedom. Firm limit-setting, however, is important. The exact determination and enforcement of these limits are sometimes difficult and evolve from experience. The adolescent must be allowed to participate in his own treatment to the extent allowed by the stated limits. The staff should be able to accept the patient's occasional failure to follow rules or instructions precisely.

The patient who is angry about his treatment

A patient may refuse treatment because he is angry about the way he has been treated by the medical or nursing staff. Such a patient begins to turn bitter and belittles or criticizes the actions of the staff. The anger and bitterness soon lead to resistance to further procedures and initial attempts to leave the hospital.

The first rule in the management of this patient (as it is for all patients) is to *listen to the patient*. The complaints may be absolutely legitimate. The emergency department may resemble chaos, the patient may have been slighted or injured, and personality conflicts between emergency staff and patients can occur. The system may appear to be inhuman, indifferent, and wrong to any normal person, certainly for those who are sensitive and always in a hurry. When listening to the patient, the physician should identify areas of congruence between the patient's expectations and the medical treatment plan. Those areas that represent incongruence should be discussed until some sort of compromise is reached.

A typical example of unsatisfied patient expectation is represented by the patient who comes to the emergency department expecting an x-ray film of his injured ankle or back. A physician who finds no clinical signs suggesting fracture or injury detectable by an x-ray film may refuse to order the radiograph. Another patient may submit to inspection of his sore throat because he expects an injection of penicillin. When the medication is not provided, he reacts with anger because "nothing is being done, and it's costing me a lot of money." A patient with chest pain who fears cardiac disease may desperately await an electrocardiogram (ECG). When the ECG is not taken because the examination suggests chest wall pain to the physician, the patient's expectations are not met and his hidden fear of heart disease goes unabated.

In nearly all of these situations a compromise can be reached. Compromise requires that the physician orders the x-ray film, penicillin injection, or ECG or that the patient be educated enough to accept the clinical reasoning behind the decision not to order the expected procedure. If the patient accepts the physician's reasoning, it is extremely important to offer him future access to the system at any time if he feels that his condition has worsened. This generally mollifies the patient's anxiety about undetected and untreated illness.

In certain instances cultural biases interfere with congruence of expectation and result. The patient from Puerto Rico, for instance, may believe that a duodenal ulcer is a "hot disease" that needs a "cold treatment." A patient with such beliefs will not take a warm liquid after he leaves the emergency department, even though it has been prescribed. Such a patient is ideally given treatment that is reasonably in line with his prejudices and beliefs.

A patient must be encouraged to be truthful about his reasons for being angry. He may have been offended by a receptionist, a nurse, or the examining physician, and he may be afraid to admit it. When he does admit it, the physician must at least sympathize with the patient's feelings of anger. An apology for the patient being hurt and agreement about the validity of his complaint certainly promote future patient cooperation and probably markedly decrease the threat of subsequent malpractice actions.

Another way to seek out patient compliance is to specifically ask if he agrees with the proposed treatment plan; if he does, are there any other ideas about evaluation or treatment that should be considered? Encouraging the patient in such a manner helps prevent him from leaving the department and immediately going to another hospital to seek the help he really requests. The essence of dealing with the angry patient is listening and compromising.

Refusal of treatment for moral or religious reasons

Patients at times have moral or religious convictions that run counter to generally accepted and reasonable medical treatment. Such a patient needs to be approached on several different levels. One of them is to educate the patient as to his illness and treatment. He must be fully informed about the hazards of letting the condition go untreated, and he should also know the benefits of treatment. If he continues to refuse treatment, asking him for the name of his religious leader and for permission to talk with this person might be helpful. Ideally the physician might convince the religious leader to come to the emergency department or discuss the situation on the phone with the patient. This can sometimes result in compliance to treatment when there has been a misunderstanding in religious dogma or standards. Such a conflict must be carefully documented in the chart, which should be signed by the patient before leaving the emergency department if he continues to refuse treatment.

Since laws vary in different states, the eventuality of a patient refusing treatment for moral or religious reasons should be discussed with the hospital attorney and representatives from various religious groups within the community. A plan should then be drafted to handle this situation in its various forms in a general way. This is a common situation and occurs time and again to anyone working in an emergency department setting. Ruling out a major psychiatric disorder with religious or philosophical delusions is important. Patients with a bipolar affective disorder, particularly when they are manic, or with a schizophrenic disorder often have such delusions. The usual mental status examination should clearly differentiate these patients from those with firmly held beliefs.

MENTAL COMPETENCY

The question of whether or not a patient is mentally competent to refuse treatment may arise. Several tests may be used to determine mental competence in a patient with a life-threatening illness. The following list is the suggested procedure.

1. Is the patient in imminent danger of death from a medical illness?
2. Does the patient understand the nature of the illness; can he repeat it to the examining physician?
3. Does the patient understand the nature of the proposed treatments, the hazards, and the benefits?
4. Does the patient understand the medical consequences of refusing treatment?
5. If the patient does not comprehend the above, he can be committed to the *least restrictive* medical treatment environment.
6. A probate court hearing must be held within 24 hours (this may vary from state to state).

The physician's initial decision must be whether or not the patient is in imminent danger of dying within several days if adequate treatment is not provided. For example, this could involve a patient with severe renal failure with hyperkalemia, a patient with bacterial meningitis, or a victim of an automobile accident who also has a distended, tender abdomen. When the threat to the patient's life is not as obvious as in these examples, the physician's best judgment must be used to determine the real threat to the patient.

Once it is determined that the condition presents an imminent threat to the patient's life, the physician must decide if there is an effective treatment available for such a condition. If there is an effective treatment, the patient is asked if he understands the nature of his condition. A "yes" answer is not sufficient; the patient must repeat it clearly to the physician and a witness. An acceptable answer, for instance, could be the following: "Yes, I know that my kidneys don't work any more and that poisonous substances are accumulating in my blood."

The next determination is whether or not the patient understands the nature of the proposed treatment, including its benefits and hazards. The patient should be able to repeat this to the physician. The final determination is whether or not the patient understands the medical consequences, including death, of refusing treatment. The patient could say, for instance, "I understand that my heart could stop beating within several days if I refuse treatment for any kidney problem."

If a patient is deemed to be mentally competent, the physician should involve the relatives to determine a proper course of action. The patient may, in fact, be deemed mentally competent and allowed to sign out against medical advice. If the patient does not understand his illness, the treatment, or the consequences of treatment refusal, he may be held involuntarily in the least restrictive environment that can provide proper treatment. A probate hearing regarding the patient's competency should be held within 24 hours. Since the state laws regarding such cases vary among states, the department's policy must be in accord with the state's statutory specifications.

Sometimes a severe mental illness makes the patient mentally incompetent. One who is psychotic, for instance, is not mentally competent. Great difficulty arises, however, when the patient is suspected of suffering from a major depression but still remains mentally alert. In these difficult cases, the help of a psychiatrist may be warranted, and the patient can probably be held a few hours for psychiatric evaluation. Since detaining the patient is complex, it is often helpful to share this responsibility with others, including the hospital administrator, the hospital attorney, and the patient's family.

Documentation of the patient's feelings about himself and the decision to refuse treatment is absolutely essential. The note in the report should always be one that reflects concern and compassion as in the following statement: "I am concerned that this patient has impaired judgment regarding the nature of his illness. I have taken steps to detain the patient against his will because I believe it is in his best interest."

If the patient leaves the hospital, the following statement might apply: "I am concerned about the seriousness of the patient's injury and informed him that it may cause his death within a matter of days. He understands this clearly and has exercised his right to refuse treatment. He has released the hospital and myself from any liability that might result from his decision." These statements are much more satisfactory than an abrupt "the patient refuses treatment."

SUMMARY

The conscious competent adult can refuse medical treatment and leave the hospital. Competency can be determined by various tests of the patient's comprehension of his illness and proposed treatment. In certain cases the patient's decision to leave the hospital can be explored and reversed by proper communication, concern, and family intervention.

Since this can be a difficult ethical question, there are times when the physician's proper course of action cannot be precisely determined. In these cases the safest position is the one that acts in the "best interest" of the patient and preserves his life and function.

16 PSYCHIATRIC EMERGENCIES ASSOCIATED WITH DEATH

The death of a loved one is the greatest stress a person or family can bear. The death of a patient is one of the most stressful events felt by the staff of an emergency department. Since death is such a common event in the emergency department, the staff should appreciate and benefit from training that deals with the family of a patient who has died. One of the first steps in helping the staff to assist others in dealing with their grief is to plan an open discussion in which staff members can work through their own feelings about death and dying.

GRIEF

Grief is a normal human response of close family and friends to the death of a loved one. Grief occurs in members of the emergency department staff in response to the death of a patient albeit in a much briefer way. Grief involves several stages (Table 16-1). Although family members and friends of a deceased person may react to death in various ways, most people experience a predictable series of stages and eventually resolve their grief.

When the grieving process is rapid, the emergency physician may see several of these phases if he remains with the patient after relating news of the death. When the phases last hours to days, the emergency physician may see the grieving survivor at various stages of the grief and recovery process. The patient appreciates the physician's reassurance that his response to grief is a normal reaction. When the grief reaction falls outside the bounds of normalcy, psychiatric consultation may be necessary.

One of the most common responses to death is an "affective anesthesia." When a family member is told of the death of a patient, he may not react at all. He appears to be numb, unresponsive, and quite withdrawn. This initial response to the loss of a loved one involves a normal denial and dissociation of feelings from thoughts. It is a common response to sudden death. When the patient appears numb, it may be necessary to repeat the information several times. This anesthetic period is usually followed within moments or hours by a sense of yearning or protest. The person may refuse to believe the news and may loudly protest the death as something that is impossible; he may deny entirely what has happened. This denial is an attempt to disavow the enormity of the change in the survivor's life and feelings and a normal emotional response to a severe stress. The

TABLE 16-1. Stages of grief

Stage	*Normal time period*
I. Affective anesthesia (''numbness'')	Immediate
II. Yearning or protest (''crying out'')	Minutes to hours
III. Disorganization (''falling apart'')	Hours to days
IV. Reorganization	6 months to 1 year
V. Pathological grief	More than 1 year

response typically lasts from a few moments to hours. When possible, a staff member can sit with the family during this phase until it subsides. However, it is not necessary to talk to them while they are in this stage.

The stage of denial is often followed by disorganization during which survivors have difficulty following through in everyday activities. They seem to ''fall apart.'' They may not be able to work or function within the family or society; they generally ''shut out the world.'' It is not at all unusual for the bereaved to be totally preoccupied with and to ''talk to'' the image of the deceased. This is a normal human response and a way of incorporating the monumental loss into reality. During this phase the survivors may concentrate on details and trivial questions about ordinary events. The answers should be straightforward and calm and need to be given by attentively listening and gently encouraging them to ask more questions. The period of disorganization may last for hours or days. Eventually this phase gives way to a period of reorganization during which the survivors ''pull together'' and begin resuming normal life-styles. The time period required for reorganization is usually 6 months to 1 year after the death of a loved one. The normal recuperative process takes time. The reorganization, however, may result in a level of social, intellectual, and physical functioning lower or higher than the level maintained before the death of the loved one. The bereaved may form permanent pathological responses to the death.

Pathological grief is defined as severe mourning and a reduced level of function that persists for over a year following the death of a loved one. Pathological grief is a crippling and disabling problem. It often results from an inability to accept and work through the death of a close family member or friend. The syndrome can generally be prevented by brief and repetitive intervention in an emergency setting, followed by competent psychiatric care.

CONTACTING THE FAMILY

If the family of the deceased is present in the emergency department, they should be taken to a quiet comfortable private room where they can be told of the patient's death by the emergency physician. When they are not in the department, they are usually contacted by telephone. Since the telephone conversation is an important first step in dealing with the family's reaction to death, the person calling should be an experienced emergency nurse or physician. A few nurses may elect to receive training in notifying family members. One clinician from specially trained groups may elect to notify the family when any death occurs. The conversation with the family in some ways is an art. The nurse or physician should identify the family member, give the name of the hospital, and clearly state his or her name to the family. They should then be informed that their relative is seriously ill or injured and that they should come to the hospital. If possible, another member or close friend should accompany the relative to the hospital, and someone other than the close relative should drive the car. In most cases the family member should not be told over the telephone that the patient has died. This is not practiced, however, in some cases in which the family member is hundreds or thousands of miles away and cannot get to the hospital for many hours or days. In cases in which it is necessary to tell the family about the death of the patient over the telephone, the caller from the hospital should be sure that the relative has an adult with him who can summon help or assist him if his reaction incapacitates him. The caller's manner and approach should be calm, gentle, and professional; bluntness or curtness is inappropriate and unkind.

Telling the family about a death

Once the family member is in the emergency department, a quiet area should be provided for him. Ideally the area is a room that allows privacy and no interruptions. The emergency physician should always tell the relatives of the patient's death. The physician has the most authority, can answer pertinent medical questions, and is the one who was in charge of the medical treatment. It is rarely appropriate that a nurse or other staff member should tell the family. Before talking with the group, each person should be identified by the physician as a member of the family. Even close friends or family intimates should be asked to wait outside until after the news is revealed. The discussion of a family death is a private affair until the family decides otherwise.

As with an initial psychiatric interview, the physician should allow about 5 minutes for interaction with the family when telling them of a death. A satisfactory approach in many cases is to ask the family what happened from their perspective. They may relate, for instance, that the patient "just couldn't get his breath," and they called the emergency service. This can help to bring the family and the physician up to the time the patient entered the hospital. This is followed by an explanation in several terms of what was wrong with the patient and the news that the patient has died. The physician need not say much at this point but should not bolt out of the room merely because he is uncomfortable.

Seeing the body

Generally if a family member wants to see the body of the dead person, he should be allowed to do so. This is often an important issue later; failure to see the body of the dead person may result in prolonged grieving and disbelief of the patient's actual death. Usually the staff members are the ones who are overprotective of the relative and are squeamish about having the person see the body. Children may also need to see the body if an older family member agrees to it and actively seeks it. Families have their own ways of dealing with crises, and generally it is best to allow this style to take precedence. If it appears that a member of the family is making a gross misjudgment concerning the handling of the death, he can be confronted with the observation in a very gentle way, but this is rarely necessary.

Whenever possible, a member of the clergy should be contacted. This can be very helpful in dealing with the family. It really does not matter which religion this person represents, since any member of the clergy can provide religious support at a time of emotional crisis. The member of the clergy may also begin discussing necessary details regarding funeral arrangements if this has not already been done by one of the emergency department personnel.

The body should be prepared as well as possible to be seen by the family members. The patient's eyes are closed, blood is wiped from the face, and all excess debris from a resuscitation should be removed. The body is generally covered; the face and hands are left exposed. Tubes, medical equipment, and intravenous catheters must be left in place in most states until the coroner or medical examiner has completed any necessary postmortem examination. These devices may show the family that every effort was made to keep the patient alive. A family member may need to be left alone for a few moments with the body of the deceased. A staff member may remain nearby, just outside the room, to be available for support. However, a few moments of privacy in such a situation are often highly valuable later, and no harm is done in such a situation.

Sending the survivor home

After the survivor has been told of the patient's death, someone should stay with him for the next 24 to 48 hours. Suicide is certainly a possibility for the survivor, especially the spouse who has been married for many years. Such a person should *never* go home alone. Survivors have been reported to have returned home to commit suicide within 48 hours. This is often prevented with support from another person, allowing ventilation of grief, expression of desperation, thoughts of suicide, and feelings of guilt. Verbally discussing such feelings tends to prevent people from acting on them. It is not necessary for a physician to tell such a person that he should not kill himself, but it is important that the person expresses the feelings of despair and even a suicide wish to someone else. The best response to self-destructive comments is "I can understand how you feel" or some similarly empathetic phrase. The components of survivor treatment are presented in the following list:

1. A charge nurse (or experienced nurse) calls the survivor when possible.
2. The survivor is brought to the emergency department by someone else.
3. The physician informs the survivor.
4. The survivor is allowed to see the body if requested.
5. The survivor is encouraged to discuss his grief and other feelings.

6. The survivor is sent home with someone or possibly admitted if his reaction is severe.
7. Follow-up calls are made, when possible, 24 hours later, 3 days later, 1 week later, and 1 month later.

Discussing the death with children

The survivor should be encouraged to discuss the death with any children who may be at home or with the family. A free and open discussion helps to encourage sharing of this emotional experience and helps to decrease the fantasy and distortion that children may produce. It is best to begin by asking the family how they plan to handle telling the children. The main goal is to encourage them not to lie or distort the truth to the children. Encouraging religious interpretations is fine. Assuring the children that everything was done to save the patient is important. Encouraging the family to have the children discuss their feelings without trying to change them is the most important issue. Telling the family members to ask the children how they feel and to allow and even encourage them to cry and express their grief is important.

The adult should also be encouraged to express his own sense of grief and loss in front of the children, rather than doing it privately. This allows children to do several things. For one thing they see a model for expressing grief, and they see it as an acceptable thing to do within the family. It also allows them to discuss their own fantasies, sometimes greatly distorted, with others who understand and can explain reality. Finally it allows the children to begin accepting the concept of death as reality. This is always a valuable step for children. The following are methods of approaching the subject of death with children.

1. Tell children of the death.
2. Encourage children to discuss their feelings and beliefs.
3. Correct distortions if necessary.
4. Allow children to see adults' grief.

Follow-up care

Superior hospital care of a grieving family member entails a series of telephone calls to the survivor following the death of a patient. Calls to a family member 24 hours, 3 days, 1 week, and 1 month later may be enormously helpful to the person surviving. The caller represents the institution as well as an individual. If emotional problems arise in the future, the survivor is much more likely to return to the emergency department for continued care when this kind of follow-up procedure is in effect. Follow-up protocol is probably rarely used in most emergency departments.

If a close family member (spouse, parent, child, etc.) has no friends, relatives, or anyone else to accompany him, the social service may be of help in finding someone to stay with the person. A severely distraught individual with no friends or family may even need hospitalization.

Supportive treatment

Immediate supportive treatment should begin with the family member of a dead patient. This person has a very high risk for future medical and psychiatric problems. It is common to find medical illnesses occurring in the relative of a recently deceased person. There is good evidence to show that a woman recently widowed, for instance, is more likely to die within the next few months than one who has not been widowed. The survivor needs to be warned that medical problems may occur in the next few months and that he should have medical attention available. He may be referred for a medical evaluation within a few weeks and told to be particularly watchful for any physical problems. Immediate medical treatment serves to reduce the aftereffects of the tragic event in the life of the survivor.

When devising a treatment plan for the bereaved, the mode of death must be taken into consideration. The patient may have committed suicide, been murdered, died in an accident, or died of medical complications. For example, if the patient died in an automobile accident, it is most important to determine who was driving and how the spouse or family member feels toward the driver, particularly if he were not killed. Sometimes a sense of rage or blame emerges, but these feelings can be dealt with in a realistic and open manner. This provides an excellent model for accepting one's own feelings and examining them fairly dispassionately in the future. The events surrounding any death should be brought up with the family member to see if he has any highly charged feelings in the matter.

The bereaved often feel guilty or abandoned and, therefore, feel anger and despair. These feelings should be dealt with as normal developments. The patient should not be falsely reassured but should be given permission to have these feelings. Telling the patient that these feelings are normal is more helpful than telling him that he should not have them. Over the next few months the feelings should fade, and more positive emotions should develop. The patient usually benefits from this prediction.

TRAINING PROGRAMS FOR STAFF

The staff of the emergency department should have an ongoing in-service training program. Such a program helps to meet the emotional and educational needs of the staff. Several of these programs can discuss specific patient deaths, the staff's overall management of the surviving family, and the staff's own reaction to death. These sessions could involve discussion of the staff's feelings about recent patient deaths and the policies and procedures for handling death in the emergency department. A prescribed period of time, such as 45 minutes or 1 hour, should be available and as uninterrupted as possible. It may be that compensation time should be given for those who come to such programs on off-duty hours or before their regular shift. This usually encourages better participation.

A group leader may be quite helpful and can easily be trained to facilitate this group experience. It is often helpful to have a group leader from outside, although a member of the staff can be trained for such a position. Staff members who are not allowed to discuss their feelings about death and other stressful events that occur in an emergency department frequently have more oblique difficulties. This situation is comparable to a pressure cooker where any weakness in the wall of the container eventually blows out. Such a situation causes seemingly irrational divisions within an emergency department staff and leads to less efficient and effective medical care. Staff turnover is increased when individual members are chronically unhappy.

The in-service training programs should help prepare the emergency department staff to handle the problems that arise when members of the family or close friends are told of the death of a patient. The types of emergencies that occur include hysteria, suicide, legal retaliation, drug abuse, alcohol abuse, future medical complications in survivors, and future psychiatric sequelae.

Hysteria

The person who has been told of the death of a close friend or relative may sometimes become "hysterical." This usually means that he screams, cries, thrashes about, falls to the floor groaning or moaning, generally makes a great deal of noise, and causes some disruption. This reaction is not necessarily a psychiatric problem but is a style of expressing grief. The most common reaction to this form of behavior is to prescribe a sedative, given intramuscularly, if necessary. In general, however, the patient is expressing grief even if it is loudly, and he benefits from this expression. A room that allows some privacy and does not disrupt the emergency department waiting room minimizes the overall disturbance. If medication is given, it should be a small dose of an antianxiety agent that has few complications or side effects. Suggestions, sympathy, and firm gentle handling of the survivor, however, usually overcome these disruptions much better than medication. The only effect medication usually has on such a distraught person is that of psychological suggestion through the dramatic use of a pill or "the needle." In certain cultures and among some types of personalities, screaming, crying, and thrashing about are normal demonstrations of grief. The staff's negative reaction to this demonstration probably stems from embarrassment.

Suicide

Suicide is something that must be a concern about anyone who has recently been told of the death of a loved one. If the patient begins speaking in an extremely negative way or intimates that he is considering self-destruction, the threat should be taken seriously. The patient should be asked about suicidal thinking and the means of self-destruction he has available. This patient should never be sent out of the emergency department alone and may require hospital admission. The family of the patient should be informed that he has suicidal thoughts; they can be enlisted as therapeutic allies. They should be encouraged to allow the patient to discuss suicidal thoughts with them over the next few days or weeks. An open discussion helps prevent withdrawal and suicidal rumination. Isolation and emotional withdrawal often result in repeated suicide attempts.

Retaliation

A relative of a deceased patient may threaten legal action for professional malpractice, reports to professional licensing boards, complaints to the hospital administrator, public disclosure in newspaper, or even (but rarely) physical harm to the medical staff. This is an attempt by the family member to project the blame onto the staff for the guilt he feels. Whenever such threats are made, the physician's best option is to sit down with the bereaved person and discuss his anger. The physician should listen calmly and not rebut each remark. After the person has thoroughly ventilated his anger, a calm, rational response, listing the types of medical treatment provided, is helpful. Under certain circumstances the family member even understands when heroic efforts have not been made to save the patient's life at any cost. Families of the terminally ill or mortally wounded usually respond positively to a discussion about sparing their loved one the pain and indignity of dying on a ventilator in the intensive care unit. The families generally appreciate not having to make such decisions. The discussion should be gentle, not harsh, and caring, not threatening. Taking a calm, professional, and thorough approach to this problem usually prevents retaliation. The most important aspect of the communication is to demonstrate to the bereaved that a concerned staff is available to listen and respond to their feelings. One of the most frequent causes of malpractice litigation and other retaliation in this situation is an apparent callous disregard for the bereaved family's feelings by the professional staff.

Drug abuse

The person accustomed to modifying his mental environment with drugs tends to opt for this solution to the pain of bereavement. Sometimes this solution is suggested by a physician; the resulting drug abuse then becomes iatrogenic. When possible, the patient should be given emotional support and counseling rather than drugs so that he can experience the normal stages of grief that eventually end in resolution and can return to his previous life-style and emotional state.

When the grieving patient comes in for care 6 months after a death and requests drugs, they should be withheld unless they are part of some clearly defined therapeutic program. The emergency physician is best advised to withhold these drugs under most circumstances.

Alcohol abuse

For some families and cultures alcohol is a part of the grieving process. The gathering of bereaving family and friends after the death may include drinking. Sometimes an open sharing of emotions results from a lessening of tension induced by the alcohol. These reactions are generally mediated by family tradition.

A real danger for each grieving individual, however, is that the use of alcohol may continue or escalate until a pattern of alcohol abuse develops. The emergency physician should have little hesitation in referring the patient for detoxification when such a pattern is detected sometime after the death of a relative or close friend.

Future medical complications in survivors

There is evidence to suggest that all people who have suffered a recent death in the family may benefit greatly from a thorough medical evaluation within a few weeks after the death. Physical illness like hypertension, ulcer disease, or diabetes may develop under the stress of grief. Survivors can be warned about this; it makes sense to most people. Careful subsequent followup evaluations by their physicians ensure optimal medical surveilance and management.

Guidelines for the immediate treatment of crises surrounding death

The most important aspect of a survivor treatment program is for emergency physicians to know that treatment should begin within 72 hours and ideally in the emergency department (p. 240). The patient is encouraged to talk about his feelings regarding the death of the loved one. "What is the most difficult aspect of this for you?" and "What was the person like?" are two helpful questions to start a discussion. The patient should be advised that working through grief takes time and that this does not make the patient odd or unusual. Medical evaluation and follow-up care are important and should be encouraged in the emergency department.

Generally, listening is difficult. It is much more tempting to do something than to listen to someone. In the listener feelings of boredom or fatigue may occur. This is a natural response to anyone who is suffering a severe emotional shock. It is a way of avoiding identification with the patient and, therefore, suffering a personal sense of depression and grief. Nonetheless, learning to listen provides a sense of compassion in a sometimes inhuman environment. Compassionate listening is a highly valuable skill. The technical aspects of the skill can be learned just as can any manual skill like suturing. The building of the skill begins with normal human compassion for the grief stricken and then remaining relatively silent while they talk.

DRUG TREATMENT

Drug treatment is rarely indicated in the emergency department when the bereaved are expressing emotion. Medication is often overused and is really used to treat the staff rather than the bereaved. All bereaved need to express their grief and work it through. In general, the more emotion that is expressed, the better it is for the patient, even though it may be embarrassing or irritating to the staff.

If a patient is unresponsive to the approaches described in this chapter, medication may be useful. An intramuscular medication has symbolic meaning to the person because it appears to be a dramatic way of changing behavior. In such a situation, hydroxyzine (Vistaril or Atarax) may be useful in low doses of 25 or 50 mg intramuscularly. These drugs provide mild sedation, are generally safe, and can be given in an injectable or oral form. A placebo should never be used, since this consciously and unconsciously encourages the staff of the emergency department to view the patient cynically and establishes trickery as a valid form of medical treatment.

GUIDELINES FOR TREATMENT OF CRISES SURROUNDING DEATH AND INDICATIONS FOR PSYCHIATRIC REFERRAL

1. Begin treatment within 72 hours. Ideally treatment of the bereaved should begin immediately within the emergency department with close follow-up.
2. It is important to recognize that the bereaved want to talk. They need to talk. They want to discuss their own feelings about the death of the relative. Talking to an anonymous person is often helpful and allows things to be said that otherwise might be screened out. Patients may need to review their own lives as a summing up process and an attempt to begin anew. They should be listened to without interruption.
3. Negative feelings that the bereaved hold need to be explored. However, this does not need to be done immediately. The bereaved should be given permission to have feelings of whatever kind but need not necessarily be guided toward the more negative feelings. As an example, if a person feels quite angry toward a spouse or loved one who has just died, he should be listened to carefully. Statements should be made to him that this is a normal feeling. It may be quite helpful to introduce the idea that in any loving relationship, both love and anger are normal feelings. This will allow subsequent emergence of other more positive feelings without experiencing guilt over these negative ones.
4. The emergency department staff members should remain voices of reason. They should be calm, reassuring, and assured. They should interpret medical information to the bereaved. They should maintain a sense of calm.
5. Medical evaluation and follow-up care should be recommended to the bereaved. The possibility of medical problems occurring in the survivor within 6 months is high. This fact can be related to the bereaved person, and he should be urged to get an appointment with his family physician.
6. False reassurance is useless when dealing with the bereaved. In fact, falsely reassuring the bereaved or predicting a bright future tends to cause the bereaved to doubt the credibility of the person saying these things. It is a tempting thing to do, but listening is much more helpful. No response is necessary when the bereaved express their fear or doubt about the future.
7. Working through grief takes 6 months to 1 year. This can be predicted to the bereaved person so that he will not feel that he is odd or unusual. Discussing some of the stages of grief may be worthwhile and may need to be repeated several times over the next few days or months.
8. Follow-up contact of the bereaved should be part of a good hospital emergency department. This can be done as a routine procedure by someone who is expert in this area.

Adapted from Shneidman, ES. *Death of man*. New York: Quadrangle, 1973.

LOSS OR TURNOVER OF STAFF

Many people have difficulty dealing with death, particularly in patients cared for intensively by the professional staff. If these feelings of loss and grief are not discussed and given credence, it is likely that there will be a higher turnover of staff. This is because strong feelings of guilt and anger, as well as questioning of medical judgment, must come out into the open, or they result in an increasing sense of frustration, impotence, and projected anger. The emergency staff, whose major training is geared toward *saving* lives, feels inadequacy or frustration when the patient dies. Rather than face feelings of inadequacy and frustration and work these through, staff members tend to resign. In their own mind they place the blame on the emergency department personnel or facility, rather than dealing with the actual stressful issues facing the entire staff.

SUMMARY

If family members and friends of a dead patient are approached in a therapeutic way, fewer emotional sequelae occur in the future. Fewer legal threats are made toward the emergency department personnel, and the hospital and emergency department receive the gratitude of the bereaved. The skills mentioned in this chapter are simple to teach and reap great rewards.

17 PSYCHIATRIC EMERGENCIES ENCOUNTERED IN DISASTERS

Disasters such as airplane crashes, floods, tornados, fires, or wartime attacks have left many physical and emotional scars on survivors. Disaster plans are frequently developed to be efficient; they are concerned with the medical and technical problems of disasters. Too often, however, the appropriate psychiatric care and treatment of survivors of these disasters are overlooked.

Disasters have been studied by psychiatrists for years. Investigators have looked at the responses to disasters by survivors, family members, volunteers, and professional staff helping the survivors. The psychiatric sequelae in all of these groups are significant. The concept of psychiatric ill effects from disaster was given legal credibility in 1974. A 13.5 million dollar lawsuit against a coal mining company was settled out of court. Approximately half of the settlement was based on "psychic impairment" claimed by the survivors of a flood caused by the collapse of a faulty dam built by the defendant company.[1]

The calamity was known as the Buffalo Creek flood. The physical impact of the flood was almost immediate. Within 15 minutes 125 persons were killed and 4000 were left homeless. Ninety percent of the survivors suffered disabling mental and emotional symptoms. Most of the symptoms included anxiety, depression, changes in personality and life-style, and developmental problems in children.

It has become clear that there are immediate and long-range effects that are important considerations when treating victims of disasters in the emergency department. Good medical intervention in the early stages of treatment helps prevent tremendously disabling sequelae in the survivors. Certain skills and techniques that can be learned by the emergency staff are useful in recognizing disaster participants like survivors and rescuers and their families who are at risk for future psychiatric problems.

EXPECTED REACTIONS TO DISASTER

Nearly all survivors of a disaster experience some psychological effects. Some of these effects are to be expected and can be considered a "normal" part of one's psy-

TABLE 17-1. Stages of psychological response to a disaster

Stage	*Time*	*Symptoms*
Psychic numbness	Hours to days	Apathy, interest in minute details, sluggishness, disorganization, difficult decision making
Depression	Few days to 18 months	Hopelessness, loss of identity
Anger	Months to years	Anger at those perceived to have caused disaster

chological adaptation to a massive stress. Survivors are generally quite reassured to learn about these predictable effects from their physician or from fellow survivors. The three basic stages of the reaction to a disaster are psychic numbness, depression, and rage.[2] These stages are outlined in Table 17-1.

The first phase is usually psychic numbing or emotional anesthesia. The survivor typically feels dazed and initially may feel no emotion whatsoever. The psychological goal in this early stage is to live through the experience. The theory behind this response is that the psyche has taken all the trauma it can, and the individual must immediately stop any further incoming emotional stimuli. This has been called *psychological conservation* by Titchner.[3] The patient experiencing this stage appears withdrawn, sluggish, or apathetic.

Sometimes patients who experience a sudden unexpected disaster become acutely concerned about minor details. One psychiatrist reports, for instance, that following a train accident in Great Britain many of the passengers (survivors) were observed wandering around quite concerned with the state of their clothing and whether or not they would be able to go to work with torn clothing.[4]

In the emergency setting these patients seem excessively concerned about details like minute aspects of their appearance, finding a lost article of clothing, or having a meal. They seem to ignore the enormity of the experience and in so doing protect themselves from further emotional trauma.

The psychic numbing phase typically lasts for moments to several days immediately after the event. During this period the survivors find that they are disorganized and have difficulty in decision making. As the survivors emerge from the "anesthesia" they may experience emotional lability and have difficulty controlling their emotions.

The second stage is typically one characterized by sadness or depression. The survivor begins to realize the full impact of the disaster and the extent of social loss. In some cases the event causes complete disruption in the victim's social network and community.

Some victims are constantly reminded of their loss if the environment has been destroyed or altered in a drastic way. After a tornado, for instance, trees and buildings have been devastated throughout the community, and the survivors need only to look outside the window or walk through town to be reminded of the impermanence of their

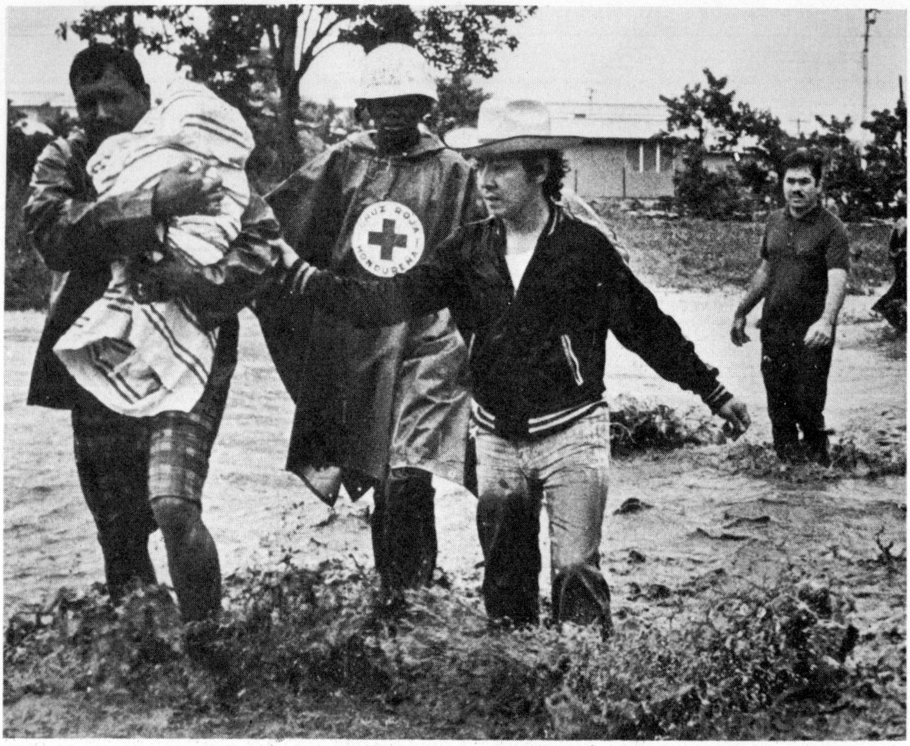

FIG. 17-1. Serious natural disasters can result in psychological injury to survivors. In September 1974 at San Pedro Sula, Honduras, Red Cross volunteers helped Hurricane Fifi victims evacuate to one of 63,000 storm shelters. Thirty-four National Red Cross Societies responded and sent teams of disaster personnel, food, clothing, radio equipment, and other supplies to stricken country. (LORCS photograph courtesy American Red Cross.)

community (Fig. 17-1). Such a realization predictably causes a sense of loss, sadness, and despair. This stage is usually most acute within the first few days following the disaster but may last as long as 24 months.[5]

A third stage of reaction following a disaster may be anger. The individual may experience feelings of rage, aggression, or retaliation. This reaction is especially prevalent if the event has been to some extent man-made, such as an airplane crash, the bursting of a man-made dam, or the entrapment of workers in a mine. Survivors or their relatives may continue to think obsessively of how they might retaliate against those who have caused the disaster. Such a reaction may go on for several months to years. When the individual becomes involved in litigation, the feelings are reinforced for the duration of the proceedings. When reactions become severe enough to cause the patient pain or bring him to the attention of a psychiatrist, a more serious condition may be present. Some of these conditions are listed in Table 17-2.

TABLE 17-2. Disorders seen after a disaster

Disorder	*Symptoms*	*Timing of appearance of symptoms*
Posttraumatic stress disorder	Reexperiencing the trauma	Acute type—immediate, lasting no more than 6 months Delayed type—6 months after disaster, lasting longer than 6 months
Organic mental disorder	Malnutrition, dehydration, infection, unavailability of usual medication, other untreated medical illness	Soon after or concurrent with rescue
Conversion disorder	Loss of sensory and voluntary motor system (blindness, etc.)	Immediate to several days
Obsessive compulsive disorder	Unpleasant persistent thoughts, images, or impulses	Immediate to weeks
Anxiety disorder	Jittery, tense, hyperactivity, hypervigilance	Immediate to days

Specific disorders

Posttraumatic stress disorder. The posttraumatic stress disorder is a syndrome of emotional and psychological response to a traumatic event. The event must be one so extraordinary that it is outside the range of usual human experience. The event may be one of the following: a natural disaster like a flood, tornado, or earthquake; military combat; human torture; a terrorist bombing; an airplane accident; or a prolonged experience in a death camp. More common traumatic stressors for patients frequently treated in emergency departments include sexual assault, mugging, or serious motor vehicle accidents. These incidents are more likely to bring patients to the emergency department each day. The more serious natural or man-made disasters that result in the posttraumatic stress syndrome can cause significant stress for both patient and staff. Events that may be stressful but do not fall outside the range of normal human experience do not qualify as causes of the posttraumatic stress disorder. Such common stresses include divorce, job change or loss, death of a spouse, or serious medical illness. When the patient has a maladaptive response (interferes with job, family or social life or causes pain) to one of the more common life stressors, the disorder is termed *adjustment disorder*.

The posttraumatic syndrome seems to be most severe when the traumatic event is a stress caused by other human beings or purposefully inflicted pain. Torture victims, for instance, commonly experience the syndrome, whereas victims of automobile accidents experience it much less often. A major feature of the disorder involves reexperiencing the event in various ways that include recollections, dreams, and reliving of the stressful moments.

DIAGNOSTIC CRITERIA FOR POSTTRAUMATIC STRESS DISORDER

A. Existence of a recognizable stressor that would evoke significant symptoms of distress in almost everyone.
B. Reexperiencing of the trauma as evidenced by at least one of the following:
   1. Recurrent and intrusive recollections of the event
   2. Recurrent dreams of the event
   3. Sudden acting or feeling as if the traumatic event were reoccurring because of an association with an environmental or ideational stimulus
C. Numbing of responsiveness to or reduced involvement with the external world, beginning some time after the trauma, as shown by at least one of the following:
   1. Markedly diminished interest in one or more significant activities
   2. Feeling of detachment or estrangement from others
   3. Constricted affect
D. At least two of the following symptoms that were not present before the trauma:
   1. Hyperalertness or exaggerated startle response
   2. Sleep disturbance
   3. Guilt about surviving when others have not, or about behavior required for survival
   4. Memory impairment or trouble concentrating
   5. Avoidance of activities that arouse recollection of the traumatic event
   6. Intensification of symptoms by exposure to events that symbolize or resemble the traumatic event

From American Psychiatric Association. *Diagnostic and statistical manual of mental disorders* (3rd ed.). Washington, D.C.: The Association, 1980, p. 238.

The patient may have recurrent, painful, and severe recollections of the event in dreams or nightmares during which it is reexperienced. In rare instances there are dissociative-like states, lasting from a few minutes to several hours or even days, during which components of the event are relived. The individual behaves as though he were experiencing the event at that moment. This can be seen occasionally in combat veterans who may suddenly grab a rifle, pistol, or knife, go out in the streets of the community, and behave as though they were back in South Vietnam fighting the war. This phenomenon may also occur in a woman who hears noises in the house or someone walking behind her and relives a sexual assault or in someone who hears a loud crash and remembers a serious automobile accident. Someone who has been through an avalanche or earthquake may hear thunder or another loud noise and respond by running out of doors or down to the basement, as though the disaster were happening again. A patient who hears the gentle rain of a summer storm may relive a terrible flood.

Patients who react to certain things that simulate the original stress may go to great lengths to avoid the stimuli. A victim who has been sexually assaulted inside the house, for instance, dreads being inside and fears being alone. The victim attacked outside prefers to be safely inside behind a locked door. Nightmares about the event may be extremely disturbing. Through the dreams the patient relives the trauma repeatedly and may wake up screaming. Disturbance of middle sleep or end sleep is a common result.

With psychic numbing or emotional anesthesia (defined earlier in this chapter) the patient shows diminished responsiveness to the external world. He may complain of feeling detached or strange and different from other people or that he has lost the ability to become interested in previously enjoyed activities. He frequently complains about the inability to feel emotions of any type, especially tenderness or sexuality. This numbness, following severe emotional trauma, should not be confused with major depression. The emotional coolness and detachment can cause significant impairment in a marriage. The unaffected spouse can easily feel hurt, unloved, and rejected.

This aspect of the disorder may be severe. The impairment may affect every part of the patient's life. He may be unable to work, or he may find his family life disrupted because of his own behavior. Intimacy is difficult, and a sense of "why bother?" pervades the patient's life.

Other symptoms of posttraumatic stress disorder may be present. Patients may appear hyperalert and vigilant. They show exaggerated responses to stimuli. This is particularly noticeable in combat veterans. They may be jittery, jumpy, and extremely nervous. Some patients have difficulty falling asleep or suffer impaired sleep or early awakening. They may complain about impaired memory and difficulty in concentrating or about having strong feelings of guilt at having survived.

Acute and chronic posttraumatic stress disorder. The posttraumatic stress disorder may be acute or chronic (delayed). The acute type has an onset of symptoms within 6 months and a duration of symptoms of less than 6 months. The chronic type has an onset of symptoms at least 6 months after the trauma and a duration of symptoms for more than 6 months.

Symptoms of posttraumatic stress disorders usually begin during and immediately after the disaster. Symptoms occasionally emerge after a period of months or years following the disaster. This is particularly true of responses to wars occurring in veterans many months or years after they have returned home. Symptoms that do not appear for several months after the event or that last longer than 6 months suggest a poor prognosis.

Organic disorder. Following a disaster, the diagnosis of an organic mental disorder must be ruled out because many people involved in disasters have suffered physical insult like head injury. Malnutrition, vitamin deficiency, and untreated medical illness and infection may be present in the victim, depending on the circumstances and duration of the disaster.

Conversion disorder. Conversion disorder is sometimes seen following disasters and involves the loss of a sensory or voluntary motor system without evident organic cause. A loss of function may not correspond to known anatomical pathways or pathological mechanisms. An example of conversion disorder might be blindness, paraplegia, or paralysis of the hand following a disaster. These symptoms usually occur immediately after the event or within a few days. Once organic disorder has been ruled out, immediate treatment should begin. For the psychiatrist the use of hypnosis or amobarbital (Amytal) is quite valuable in diagnosing and treating the patient with conversion disorder precipitated by severe emotional trauma. Psychiatric consultation should be obtained early in the patient's evaluation and management.

Obsessive compulsive disorder. The obsessive compulsive disorder that may develop in survivors of trauma usually involves unpleasant and persistent thoughts, images, or impulses. Typical impulses include an almost uncontrollable desire to scream out or a need to perform rituals like lining up one's shoes before going to bed, arranging personal items on the dresser in a certain way, or checking doors and locks repeatedly before going to sleep. These reactions are *ego dystonic* to the patient, which means that they cause him discomfort; they are not part of what he perceives to be his personality. The patient does not know why he is feeling these things or having these thoughts. He may have recurrent images of the disaster. Obsessive compulsive symptoms occur immediately to within several weeks following the disaster.

Anxiety. Anxiety is obviously a common problem following a disaster. Patients may feel jittery, tense, and nervous. They may experience an increase in autonomic activity with sweating, hyperventilation, and elevated blood pressure. They may appear to be hypervigilant and constantly scanning the room as though fearful of attack. These symptoms usually occur immediately to within a few days after the disaster. Since elements of anxiety occur in many patients following a disaster, only those who are severely anxious may require treatment.

Medical illness associated with stressful events. Disasters are as stressful as any event can be. There is a well-documented increase in incidence of various medical illnesses following stressful events. For example, British physicians noted increased morbidity from perforated peptic ulcer following the World War II bombing of London and a 50% increase in the death rate as a result of malignant tumors among survivors of the Bristol floods.[6] After hurricane Agnes roared through Pennsylvania, there was an increase in physical symptoms in the survivors who then sought medical treatment.[7] Women suffered more physical symptoms and continued to have them longer than their husbands.

The relationship between stressful events and medical illness is well known, and actuarial tables that show a link between clusters of stressful life events (good and bad) and physical illness have been developed.[8] The magnitude of the stress is generally proportional to the severity of the physical illness.

Dynamics (causes)

Disasters can be devastating events for the psyche. The survivor realizes in a vivid and forceful way that life is fragile and that all things can be instantly destroyed. When interpreted in a personal way, survivors and rescue workers realize that they can be separated instantly from loved ones. Abandonment, impermanence, and a feeling of fragility result.

The immediate possibility of death brought about by an awesome natural event generates great psychological needs. The treatment team becomes truly expert when the professionals acknowledge their own needs in the event, yet are able to go beyond the strict medical management and pay attention to the victim's psychological needs.

The survivor predictably does several things to protect himself from feelings of complete and utter annihilation. One common reaction is to project anger at anyone available. The victim tends to blame others for the disaster. Sometimes prolonged anger results in lawsuits against anyone presumed to be responsible for the event. Anger and retaliation sometimes make the patient feel that he is mastering his future fate and that he is on a rational course once again.

Some survivors change their memories of the event or block it out almost entirely. They frequently distort the details concerning the disaster or have trouble remembering the specific sequence of events. The survivors may dream about the disaster for several weeks or months. Sometimes the dream's outcome is better than that of the real event. Survivors tend to be quite reluctant to enter any situation that stimulates or increases their level of excitement. They may explain this "dampening" of emotional response by saying, "It is better to live without hope than not to live at all."

Survivors may feel a sense of dehumanization; the individual is merely a pawn of fate. The result of such an attitude is a sense of hopelessness that can become a deeply ingrained personality trait for many years.

Characteristics

Certain general characteristics of the disaster influence the psychological response of the survivors.[1] Characteristics that seem to be important in this regard include suddenness, unexpectedness, irresponsibility of other persons, pain inflicted intentionally by another human being, a preventable disaster, isolation of the community, and the extent of destruction.

When the event is gradual and predictable, persons seem to have more time to build up psychological deficiencies in anticipation of its occurrence. When the event is sudden and unexpected, however, the individual is shocked. When the dam collapses and the valley is immediately destroyed by a flash flood, the psychological impact is far worse than if the town floods gradually from weeks of heavy rain.

When preventable disasters seem to have been caused by another's irresponsibility or negligence, the result generates considerable bitterness within the survivor. An explosion in a coal mine, for instance, caused by correctable factors that the company knew about is harder on the survivor than a mine accident caused by an earthquake.

If the environment is totally devastated and the victim remains in the area, there is a continuing reminder of the event. Landscape around the community that remains flattened and scarred tends to create a longer illness than the environment that is returned to normal fairly quickly. A disaster area that is geographically isolated tends to result in prolonged symptoms more than one that is a part of a larger, undamaged community.

Management

The dynamics of disaster reactions provides clues to their management. Treatment plans can be considered in the following three categories: immediate, intermediate, and long-term (Table 17-3).

Immediate treatment. The immediate psychiatric treatment of a disaster victim is the most important aspect of the patient's treatment for the emergency phsycian. It is also the most crucial to the patient's subsequent recovery because the events are fresh in his mind, and he has not yet dampened his emotional responses to the event or repressed his recollection.

Active listening. Active listening with concern and sympathy for the patient is by far the most effective first step in the management of stress reactions. Active listening means that the physician or staff member encourages the patient to recall the events of the disaster and put names to visual images. The recollection of the event brings up painful memories of helplessness, separation, or fear of death. The survivor must be encouraged to describe his feelings in detail. The flood victim, for instance, must be encouraged to describe how the water rose, what structures were destroyed in what sequence, how others reacted, and what specific feelings were generated. This process usually requires that the patient repeat the recollections several times. By becoming involved once again in the event, the patient becomes more of an active participant than a passive victim, and this provides an avenue for healing and growth. Repeated remembering, naming, and talking about the details of the event gradually give the patient a sense of mastery over the situation.

It is unlikely that the emergency physician can do much of the active listening; the department is responding to a disaster in which the patient load is greater than normal. The skill of active listening can be fairly easily taught to aides, orderlies, clergy, administrators, or other volunteers. Such training may be carried out in advance as part of

TABLE 17-3. Treatment of survivors of a disaster

Immediate	Practice active listening with concern
	Encourage reliving and describing the experience
	Discuss feelings the patient had during the disaster
	Encourage labeling of recollections and feelings
	Stimulate repetition of story
	Prescribe no drugs
	Keep survivors together
Intermediate	Encourage survivors to use their experience to teach others
	Refer to agencies for support (give victims a list and make appointments)
Long-term	Make routine follow-up appointments
	Maintain a regular counseling schedule
	Recommend psychotherapy

the overall disaster response plan of the hospital. If the physician or nurses have time, they may be able to initiate the process.

Empathy. One of the most important aspects of care for the disaster victim is an empathetic or concerned attitude toward the victim. Since the proper treatment provides a corrective emotional experience, the patient must sense that people in the helping profession still care about him. The human link must be preserved, but this is often difficult because the staff's own feelings may come into play. It is usually quite difficult to face the enormity of a massive disaster against which we are impotent. To avoid these feelings we tend to become mechanized and focus on the strict medical management of the case.

Avoidance of medications. Drug treatment should be avoided when possible. Alcohol and drug abuse are traditional human responses to disasters because these agents lower the victim's anxiety. The result, however, is not a therapeutic reexperiencing of feelings and events of the disaster, but denial and drug dependence. Since there may be many survivors, a drug-prescribing response could mean that a large number of patients would begin using antianxiety agents. Drugs are hardly an alternative to a process of working through the difficulties, and they provide a poor model for future responses to stress.

Keeping survivors together. The survivors should not only be allowed to talk to one another, they should be encouraged to do so. The contact with other survivors allows the patient to see that his own reactions are quite common and shared by others in the same situation. The survivor can discuss feelings of fear, helplessness, impotence, and guilt openly and share these feelings with a sympathetic group. The group discussion may persist for some time after leaving the hospital. Children should not be separated from their parents if possible. The children must be encouraged to express their feelings and perceptions of what happened. Keeping the group together may also speed the development of positive attitudes like planning to repair the damage and reconstruct the community.

Patients with previous psychiatric illness. The manifestations of preexisting psychiatric illness may be suppressed, and patients have symptoms typical of the posttraumatic stress reaction. Their previous symptoms may recur, however, within 12 to 48 hours following the disaster.

Intermediate treatment or referral. Since it is usual for survivors to have psychiatric sequelae,[9] most of these patients should at least be provided with instructions for seeking appropriate psychiatric counseling. Most of them should plan to attend at least one counseling session. When the referral agency or office is informed in advance, the patient can be notified if several days elapse without any contact. As in the immediate management of these patients, the earlier the follow-up appointment, the more beneficial the counseling is, since the emotions associated with the disaster are still alive.

Another feature of intermediate treatment is the assurance of adequate social support. Most persons are supported by a social network that includes their family, friends, work associates, and church groups. For survivors of a disaster, community agencies may need to be involved as well. The social service office of the hospital should be able to work out some referral details well in advance so that the patient's social supports are maintained. Social workers may also need to help survivors find temporary housing, food, and perhaps government disaster aid for temporary subsistence.

Long-term management. Long-term psychiatric management of these patients continues the basic treatment strategy initiated in the emergency department. It involves attentive listening, empathizing, and maintaining a human link with the survivor. Psychotherapy may be needed to regularly reinforce reality and the survivor's strength to deal with the loss and go on. Regular appointments are important for patients who seem severely impaired.

EFFECTS OF DISASTER ON RESCUE WORKERS AND MEDICAL STAFF

People who have worked with disaster survivors often find the development of some symptoms of the posttraumatic stress disorder among themselves. They may have decreased concentration, feelings of irritability, depression, fatigue, and a sense of hopelessness about life. The symptoms may be most intense in those who are actively involved in the rescue effort at the scence. The syndrome has developed in rescue teams that have been involved in sifting through the remains of aircraft wreckages, for example. The symptoms generally develop within a few days or weeks following the rescue efforts. The syndrome is treated in a way similar to the treatment of the survivor. The worker should be encouraged to relive and relate the experience and to place names with feelings and images. Empathy and concern from the active listener provide emotional support. Some sort of continuing psychological counseling may be necessary. Because the syndrome may develop in certain rescue workers, it might be appropriate to routinely provide some sort of psychological support for front-line workers who have directly aided the victims. In-service sessions in the emergency department could accomplish similar goals for the emergency staff.

SUMMARY

Mental and emotional problems arc quite common in both survivors and rescue workers following a disaster. Most survivors are stunned or dazed (75%), some panic (12% to 25%), and a few remain capable of effective actions (12% to 25%).[10] The immediate psychiatric treatment of these individuals is extremely important because the intervention comes at a time when the memory and emotional impact of the disaster is fresh in their minds. During this early stage the mainstay of treatment is active listening and empathizing. Survivors are encouraged to stay together and relate their feelings to one another. The group may elect to meet subsequently for mutual reinforcement. Psychological and social resources should then be made available to the survivors. Psychiatric hospitalization is rarely necessary. Early intervention by the emergency staff or trained volunteers should be enormously helpful in preventing future emotional pain, psychiatric impairment, and medical illness that develops in survivors of a major disaster.

REFERENCES

1. Lifton, RJ and Olson, E. The human meaning of total disaster. *Psychiatry*, Feb. 1976, *39*, 1-17.
2. Rangell, L. Discussion of the Buffalo Creek disaster: the course of psychic trauma. *American Journal of Psychiatry*, March 1976, *133*(3), 313-316.
3. Titchner, JL, and Kapp, FT. Family and character change at Buffalo Creek. *American Journal of Psychiatry*, March 1976, *133*(3), 295-299.
4. Boman, B. Behavioral observations on the Granville Train disaster and the significance of stress for psychiatry. *Social Science and Medicine*, 1979, *13* (A), 463-471.
5. Gleser, G, Green, B, and Winget, C. Quantifying interview data on psychic impairment of disaster survivors. *Journal of Nervous and Mental Disease*, 1978, *166*(3), 209-216.
6. Kinston, W, and Rosser, R. Disaster: effects on mental and physical state. *Journal of Psychosomatic Research*, 1974, *18*, 437-456.
7. Logue, JN, Hansen, H, and Struening, E. Emotional and physical distress following Hurricane Agnes in Wyoming Valley of Pennsylvania. *Public Health Reports*, Nov.-Dec. 1979, *94*(6), 495-502.
8. Holmes, TH, and Rahe, R. The social readjustment rating scale. *Journal of Psychosomatic Diseases*, 1967, *11*, 213.
9. Sims, ACP, White, AC, and Murphy, T. Aftermath neurosis: psychological sequelae of the Birmingham bombings in victims not seriously injured. *Medical Science Law*, 1979, *19*(2), 78-81.
10. Kentsmith, DK. Minimizing the psychological effects of a wartime disaster on an individual. *Aviation, Space, and Environmental Medicine*, April 1980, *51*(4), 409-413.

18 PSYCHIATRIC PROBLEMS IN THE ELDERLY

In the past 10 years the overall number of elderly people living within our society has increased; the average person lives longer partly because the treatment for many serious diseases of the elderly has improved. In addition to this overall increase, changes in laws regarding commitment, competency, and the right to refuse treatment have resulted in the transfer of elderly persons from mental institutions to nursing homes and other facilities like "group homes" that usually do not provide psychiatric or medical services. For many elderly persons the emergency department thus constitutes their main source of care, especially "after hours" and on weekends.

Of the elderly population 20% to 30% show evidence of a psychiatric disorder; dementia and depression are the most common problems. The elderly patient is no different from younger individuals, however, in the respect that both can develop acute psychiatric or medical disturbances that may be superimposed on a chronic medical or mental condition.

Most acute psychiatric emergencies among the elderly are *not* the result of irreversible organic brain damage. Elderly patients with these behavioral disorders need aggressive investigation and acute care. An acute medical disorder must be suspected first and an acute psychiatric disorder second. Failure to consider acute and reversible causes of deterioration can result in unnecessary referrals to a chronic care facility or nursing home. The resulting temporary institutionalization can result in medical and/or psychological deterioration. If the patient survives such mismanagement, the temporary confinement often results in a premature permanent institutionalization of the elderly patient. A vicious cycle resulting in increased dependency and regression then develops. The final outcome is increased mortality and morbidity. Competent medical treatment and crisis intervention in these cases may prevent further deterioration and actually delay the onset of chronic dementia.[1]

There are many reasons why the elderly patient has difficulty getting emergency medical care. He is often indifferent to his own medical status; frequently the staff or the family also feels this way toward the elderly patient. These participants in the patient's care (including himself) may believe that he is going to die or that psychiatric illness is an expected consequence of old age.

EMERGENCY EVALUATION

A geriatric patient can present a confusing array of symptoms to the emergency physician. The patient may or may not be able to relate any significant history. The family or nursing home personnel who could relate a history may leave the patient at the hospital and return home. When the patient can give a history, it may be a long, rambling tale with frequent digression. This can be maddening to an emergency physician who feels the pressure of time. The emergency staff's predictable response is an outcry about nursing home transfer policies and the Friday night deposit of an elderly relative at the emergency department registration desk just before the weekend.

When the situation arises, it should be helpful to know that there are three major clinical portraits presented by elderly patients who appear to have mental or behavioral disorders. These three patterns are cognitive dysfunction, depressive disorder, and paranoid psychosis. Personality disorder may appear as an isolated ailment or in combination with one of the three major portraits just mentioned.

Cognitive dysfunction

If the patient has unimpaired senses and communication skills, it should be fairly easy to test rudimentary cognition in a simple mental status examination. The examination need not and cannot take all afternoon or evening to perform. The physician should be able to ask several questions in 1 or 2 minutes that determine the patient's impairment in the following areas:

Areas	Questions
1. Orientation	Do you know where you are? Do you know the month—the day?
2. Memory	Try to remember three things—a blue book, a red apple, a brown chair.
3. Intellect	Can you subtract 7 from 100?

Affect, judgment, and other components of the mental status examination can often be assessed during the patient's conversation. A sense of general intellectual functioning should be determined fairly easily and quickly during the initial interaction with the patient.

Dementia is one of the two most common mental disorders in the elderly. It is caused by various processes; the most common is Alzheimer's disease. Dementia can occur at any age from the 50s on. If it occurs before the age of 65, it is called presenile dementia, and if it occurs after the age of 65, it is called dementia. Dementia is a chronic process with a loss of intellectual abilities that interferes with social or occupational functioning. Actually it only occurs in about 10% of geriatric patients and is overdiagnosed so frequently that other causes of the dementia-like picture are overlooked. It is often, but not always, irreversible. Dementia may be quite apparent to the emergency physician soon after the patient's arrival, or it may be more subtle. The patient is often able to carry on social chitchat, but as soon as a few mental status questions are asked, he begins to become disorganized. Therefore brief mental status questions concerning orientation, memory, and intellectual functioning should be asked of all geriatric patients. Having made the diagnosis of dementia, the physician must discover if a second acute process has developed to cause further deterioration in the patient's mental or behavioral functioning.

Delirium is an acute process characterized by reversible interference with brain functioning and difficulty in focusing and sustaining attention. It differs from dementia in that the patient's attention shifts rapidly, as does his level of consciousness. The waxing and waning of symptoms of intellectual impairment should always alert the physician to delirium. Often patients can "hold it together" for brief periods and then become confused and rambling. They may appear more anxious partially because they have some insight into their own confusion. Demented patients, by contrast, may lose insight into their problem and, therefore, appear less anxious.

Medical illness

Delirium must be considered to be the result of an organic mental disorder (Table 18-1). Even minor illnesses can impair behavior and thinking in the elderly patient. A urinary tract infection that is well tolerated in a younger person can initiate mild delirium in the elderly. The mildly febrile elderly person may begin to hallucinate, especially at night. Confusion increases as the patient begins to misinterpret stimuli that normally serve an orienting function. A common concomitant feature of abrupt disorientation in the patient is a severe anxiety that develops when he cannot trust his perceptions. When these symptoms develop in a chronic care facility like a nursing home, they could erroneously be interpreted as a sign of senility and treated with an antipsychotic agent like haloperidol (Haldol) instead of being seen as signs of an organic disorder that requires evaluation with an adequate history, vital signs, physical examination, and urinalysis.

A respiratory infection is a notorious problem for the elderly patient because he sometimes lacks the inflammatory response mechanisms of the younger patient. The elderly patient may develop a pneumonia characterized only by mental changes, a mild fever, and perhaps a slight cough. The hypoxia that results from a pneumonia in the elderly patient causes confusion and agitation, but because he does not have bed-rattling chills, high fever, and rusty sputum, the diagnosis may be overlooked.

Congestive heart failure results in hypoxia and poor cerebral perfusion that can cause insomnia, agitation, and confusion. The patient with cardiac difficulties is often treated

TABLE 18-1. Causes of mental or behavioral disturbances in the aged

Category of stress	*Examples*
Medical illness	Congestive heart failure, respiratory insufficiency, infections, decrease in vision or hearing, drug toxicity, intracranial mass lesion, recent stroke, anemia, electrolyte imbalance, dehydration
Stressful life event	Relocation, robbery or assault, financial problems, loss of pet, death of family member or friend

with diuretics or has fluid loss from other sources, like diarrhea. He can develop severe electrolyte disturbances that produce mental and behavioral changes. Any older person with these acute changes deserves an evaluation of fluid and electrolyte status.

Occult bleeding can result in hypoperfusion and hypoxia in the elderly patient. The first indicators may be confusion and disorientation. Incontinence may be the result of the stimulating effect of blood in the gastrointestinal system; the patient may be passing melanotic stool. A rectal examination that includes testing for occult blood is important in the evaluation of the elderly patient who becomes delirious.

An acute neurological process can certainly produce mental and behavioral changes. A cerebrovascular accident is common in the elderly patient, and a focal neurological deficit may not be immediately apparent in a rather inactive person. Chronic subdural hematoma, cerebral neoplasia, hydrocephalus, or meningitis can produce mental and behavioral changes. A neurological examination is required for evaluation of the patient. A computerized tomography (CT) scan and even lumbar puncture should be strongly considered for the elderly patient with sudden deterioration in mental function. Sometimes decreases in vision or hearing cause confusion and obviously impair the patient's sensory input and ability to respond to questioning.

The patient's medication may be the cause of delirium. Medication side effects, dose-related toxicity, or drug interaction can cause all types of mental disturbances in the elderly patient, including confusion, paranoia, tactile and visual hallucinations, and combativeness. Nearly all medications are capable of producing side effects in some patients. Reserpine classically causes depression and may produce psychotic symptoms. Antianxiety agents like diazepam (Valium) and chlordiazepoxide (Librium) may also create psychotic behavior in the elderly patient. Antipsychotic agents like the phenothiazines may cause anxiety, insomnia, tachycardia, and psychosis in the geriatric patient. Bromide and methylphenidate (Ritalin) intoxication cause psychotic symptoms in the aged person. Cimetidine may also cause confusional states. Combinations of drugs often cause unpredictable psychiatric crises in the elderly patient. A few drugs that can cause psychiatric symptoms are listed in Table 18-2.

A thorough drug history unravels a sometimes complex pattern of medication for the

TABLE 18-2. Drugs that may precipitate an acute psychiatric emergency

General	*Psychotropic*
Hypoglycemic agents	Antipsychotic agents
Steroids	Antianxiety agents
Antituberculous agents	Sedatives
Sulfa drugs	Antidepressants
Penicillin	Antiparkinsonian agents, including L-dopa preparations
Anticholinergics	Anticonvulsants
Diuretics	General anesthetics
Reserpine	Alcohol

preceding months. Sometimes the patient increases the therapeutic dosages of medication or adheres to an inaccurate dosage schedule that provides more medication than needed. Dosages of many drugs must be adjusted in the elderly patient and in the person with impaired renal or hepatic function. A change in the patient's drug metabolism may follow the initiation of a new cause of medication or an illness that alters the patient's metabolic function. Since the patient may not be able to provide a lucid account, the history must often be obtained from family members, nursing home personnel, or even the emergency medical service team that brings the patient from his living quarters to the emergency department.

From the preceding discussion it should be clear that the emergency physician's first consideration in the evaluation of the elderly patient with acute mental or behavioral change must be that the alteration is caused by an acute medical illness, sensory impairment, or medication effect. The proper evaluation, therefore, includes a history of drug use as detailed as possible, a physical examination (including vital signs and rectal check), and appropriate laboratory tests that usually involve a complete blood count, electrolyte concentrations, glucose tolerance, blood urea nitrogen (BUN) level, and arterial blood gas levels. Other tests can include an electrocardiogram and chest radiograph. Occasionally a drug screen is necessary. A patient, for instance, who is ill enough to be hospitalized on a psychiatric service may give little information about possible drug intoxication. Another patient may have a history that suggests ingestion of excessive amounts of medication. The care of such patients is usually improved if drugs can be identified and quantified in specimens of urine and blood. Some authorities believe that these tests should always be part of the evaluation of a patient admitted to a psychiatric service. Because of the costs involved in such a routine, however, perhaps toxicology screening should be reserved for high-risk groups like those of the elderly who develop acute changes in behavior or thought.

Reaction to stressful events

Under the right circumstances cognitive dysfunction may also be associated with personal loss, separation, or relocation. The elderly patient is at high risk for stressful events for obvious reasons. He often suffers a decline in his financial, physical, and psychological resources. Friends and pets die, and family members may move away. These losses can cause a deterioration in the mental functioning of the geriatric patient and may precipitate an emotional crisis. The chief characteristic of such a crisis is disorganization severe enough to cause failure of the person's usual problem-solving techniques. If an elderly patient who is used to a structured routine becomes even mildly disoriented, a vicious cycle of fear, "adrenalin rush," physiological disequilibrium, disorientation, and increasing fear may develop. This usually occurs in a state of mild or very minimal senility or dementia that would not be a problem in a familiar and structured setting without stress. Some life events that may precipitate acute psychiatric emergencies in the elderly are listed on p. 259.

Relocation stresses the elderly tremendously. Movement of living quarters causes serious physical and emotional disorders in many patients. Several studies have demonstrated that relocation of old people results in high mortality. One study assessed the result of a fire in a geriatric ward that necessitated the relocation of patients. The mortality of the relocated patients was 20%; in the 3 months preceding the fire the death rate had been 7.5%. The authors concluded that the cause of the increased death rate was the disruption of the social milieu, separation, change of routine, and stressed emotional reactions of the caretakers.[2] Plasma cortisol levels in psychotic elderly patients stressed by relocation were higher than in the control group, and the cortisol levels of the relocated men were higher than those measured in the women.[3]

Relocation strsses elderly patients who have impairment of recent memory. They have difficulty adjusting to new places and lose the orienting stimuli provided by common paths to their usual activities. This loss and the resulting confusion cause acute and chronic anxiety, agitation, depression, and a sense of dislocation.

Robbery, assault, or the threat of either in old people brings about a severe sense of anxiety. The elderly often feel severely threatened by youthful pranksters or joking threats. Frequently seen after the assault or robbery of elderly persons is acute confusion, disorientation, and possibly severe depression. They may not be able to return to their living quarters for fear of reattack. Such patients may need to be moved to a different location. Sometimes psychotherapy is required. The object of the therapy is desensitization; the patients' fear must be controlled before there can be a return to previous levels of mental function.

Another common stressor of the elderly is financial concern. The elderly are at great risk for severe financial difficulty, and the stress of economic worries added to their preexisting confusion can precipitate severe depression or anxiety. Even minor financial problems may seem to balloon into insurmountable debt for older persons. Social service counseling regarding these issues must be undertaken at once to prevent a spiraling sense of anxiety, fear, and disorganization. Financial concerns may form the basis of psychotic delusions; for example, patients with financial problems may become paranoid and believe that others are taking money from them. They may suspect that their children are trying to take away their house or that a neighbor is stealing from them. Questions such as the following may be helpful in discovering some of the more common stresses that can affect the elderly.

1. Has the patient been moved from his room or usual living quarters recently?
2. Has the patient been robbed or assaulted recently?
3. Does the patient have financial problems?
4. Has the patient lost a pet recently?
5. Have their been deaths or illnesses in the family or among friends recently?
6. Are relatives visiting the patient as often as they did previously?

Management of cognitive dysfunction, medical illness, and reaction to stressful events. The proper treatment of cognitive dysfunction depends on the underlying cause. Medical illnesses are managed appropriately, and the patient's medications are adjusted as needed.

Problems that involve a major life stress are sometimes best handled by the hospital or community social service agency. Problems like these constitute some of the best reasons for having 24-hour social service coverage or a separate psychiatric–social service component of the emergency department. When the patient lives in a nursing home, the social service offices of that home can be contacted to help him deal with the life stresses effectively.

More personal attention and involvement of the family would be helpful. This kind of intervention may be enough to get the patient reoriented and cause gradual improvement over the next 2- to 3-day period. If the patients symptoms do not clear, he should return to the emergency department for consideration of more intensive evaluation, including a brief hospitalization.

A low dose of haloperidol, such as 2 mg at bedtime, may be helpful in getting the patient back to normal. It is important to be sure that this order is written for 2 to 3 days only. It is common that once an order is written, it continues forever on an elderly patient's chart.

Paranoid psychosis

Elderly patients can suddenly develop persecutory delusions or vivid auditory or visual hallucinations. At the other extreme they may become withdrawn. Patients who become delusional and fearful, believing that others are trying to harm them, may develop outbursts of belligerence in an attempt to protect themselves. The rapid development of agitation associated with paranoid psychosis generally causes great concern among patients' families or nursing home workers. The result of their concern is often a trip to the emergency department, particularly during the nighttime hours. Medications, especially those taken to induce sleep can cause behavioral storms during the night, and patients with underlying organic pathologies can become agitated and paranoid at night when their orienting stimuli are removed. The latter patients are often called *sundowners*.

Treatment. When the patient's medication seems to be the cause of the disturbed behavior, it can be stopped temporarily at least until the individual sees his regular physician. Hypoxia is a well-recognized cause of agitation, and the patient with chronic lung disease and sudden agitation should be evaluated by obtaining an arterial blood gas level and a chest x-ray film. The treatment may require low flow oxygen and bronchodilators. The elderly patient who develops pneumonia is at great risk and may experience severe hypoxia. Such a patient requires hospital admission and aggressive management.

The paranoid, suspicious, belligerent, or withdrawn patient can be treated quickly with antipsychotic medication. Haloperidol or thiothixene (Navane) may be used in small doses. Administration of either of these medications results in the rapid disappearance of paranoid thinking with its resultant bizarre behavior. Haloperidol may be given in an initial dosage of 0.5 to 1.0 mg two or three times a day. After this medication is initiated, the patient should be reevaluated in 12 to 24 hours. At no time should this medication be ordered without defining a time to stop it. The patient could conceivably return to the nursing home from the emergency department and continue taking the prescribed medication indefinitely. Any such orders should be written for no more than 72 hours under most circumstances. If the hallucinations, delusions, and other symptoms of a paranoid psychosis do not disappear within 2 or 3 days, further psychiatric evaluation is needed.

Depressive disorder

Depression is one of the most common problems of the aged. It has been estimated that as many as 20% of patients in nursing homes are debilitated because of severe depression. These patients may have been misdiagnosed and may still be able to recover with treatment if the correct diagnosis is made. Depressed elderly patients usually experience fatigue, listlessness, constipation, and decreased appetite. They typically have disturbed sleep and may actually appear to be quite sad. Their sadness may be overlooked by a young, healthy caretaker who believes that anyone would be sad about being that old. Even brief conversations with those severely depressed may reveal sad content or themes. They have recurrent thoughts of death, illness, and hopelessness. They see their lives as futile and separation from their families as lonely and unending.

Depression is so common in the elderly that this type of conversation may be heard often. It is not the ordinary picture of the elderly, however, and such patients may be helped significantly by proper treatment.

Management

Activity. Depressed elderly patients should be encouraged to increase their activities. Increased mobility and social interaction can be promoted at patients' nursing homes by activities directors, social services workers, or administrators. The expansion of patients' activities is easier once the full effects of antidepressant medications are seen.

Medications

Antidepressants. The tricyclic antidepressants most frequently prescribed for depression in the elderly are doxepin (Sinequan), amitriptyline (Elavil), and imipramine (Tofranil). Amitriptyline is quite sedating and should be tried after doxepin has been attempted. If the patient is "knocked out" with a relatively small dose of amitriptyline, for instance, he may be resistant to any other kind of medication and, therefore, noncompliant.

In the elderly population tricyclic antidepressants should be initiated at low doses, such as 25 or 50 mg at bedtime. The clinical effects of these medications must be monitored quite carefully in elderly patients. Hospitalization may be necessary to provide this kind of close scrutiny. As the dosage of tricyclic antidepressants is raised to appropriate therapeutic levels (generally between 75 to 200 mg per day), serial electrocardiograms (ECGs) and repeated clinical examinations help monitor the effects of the medication. Flattened T waves, prolonged QT intervals, and depressed ST segments are effects that have been seen in patients taking therapeutic doses of tricyclics. A prolonged QRS complex (greater than 100 m per second) usually indicates toxicity. When this is noted, the drug should be stopped, and the patient probably needs to be hospitalized. Adverse cardiac side effects seem to be more prominent in patients who have preexisting cardiovascular disease. A tricyclic antidepressant should be prescribed for a short, limited period like 4 to 6 weeks. If no improvement is noted after that period, psychiatric hospitalization should be considered.

Antipsychotics. Antipsychotics are occasionally useful for the patient who is agitated or so depressed that psychotic symptoms are present. An antipsychotic agent like haloperidol should be given in a relatively low dosage, such as 0.5 to 1.0 mg once or twice a day. The elderly patient does not seem to require as large a dosage of antipsychotic agents as does the younger patient. A typical elderly patient who might benefit from an antipsychotic agent is the one who is agitated, tearful, and not sleeping through the night. A small dose of an antipsychotic drug in such a patient encourages orientation and reduces agitation. It is often enough to get the patient "back on track." No additional medication may be needed. If significant improvement in symptoms does not develop in several days, the medication should be discontinued, and the patient should be reevaluated. A course of antidepressant therapy is usually required at this point.

Personality disorders

Personality disorders do not develop in the elderly patient, since they represent a lifelong pattern of interpreting and responding to the rest of the world. A previous disorder may, however, become troublesome in old age because of changes in the environment that no longer enable the patient to function properly, the emergence of an additional medical or psychological problem that highlights the personality disorder, or an exaggeration of the maladoptive personality characteristics in response to severe stresses. In many people a personality disorder (like antisocial personality) tends to improve with aging. The antisocial patient over 40 years of age is much less likely to commit a violent crime than the younger patient, for instance. The more stable disorders like obsessive compulsive disorder may become worse with age. The patient may develop symptoms of depression or paranoia. Treatment may help him live with less conflict in the nursing home. No dramatic change should be expected with psychotherapy.

Management

Crisis intervention. Depressed elderly patients do not always require medication. In one study[1] the most common diagnosis in patients referred for crisis intervention was depression. Delirium or dementia occurred in 17% of these patients. Schizophrenia or paranoid states comprised only 8% of the referrals. Of the patients referred for crisis intervention 20% required no medication at all. Tricyclic antidepressant agents (31%) and lithium carbonate (6%) were cited as the most frequent medications used in the treatment of depressed patients.

Crisis intervention focuses on the patient's immediate problems and provides a framework for the solutions or adaptations to new limits imposed by the difficulties. For the severely depressed patient crisis intervention is a necessary adjunct to antidepressant medication. For the mildly depressed patient either drug therapy or crisis intervention may provide sufficient treatment.

Other medications. Certain drugs are not helpful in depression and may actually worsen the illness. Hypnotics are included in this group. Agents like secobarbital or chloral hydrate may be requested by the patient or nursing home staff to help induce sleep. These agents do not alleviate the underlying depression, however, and may further decrease the patient's ability to orient himself. They can also worsen his sense of confusion and turmoil.

Target symptoms. Because the elderly patient is difficult to diagnose and treat and

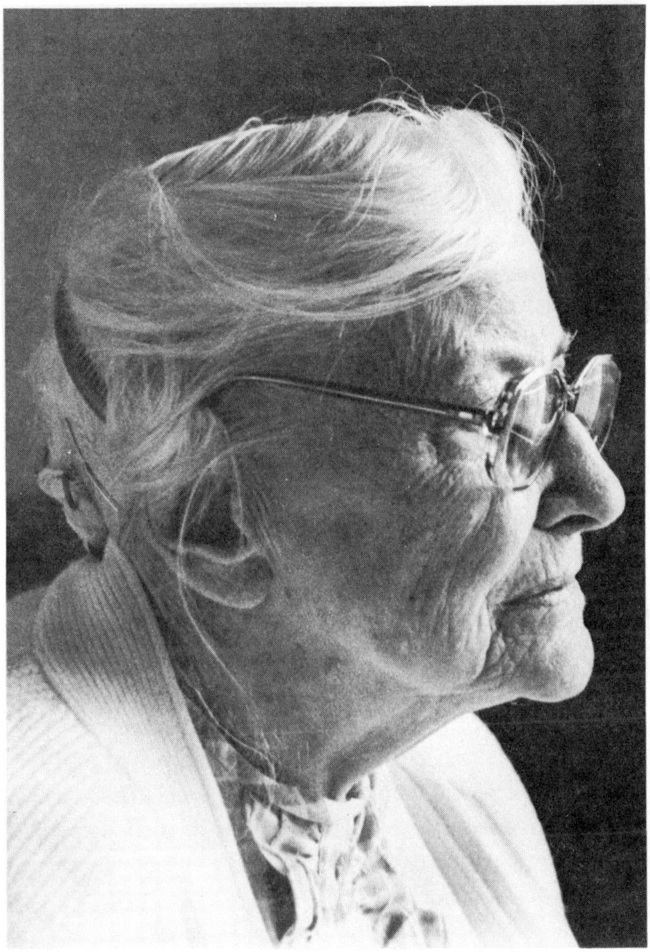

FIG. 18-1. Elderly patients can have numerous organic and functional causes for mental illness. They are at risk for serious medical disease that manifests as mental disorder, and they are at risk for major life stresses, depression, and dementia, which are problems of elderly. (Courtesy Lee Jansen, Columbus, Ohio.)

acute and chronic medical problems are often combined with a social and psychiatric problem, it is most helpful to identify certain target symptoms that seem to cause greater disability for the patient than others. A fairly good target symptom for the depressed patient is lack of sleep. The patient with sleep disturbance may remain awake at night or awaken in the middle of the night and be unable to get back to sleep. The patient or nursing staff can generally be fairly precise about this symptom, and an improvement in the depression should follow a positive change in the sleep pattern.

Hospitalization. There is a negative side to early hospitalization of the elderly patient. Once admitted to the hospital, he tends to stay there for long periods. Since the patient is likely to have several medical problems as well as psychiatric problems, the inhospital evaluation may be prolonged as consultants are called and tests are scheduled. In addition, the patient's social environment outside the hospital may not seem ideal; the inhospital setting may seem preferable. Hospitalization, however, takes away the patient's independence. As he becomes increasingly dependent on the hospital, there is a tendency for him to regress psychologically, and he may actually experience a higher risk of morbidity and mortality. Prolonged hospitalization and aggressive social treatments, such as early declaration of incompetence and guardianship, may exert a negative effect on the patient's well-being. If hospitalization is considered, it should be as brief as is realistically possible.

SUMMARY

A behavioral problem in the elderly patient is too often diagnosed as being "a natural result of old age." The least satisfactory outcome of such a stereotype results when the patient is routinely sedated and returned to his private or nursing home. Careful clinical examination generally reveals a medical illness that explains or contributes to the behavioral abnormalities in about half of these patients.[1]

The medical history must include questions about the patient's medication. The physical examination need not be inordinately long but should screen for obvious neurological signs or evidence of respiratory or circulatory difficulty. An evaluation for sepsis and a rectal examination to determine sphincter tone, prostatic enlargement, or occult gastrointestinal bleeding should be made. Routine laboratory screening tests and perhaps blood levels of selected medications may be indicated.

If a basic physical assessment does not reveal the underlying cause for the problems, the physician must look for precipitating events. If a psychiatric picture is the result of separation, loss, financial problems, relocation, or other similar stresses, crisis intervention may be undertaken in the emergency department and continued on an outpatient basis or in the patient's nursing home.

Premature hospitalization often results in increased confusion and an exacerbation of psychiatric symptoms. The emergency department is the most important place for this type of patient to receive excellent medical evaluation and treatment. These patients often respond dramatically to crisis intervention and brief medical intervention.

REFERENCES

1. Grauer, H, and Frank, D. Psychiatric aspects of geriatric crisis intervention. *Canadian Psychiatric Association Journal,* 1978, *23*(4), 201-207.
2. Aleksandrowicz, DR. Fire and its aftermath on a geriatric ward. *Bulletin of the Menninger Clinic,* 1961, *25,* 23-32.
3. Kral, VA, Grad, B, and Berenson, J. Stress reactions resulting from the relocation of an aged population. *Canadian Psychiatric Association Journal,* 1968, *13,* 201-209.

19 THE EMERGENCY DEPARTMENT REPEATER

Every emergency physician knows the frustrations of seeing certain patients return "regularly" to the emergency department. Labeled as *repeaters, frequent visitors,* or *abusers,* these patients often appear in the emergency area with trivial complaints, problems related to alcohol intoxication, self-inflicted injury, or an exacerbation of preexisting illness for which they seem to obstinately avoid obtaining regularly scheduled medical care.

Even though the problem of the "chronic" emergency patient is well recognized by experienced practitioners, only a few studies have collected data about the problem, but they suggest that it is a significant one. One study in a large university hospital indicated that of 3,044 patients seen by the emergency psychiatric service, 1,113 (over one third) had appeared on more than one occasion.[1]

Another study from Denver General Hospital showed that the repeaters often inappropriately used the public ambulance or emergency medical service (EMS) system to get to the hospital. The authors of the study point to this "massive diversion of available resources to a small percentage of the population who rarely seemed to benefit from the attention they received at the hospital."[2]

STAFF ATTITUDE

Repeaters are regarded and received in various ways. The more benign repeaters may be treated affectionately by the staff, and some may be regarded almost as "mascots." They may even have nicknames, and their complaints are familiar ones. The staff may chat with such patients for a short time and eventually discharge them, not considering that a new and serious problem could be present. Other patients may be more obnoxious and create a sense of disruption within the department. They seem to abuse the service. Such repeaters tend to anger or frustrate the emergency staff. They appear to consume health resources without any apparent benefit; the alcoholics do not seem to stay with detoxification programs, the chronically ill do not seem to find the ongoing care they need, and the psychiatrically impaired seem to discontinue their medications and psychiatric follow-up care only to return to the emergency department when a crisis arises.

The sense of frustration or anger is an understandable human response to patients who seem to abuse the system by coming to an emergency facility time and again. Such thinking, however, is both unprofessional and anachronistic. Emergency physicians have made a pledge to be "available when the patient needs them."[3] Such needs are "defined by the patient and only subsequently assessed by the physicians."[4]

Neither the emergency physician nor the patient can afford a relationship that begins with an assumption that the patient is not ill, does not deserve proper treatment, or abuses the health system. The patient perceives a need for care and uses the health system, and it may be that the patient's only perceived ready access to the system is the emergency department. Emergency physicians must care for patients who no one else wishes to see or is able to treat and for those who are unable to act in ways that the physician might perceive as best. If the emergency physician does not accept this overriding responsibility, patients with serious medical disorders are overlooked; those patients who have psychiatric illnesses or disorders, resulting perhaps from a rapidly changing society, do not receive sympathetic, nonjudgmental, professional treatment.

When the emergency physician detects a negative attitude among the staff toward these patients, it may be necessary to point out that they may indeed have serious medical or psychiatric problems (e.g., electrolyte imbalance, vitamin deficiency syndromes, subdural hemorrhage, cardiomyopathy) that require thoughtful evaluation. In such a way the physician can deliver the information as medical teaching, not as a moralistic sermon.

PATIENT CHARACTERISTICS

Despite the paucity of data about repeaters, certain general demographic characteristics and diagnoses seem to apply in most of these patients. Alcoholism, seizure disorder, personality disorder, chronic organic mental disorder, depression, and schizophrenia are diagnoses that may be applied to many of the repeaters.

Age, sex, and marital status

Though the data are limited, most repeaters seem to be single men in their middle years (30 to 50). They tend to be divorced, widowed, or never married but are rarely still married.[2] Perhaps this reflects the population of alcoholics who would tend to have difficulty entering or maintaining a marriage or an underlying personality disorder that makes success in marriage unlikely.

Alcoholism

Alcoholism seems to be the most frequent diagnosis in this population of chronic repeaters. In the study by Purdie[2] 87.5% of patients identified as "chronic emergency department visitors" were alcoholics. This chronic population visited the emergency department an average of 1.75 times per month. The alcoholic may be found intoxicated, unconscious, or sleeping in a public place. When such persons are found, the community emergency medical service is generally called to action. The intoxicated patient may be encouraged to move on, could be taken to jail, or may be escorted to the hospital for evaluation.

The following scenarios are familiar to emergency physicians: the alcoholic who stops taking anticonvulsants for seizure disorder during a binge and experiences a seizure; the alcoholic who injures himself in a fight or accident while intoxicated; the alcoholic who cannot find adequate shelter from the cold and develops frostbite or hypothermia; and the alcoholic who is depressed and threatens or attempts suicide. These scenarios are likely to involve the EMS system.

When he arrives at the hospital, the repeater is often quickly recognized by the emergency staff, which may refer to him by his nickname. The familiar face resting on the emergency cart evokes various reactions within the staff that depend, in part, on the current patient census and the degree of "cleaning up" the patient requires. He may be greeted with groans of disgust, jokes, or indifferent resignation. In most departments the overriding principle of patient management emphasizes a speedy disposition of the alcoholic repeater. The best management strategy seems to be the one that moves the patient out as fast as possible. The patient's clinical evaluation in such an atmosphere is abbreviated at best; if the patient awakens from his stupor and declares that he is ready to leave, he will be escorted out of the department with dispatch.

Alcoholics who are not brought in by public service units like the police or emergency service generally have some complaint that causes them discomfort. More common disorders are abdominal pain, gastrointestinal hemorrhage, minor injury, "nerves," or the wish to stop drinking.

The alcoholic patient can have medical disorders that are quite complex yet difficult to unravel or comprehend immediately because he may be intoxicated or in various stages of withdrawal. Because the disorders can be so complicated, the patient deserves a thorough evaluation from staff members who should be looking for conditions like hypothermia, pneumonia, metabolic acidosis, vitamin deficiency, chronic subdural hemorrhage, gastrointestinal bleeding, alcoholic hepatitis, dehydration, electrolyte imbalance, or hypoglycemia. Whether or not the alcoholic repeats, he can still have a serious medical disorder.

Schizophrenia

Schizophrenic patients and those with personality disorders may become repeaters. The familiar paranoid schizophrenic, for instance, may walk in one day rather calmly and say that he has just been attacked by dogs and that his leg has been completely torn off. On another day he may complain that his insides are rotten and decaying. The chronic, undifferentiated schizophrenic may enter with a variety of psychiatric physical complaints and may resist any referral for psychiatric treatment. Sometimes the patient seems quite simpleminded and the staff may wonder how he cares for himself at all.

The repeater phenomenon among schizophrenics is not entirely understood. Because they react to unheard and unseen stimuli, their behavior tends to be impulsive and unpredictable. It is also probably true that certain abrupt intrapsychic events generate fear and anxiety. Auditory hallucinations or an acute somatic delusion that one's body is rotting away is probably quite frightening to the schizophrenic. Since he cannot distinguish delusion from disease, he perceives that his complaints are most serious. Such a patient may react to these inner stimuli by seeking immediate medical care in a facility that he knows is always available and usually supportive.

Personality disorder

Certain personality disorders predictably cause the repeater phenomenon. Somatization disorders create a patient who knows something is wrong and wants treatment. This patient steadfastly resists a psychiatric explanation and may frustrate his regular clinic or private physician so much that the only alternative left is the emergency department. The obsessive compulsive patient may have repeated trivial complaints, or he may come for checkups to make sure nothing is wrong.

The schizoid or schizotypal patient who appears eccentric, withdrawn, and "strange" may repeat for apparently unexplainable reasons. The patient gives a history of being a "loner" and tends to talk in a formal, "stiff" language. His complaints are usually not delusional but result from "odd" thinking peculiar to himself.

Depression

The depressed patient may ask for help repeatedly in the emergency department. Since the patient characteristically experiences sleep disturbance, he may be among the nighttime repeater population.

The depressed patient commonly complains about global physical symptoms ("sick all over") or vague, neuropsychiatric signs like dizziness or weakness. The patient may be a repeater because of multiple suicide attempts. The depressed patient may really benefit from early psychiatric intervention and treatment. The screening questions for depression are so easily and quickly asked that they should probably be used for all patients when depression is suspected. Depression should be suspected in all elderly patients who have multiple vague somatic complaints.

Organic mental disorder

Some organic mental disorders render the patient so impaired that family members or friends may bring him to the emergency department for evaluation of confusing symptoms that elude easy interpretation. The patient may also experience tremendous difficulty understanding his medications and maintaining the proper dosage schedule. Such a person is at risk for developing medication side effects or therapeutic failure that brings him to the emergency department. The immediate stimulus for the visit may be the discovery of the patient by a well-meaning relative or friend. Drug or alcohol intoxication, side effects, and withdrawal are such common causes of organic mental disorder that the family must be questioned specifically about drug and alcohol use.

PREVENTION OF THE REPEATER

Even though there may be more appropriate sources of care for most repeaters, every emergency department has at least a few "regulars" no matter what corrective measures are tried. There should, however, be certain routine steps taken to give these patients an alternate, effective source of care more tailored to their specific needs.

MANAGEMENT OF THE REPEATER

Medical evaluation

The busy emergency physician is quite easily tempted to assume that the repeater has no new medical illness. For the ultimate well-being of both patient and physician, however, each visit should be viewed from a fresh perspective. This is actually quite difficult in practice, but it best ensures that a new medical event or emergency is not overlooked. One of the most important features of each new evaluation is an adequate history and examination. In the emergency setting time is a precious commodity, but an adequate examination can be conducted in a rather short time when the physician and the system are well organized.

The general appearance of the patient usually determines initial priorities. The pale obtunded patient requires rapid attention, an intravenous line, and examination for suspected bleeding, overdose, or sepsis. The head, ear canals, face, and eyes can be rapidly examined for evidence of acute trauma or other disorder. The neck is examined for mobility, masses, or distended veins. Examination of the heart, lungs, and abdomen can be completed easily. The patient's gait and coordination are easily tested by watching him walk or try to get dressed or undressed. If subdural hemorrhage or an intracranial process is suspected, a thorough neurological examination should probably be performed on all these patients.

The reason for emphasizing an interview and a pertinent physical examination as a routine is to ensure that they are done. Many of these patients, especially the alcoholics, may present a complex picture. The alcoholics who require attention repeatedly are at risk for serious medical problems that may be masked by their intoxication.

Certain common complications of disorders can be anticipated in advance and a method of treatment determined ahead of time. Hypoglycemia, thiamine deficiency, and dehydration in the alcoholic are examples. Routine administration of intravenous glucose, fluids, and thiamine to alcoholics prevents adverse sequelae that can be predicted in advance and prevented.

Interviews

A second phase of evaluation, especially relevant for the alert patient, is an interview that, when possible, includes brief screening questions for the common psychiatric disorders of repeaters. Questions about appetite, sleep, interests, and mood partially screen for depression. The content and flow of the patient's conversation and a history of psychiatric illness provide clues of schizophrenia.

The physician should try to meet and talk with those who accompany the patient. The concerns and observations of friends, family, and guardian are often invaluable and essential in determining the patient's immediate problem, underlying condition, and social support.

The patient's medications deserve review. This may be nearly impossible when an incoherent patient is brought to the department by ambulance from a public place. On certain extraordinary occasions it may be necessary to send an EMS crew or the police to the patient's home to find his medication or someone who knows what medicine he takes.

Referral

Slaby has shown that the following groups of patients tend to be referred from the emergency department to public inpatient facilities: those over 50 years of age, men, those divorced or separated, blacks, alcoholics, drug abusers, and psychotics.[1] When these patients are referred to a facility a long distance from home, they are not likely to return for subsequent care. Instead they return to the emergency department in several days or weeks for treatment. A referral to a distant state hospital for continuing outpatient assessment and treatment, therefore, is likely to fail. The repeater feels isolated, away from his own territory, and probably more welcome in the emergency department of his own community hospital. The failure of these large public facilities to provide ongoing care for the repeater is partially characterized by the "revolving door syndrome." The patient is whisked in for brief inpatient treatment, rushed out again, and the stage is set for the return trip by way of another referral transfer in the near future. Developing a liaison with a local community mental health center is important. These places often have 24-hour outpatient facilities for evaluation of acute psychiatric emergencies. If communication is kept open, these centers will not feel "dumped on" and can be of great benefit as referral sources. It is certainly in the best interests of emergency physicians and their patients to support the development of these community mental health and detoxification centers.

Social supports

Social isolation seems to be a critical factor in promoting the repeater phenomenon. The patient who has no family or lacks their support, has unstable employment, and lacks external social support like a church affiliation is at high risk for becoming a repeater. Early identification of such a patient may make it possible to include a social service evaluation and early referral to either a community support service or mental health agency.

Record system. A good record system is one that allows quick retrieval of information about the patient's most recent visits to the emergency department. Such a system allows the staff to quickly recognize that the patient is a repeater. Whether the clue is a recent stack of emergency records or a computer printout of recent dates of entry and discharge diagnoses, the physician should have access to this information early in the patient's evaluation. An ideal system, perhaps for the future, is one that allows various community hospitals to share data in a way that identifies the patient who visits regularly at more than one hospital in the community.

When the patient is not known to be a repeater, he must be treated sympathetically, but a lengthy, personal involvement with an individual who has a deep need for compassion is not appropriate. If any one staff member has become personally involved and has befriended the patient repeatedly, this action may consciously or unconsciously encourage repeated visits.[5]

Prevention of medical problems

Certain medical practices may actually cause an increase in repeated emergency visits and may need review. In some hospitals, for instance, the patient with alcohol withdrawal seizures gets a loading dose of anticonvulsants and a prescription for them. In all likelihood the patient either does not fill the prescription at all or fills it and soon discontinues the medication when he resumes drinking. When the patient decreases his alcohol consumption, the resulting fall in both alcohol and anticonvulsant levels may be more likely to precipitate a seizure than a decreased level in either one of the agents individually.

Other medical practices may cause similar problems. The patient, for instance, who succeeds in getting an injection of a narcotic for a complaint of pain and does not receive an appointment for appropriate follow-up care but is merely told to call the clinic for an appointment may soon return for similar medication. On other occasions the patient may be given a new medication, a nonsteroidal antiinflamatory agent, for instance, for his complaints of pain. When the patient returns with an allergic reaction or other side effects, he has initiated a legitimate set of subsequent visits and perhaps treatments, caused by failure to ensure adequate follow-up care or by the prescription of a medication that was only questionably indicated in the first place.

SUMMARY

The repeater, regular, or chronic patient is probably a source of at least some frustration to most emergency departments. The first consideration must *always* be that the patient has a new medical problem or previously undetected one that is worsening. The patient who returns only once or twice for the same complaint in a short time deserves intensive reinvestigation.

The inveterate repeater is likely to have a chronic organic illness like respiratory disease, a psychiatric condition like a personality disorder, poor family and social supports, and an unstable life-style. Alcoholism is perhaps the most common overall characteristic of these patients.

When the appropriate medical-psychiatric evaluation has been completed, the emergency staff must focus on an adequate referral for the repeater. The several characteristics of the referral should be that the office or center is located near the hospital or the patient's home and that access is relatively easy. The staff should arrange the appointment for the patient and document it clearly on a card that is sent home with him. Ideally the patient would be called a day ahead of time to be reminded of the appointment. The repeater who calls for an appointment and is put on "hold" for 15 minutes and then told that he cannot be seen for 2 months is likely to return to the emergency department shortly thereafter. Referral sources for psychiatric components of the patient's illness include a community mental health clinic, the hospital's outpatient psychiatric service, and community or hospital daytime programs, especially if they have "outreach" or care programs. Developing rapport with these agencies or hospital programs can be accomplished by assigning a nurse or social worker to a liaison program. This person can visit these referral sources monthly and keep open lines of communication, thus resulting in better medical care and less frustration for all.

REFERENCES

1. Slaby, AE, and Perry, PL. Use and abuse of psychiatric emergency services. *International Journal of Psychiatry and Medicine,* 1980-81, *10*(1), 1-8.
2. Purdie, RFJ, Honigman, B., and Rosen, P. The chronic emergency department patient. *Annals of Emergency Medicine,* June 1981, *10*(6), 298.
3. Riggs, LM, Jr. A vigorous new specialty. *New England Journal of Medicine,* 1981, *304,* 481.
4. Rund, DA. Emergency medical services systems: an overview. In *Essentials of emergency medicine.* New York: Appleton-Century-Crofts, 1982.
5. Fauman, JB. Current concepts in emergency psychiatry. In Rund, DA, and Wolcott, BW (Eds.), *Emergency medicine annual: 1983.* New York: Appleton-Century-Crofts, 1983.

20 INTERPERSONAL PSYCHIATRIC THERAPY

Interpersonal psychiatric therapy includes psychoanalysis, psychoanalytic psychotherapy, and brief psychotherapy. The essential features of these treatments are that the patient and physician identify the patient's major symptoms, gather information about these symptoms, and formulate a problem. When the patient recognizes the real underlying problem, he should be encouraged to try to develop solutions. Even in the emergency department the establishment of rapport and the encouragement of the patient are among the most important aspects of early interpersonal therapy.

FEATURES OF PSYCHIATRIC THERAPY

Identifying symptoms and gathering information

The most difficult part of eliciting any medical history, including psychiatric data, is gathering adequate information to formulate the problem. Therefore using a standard medical interview is most important. One of the keys to getting an appropriate amount of information is to define the chief complaint. Oftentimes the patient is unsure or vague about his chief complaint. It is important to take time to get him to identify what is "really bothering him." Once this is achieved, discovering the history of the present illness is the next most important issue. When did the symptoms begin? Were they related to any other circumstances or events? What has helped to improve these symptoms, or what has made them worse? Once these questions have been clearly answered, no easy task, doing a mental status examination becomes the next item of importance.

Once it is clear that the patient has a psychiatric problem, a decision has to be made about which type of treatment would be most helpful. Even if the patient has a clear "chemical disorder," such as a bipolar affective disorder (manic depressive illness) or a schizophrenic disorder, psychotherapy continues to be an important adjunctive treatment to the chemotherapy that should begin. Interpersonal psychiatric therapy is referred to as *psychotherapy*.

Psychotherapy is an often abused term. Despite the connotation that psychotherapy can be anything from a friendly conversation with the local bartender to "talking it over with a friend," psychotherapy is a highly specific and well-understood treatment tool.

There are various types of psychotherapy. Because it is appropriate in emergency patients, the type emphasized here is *brief psychotherapy*. Brief psychotherapy consists of a limited number of interviews (1 to 15), occurring between a physician and a patient, sometimes involving family members or friends. There are three indications for this type of therapy.[1] The three include problems with thinking, mood, and behavior; people with one of these three indicators benefit from brief psychotherapy. These patients come to the physician or emergency department in a state of crisis. It is important at this stage to break down their chief complaints into one of the three types of problems just mentioned.

Formulation of the problem

Once the chief complaint is evident, a history of it must be taken. This gives focus to the interview. All of this may sound as though it takes more time than it does. A chief complaint and a history of the present illness can be elicited in 5 to 10 minutes. Once the circumstances surrounding the present problem emerge, problem solving can begin. In these early moments of interview a skillful physician may actually begin effective psychiatric therapy. To do this it should be realized that the patient must play a large role in his own problem solving. This is different from the medical model in which the physician usually recommends a specific solution. The physician cannot and should not solve problems for the patient. This may need to be emphasized to the patient and can be done with such statements as, "I can think of several ways of approaching this problem, but they might help me and not you." This is usually obvious to the patient, particularly if it is brought to his attention. It may be that if the patient cannot come up with some answer or alternative to his problem, several possible solutions can be given to him. These suggestions should be given with the repeated warning statement, "These come to mind as solutions for me, but they might not be useful to you."

If the patient has difficulty coming up with the solutions to his problem, giving him pencil and paper and coming back in 30 minutes might be helpful. This aids him in formulating some type of alternative behavioral activity that will help solve the problem differently from the way he has been trying.

A problem arises often, however, in the heat of the moment when a patient cannot come up with any solutions. Usually this patient is demonstrating a form of resistance called the *"Yes, but . . ." syndrome*. He agrees that there are possible solutions but finds reasons why none will work. This can be extremely frustrating to the physician who is used to solving problems simply and with nearly complete resolution. If this pattern is established, the next step is to make it the patient's problem. That is, he should be told, "This seems to be a difficult problem for you to solve, and all of my suggestions are of little help. It is a tough problem, and only you are going to be able to solve it. If I can be of any further help to you, let me know, but I am stumped." This puts the shoe back on the patient's foot and requires him to enter into the process in some way. He may then try to make the physician feel impotent or guilty, to which there should be no response.

MOST COMMON TYPES OF PSYCHOTHERAPIES

Psychoanalysis

Psychoanalysis traditionally is an intensive form of psychotherapy, requiring the patient to participate in at least four 1-hour interviews per week, while lying on a couch with a psychiatrist out of view. This form of psychotherapy is extremely expensive, is time consuming, and requires a highly sophisticated patient. Psychoanalysis was popular in the 1940s and 1950s in the United States, but it has gradually faded from the forefront of modern psychiatry. It is still useful in the treatment of a mildly disturbed (neurotic) patient who has a good deal of time and money to invest in such a form of treatment.

Psychoanalysis requires that the patient learn how to use "free association." That is, he needs to identify random thoughts and feelings flowing through his conscious thinking. These are markers for unconscious conflicts that are being avoided by the conscious mind. The patient is also taught to remember his dreams, which are then used to reveal unconscious conflicts and processes. An important part of psychoanalysis is the identification of feelings projected onto the unseen, but always present, psychiatrist. The process involving these projected thoughts and feelings is called *transference* and results from early relationships with family members. Much of psychoanalysis is, therefore, involved in the understanding of this transference phenomenon, a present picture of past neurotic conflicts.

Once these unconscious conflicts (having been identified in free association, dreams, and transference) are made conscious, the patient ideally understands his symptoms, and they disappear. Psychoanalysis often takes from 6 months to many years. It is easy to see why this form of treatment is reserved for a privileged few.

Psychoanalytic psychotherapy

Psychoanalytic psychotherapy involves a psychiatrist and patient sitting face to face, usually once a week for an hour but sometimes less often. The usual time involved in this form of psychotherapy is from 3 to 12 months, but it may last longer. This is the most common form of psychotherapy used in the United States by psychiatrists today. Psychoanalytic psychotherapy involves forming a theory about the patient's symptoms.

CASE EXAMPLE 1

A 32-year-old woman had "panic attacks." She had periodic feelings of extreme fear and terror, evidently unrelated to anything that was going on in her life. In the emergency department it was determined that she did not have a mitral valve prolapse or other medical cause for her panic attacks.

In taking a history it became apparent that the patient thought she was very independent. She was currently married to her second husband who was not working. As she continued discussing her marital situation, it became evident that her husband was depending increasingly on the patient in emotional and financial ways. As a past history was taken, it became evident that she was brought up in a financially deprived household where the mother died when the patient was 13. The patient always had to present herself as very independent and competent and was never allowed to express dependency needs. The outcome was the common problem that the patient was becoming increasingly fearful that her apparently strong husband was more and more dependent on her and that she would be incapable of having her own needs fulfilled. She repressed all of this in her unconscious and developed symptoms of panic attack.

Psychoanalytic psychotherapy is the treatment of choice for this patient. In this form of therapy her present symptoms are related to her past history; she becomes aware that she was never able to express dependency and, thus, developed a "pseudo independence." Once she understands this, it is likely that she will be able to begin expressing her own needs, begin expressing some of her irritation and anger at her husband's lack of motivation to work, and begin bringing about an adjustment in her marriage and relationships with others so that they are more realistic. Her symptoms will then disappear. This is likely to take several months and requires discussing both her background history and her present situation and blending the two. The concomitant use of tricyclic antidepressants, propranolol (Inderal), or other chemotherapy helps to control her symptoms while she is undergoing such specific treatment.

Brief psychotherapy

Brief psychotherapy is related to psychoanalytic psychotherapy. However, the process is abbreviated and does not occur in such depth. That is not to say that brief psychotherapy is less beneficial or effective. It is best applied to a different type of problem that is more immediate, is not as imbedded in the patient's past history and is, therefore, more quickly overcome by the patient's normal coping mechanisms.

Conditions for successful brief psychotherapy. There are six major requirements that may seem obvious for success in brief psychotherapy.

1. The patient understands that there is some psychological basis for his present symptoms. This requires that an empathetic and authoritative professional links the patient's symptoms to psychological conflict. The physician must use words that the patient can understand. The patient who comes in with "shaking all over" as a chief complaint may have to be told that his symptoms are signs of stress.
2. The patient must trust the physician. This requires that the physician appears to be an empathetic, nonjudgmental, caring person. This can be accomplished quite rapidly in an emergency department or physician's office. It requires specific techniques and results in the development of rapport, which refers to the feeling of trust that the patient has for the physician and his belief that this person can help him get better. This can be established rather quickly by even a busy and hurried physician. The physician needs to establish privacy with the patient, a sense of calm on the part of the physician, and the ability to listen in an attentive and concerned manner without responding for several minutes. It usually involves maintaining some eye contact with the patient, listening thoughtfully and appropriately, and encouraging the patient to "tell his story."

3. The physician can arouse hope that the patient will recover. The physician needs to seem to be able to understand the patient's problem and to identify it for him. The patient can then confidently be told that treatment is available and that although it is not dramatic and sudden, it will result in his improved condition.
4. The patient has motivation to understand himself better and to change his behavior. It becomes rapidly clear that some patients need their symptoms and do not want to give them up. The classic response to any attempt on the part of the physician to involve a patient in treatment is the "Yes, but . . ." syndrome. The patient listens to the physician, and when alternatives are presented, he gives reasons why they would not work. The physician can point out this "Yes, but . . ." phenomenon to the patient, and at this point the patient either maintains it or becomes aware and attempts to stop it and to begin participating in finding alternatives. If he maintains the response, it is difficult to pursue treatment further. It is only advantageous to tell the patient in a warm and concerned manner that treatment is available when he feels that it will be helpful for him. This avoids the common problem of the physician who is irritated at a patient's refusal of help, causing the physician to reject the patient, which only increases the patient's defensiveness and prevents him from earlier intervention at a later date.
5. Another condition for successful psychotherapy requires the physician's understanding of the patient's background. A recently arrived immigrant has a different view of his own symptoms than would a middle-class suburbanite. Therefore being able to speak to the patient in his language (the cultural sense) is important in establishing trust.
6. The physical environment is important for successful treatment. The patient must feel a sense of privacy and security. He should be at an eye level or only slightly below the eye level of the physician. Therefore both physician and patient are either sitting or standing, or the patient is lying in a position so that his eyes are at the physician's eye level. The physician and patient should be sitting 2 or 3 feet apart, and the physician should appear relaxed.

Process of brief psychotherapy. Brief psychotherapy is a specific and useful tool in the emergency department or physician's office. Discovering the chief complaint or "what is wrong" is the most difficult part of a medical evaluation. With any medical condition the patient gives a chief complaint that is not always specific or exactly related to the underlying problem. Therefore it is most important to specifically identify the chief complaint before going on to the next step, which is taking the history of the present illness. Thus a patient who comes in with "vomiting" and a "bad feeling" requires a medical workup. If this is negative, sitting with the patient and reviewing his emotional status become the next most important issue. The patient's present relationships with family members is the place to begin. Is there a problem with a spouse or other family member? If so, what is it? Is this problem related to his present symptoms?

THE PROCESS OF BRIEF PSYCHOTHERAPY

A. Establish a "chief complaint."
B. Review personal hallmarks.
   1. Family problems?
   2. Work problems?
   3. Life-style problems?
C. Formulate a problem with the patient.
D. Have the patient list three ways to begin solving the problem.
E. Set specific goals (either in time or behavior changes).

Once the family relationships have been explored, the next most important area of questioning is the patient's occupation and his relationship with co-workers. Has there been a sudden change in his status on the job? How does he get along with his boss and co-workers? Is he progressing in his occupation as he thinks he should? These questions usually reveal some difficulty in this area if it exists.

The next most important issue to explore is the life-style of the patient and whether or not it is providing pleasure. Asking him what he does for fun, how he entertains himself, and what pleasure he has found in his life are important questions. As these questions are asked and the physician appears attentive and concerned, the patient feels increasingly able to discuss personal issues without needing to continue to present himself as "physically ill" only. In this protective environment psychiatric problems become evident, and an obvious chief complaint emerges.

Characteristics of brief psychotherapy. Initially in brief psychotherapy a problem is formulated, and the patient is encouraged to come up with alternative solutions to it. The physician, therefore, is doing several things. He is reassuring the patient, educating the patient about himself, and modeling ways of resolving psychological conflicts. Often the patient in conflict needs to be reassured that he is proceeding normally and doing a good job. He can be reassured that he does not have a psychiatric disorder; this in itself may be highly therapeutic for some patients.

Patients who are selected for brief psychotherapy should have some of the following easily recognized criteria:

1. The patient should be highly motivated. He should see that he has a problem or conflict and feel a need to change. He should be able to tolerate the anxiety of trying new behavior. Therefore a history of successful problem-solving behavior in the past is a good prognostic sign. A question such as, "Have you ever had a failure or problem before that you solved well?" is a good way of getting this information.
2. The patient should be psychologically minded. That is, he should show some

interest in his own psychological functioning. This is demonstrated during the interview by the way the patient responds to such questions as, "Have you ever had problems with your nerves?" If the patient shows some knowledge of his usual psychological functioning and a willingness to discuss it, this is again a good prognostic sign.

3. The patient should be able to understand interpretations of his behavior. That is, he should be able to see the link between becoming nauseated and being angry at his spouse. This is also a good sign that brief psychotherapy should work.

If these characteristics are not present, brief psychotherapy will not work. The patient then needs to be referred in the medical model back to his family physician for further preparation for psychiatric referral. The family physician would be helped if he received a telephone call or a note indicating the nature of the problem.

CASE EXAMPLE 2

A 42-year-old factory foreman enters the emergency department with "chest pain." A workup is done with no results. During a brief interview it becomes clear that he is under stress from his boss to increase production. The men under his supervision are growing resentful, and his wife feels he is "working too hard." He is near tears and becomes angry and defensive when the emergency physician suggests, "The stress of your job is tremendous. I think your body is reacting to it with this pain. Do you see any relation between this stress and your pain?" The patient accuses the physician of saying that it was all in his head and protests, "I don't have any problems at work or at home."

At this point the physician should "back off." The patient should be reassured that he is in no danger, told to rest overnight, and instructed to see his physician in the next few days. A call or note to the family physician, explaining the psychological nature of the patient's symptoms and his inability to explore them would be helpful. Asking the family physician to further investigate the stress-related factors and refer for psychiatric evaluation, if indicated later, might be helpful.

An example of a patient who should benefit from brief psychotherapy is the one presented as case example 3.

CASE EXAMPLE 3

After probing into her present history, the patient came up with the following facts. She had been a hardworking, conscientious person all her life. She recently had difficulty with her 3-year-old daughter who was crying a great deal and making constant demands. She felt unable to be a "perfect mother," and keep the house in order as her husband required. It also became obvious that her husband was quite critical, required a good deal of her, and gave little emotional warmth back. He was a highly successful executive who was involved in his own business.

She also revealed a history of having grown up in a professional family with a critical father and a somewhat submissive and socially active mother. The result of all this was that she was an extremely conscientious person who never rebelled and who never found her place in life. She constantly reacted to others, trying to get approval.

GOOD PROGNOSTIC SIGNS FOR BRIEF PSYCHOTHERAPY

A. High motivation—"I can see that I have a problem, and I need to solve it."
B. Psychological insight is present—"I usually bottle up my anger."
C. Linking symptoms with feelings—"I get dizzy when I'm around my boss."

She never expressed her anger directly and felt guilty about her sense of rage toward her daughter and husband.

As the physician listened, she became tearful and sobbed. The physician encouraged her to continue and told her that it was "all right to cry." He began reflecting that she rarely expressed some of her feelings of frustration and anger, which were quite normal and understandable. He asked her for ways in which she might modify some of her responses to others so that she could have her own needs fulfilled. In a surprisingly short time she admitted that she had felt increasingly angry and frustrated and that she needed to become more assertive. She began to feel better; she felt that there was some hope. The physician assured her that everything would not be suddenly better but that she should try to become more assertive. He suggested that she discuss her feelings with her husband and find out in what ways he might help her become more assertive. He recommended that if she continued to have difficulty after 2 or 3 more weeks of such efforts, she should consult her family physician or a psychiatrist. This example of brief psychotherapy took approximately 20 minutes.

Using this case vignette, it should be evident that most psychological problems are not necessarily complicated or untreatable. They do not automatically require large amounts of time. Often one session may be sufficient.[2] Generally an emergency department physician may wish to initiate this form of brief treatment. If this fails to provide a fairly significant change, referral for ongoing psychotherapy would be appropriate. The emergency department physician might follow a patient over four to six sessions, but this is frequently not possible. A family physician in a general medical setting can realistically spend several weeks with a patient like this.

SUMMARY

Psychiatric treatment of a brief nature involves information gathering. The information gathering is often therapeutic because it places the problem of the patient in perspective.

Once the problem has been identified, problem-solving techniques need to be encouraged in the patient. Most of the time the patient has not attempted various solutions to the problem but has only tried one, which has not worked. Helping him to find alternative behaviors to solve his problems is the most important part. Sometimes the physician loses perspective and tries to provide answers for the patient; this is often counter-productive.

Once this process has begun in the emergency department or the physician's office, referral for continued treatment might be helpful if it seems that this process may be prolonged (requiring several weeks or months of treatment). The manner in which this referral is made is most important. It should be kept in the medical model, "You have a problem for which there is a solution, and I know an expert who can help you solve it." Referral to a local psychiatrist, community mental health center, or other helping professional at this point would be appropriate. The next few sessions with one of these people involves further history taking, such as getting an extensive family history. It may also involve the use of medication and should be explained to the patient. He will then learn different techniques for solving his present problem.

All of these techniques involve four systems. The patient is being *reassured,* it is being *suggested* to him that he will improve, *environmental manipulation* may be suggested, and the use of appropriate *medication* may be useful.[3] Brief psychotherapy is not a vague or ill-defined concept. It is something that can be learned, can be used with some precision, and can provide excellent results. When used in an emergency department or general medical office, it often results in satisfied patients and a great saving in professional time and repeated medical workups.

REFERENCES

1. Groves, JE, and Kucharski, A. Brief psychotherapy. In Hackett, TP, and Cassem, NH (Eds.), *Massachusetts General Hospital handbook of general hospital psychiatry*. St. Louis: The C.V. Mosby Co., 1978.
2. Rockwell, WJK, and Pinkerton, RS. Single session pychotherapy. *American Journal of Psychotherapy,* 1982, *36*(1), 32-40.
3. Karasu, TB. Psychotherapy and pharmacotherapy: toward an integrative model. *American Journal of Psychiatry,* 1982, *139*(9), 1102-1113.

21 PSYCHIATRIC THERAPY: MEDICINAL AND ELECTROCONVULSIVE

The discovery and clinical introduction of phenothiazines into psychiatric practice in the 1950s created a whole new dimension in psychiatric care. The control of psychotic symptoms by these agents drastically decreased the need for physical restraint and allowed the eventual release of large numbers of patients from mental institutions. Their care could be transferred from an inpatient to an outpatient setting in large part because their disabling symptoms could be effectively treated with regular dosages of antipsychotic medication. The more recent introduction of the antidepressants into clinical practice has had a similarly remarkable effect on the symptoms of depression, and lithium carbonate has become the drug of choice for bipolar affective disorder (manic depressive illness). The indisputable efficacy of these medications not only changed the style of clinical practice, it reinforced the biochemical theories of psychiatric illness and nudged psychiatry more firmly into the medical realm.

In emergency practice the usual indications for initiating therapy with medications effective in psychiatric disorders are acute changes in the behavior or thought patterns of the patient. These sudden changes can be treated by the emergency physician, particularly when they are thought to create a potential danger for the patient or other people. These signs and symptoms of psychiatric disorder also cause severe emotional pain for the patient and again may require the initiation of treatment. It is also useful to know enough about psychiatric medications to recognize and manage side effects, adverse reactions, drug interactions, and overdosage of these agents when the patient's drug regimen has already been established.

The intent of this chapter is not to present comprehensive information about all psychoactive medications; rather it is to discuss a few representative medications that are effective in the more common psychiatric disorders. The objective is to provide enough information so that the emergency physician can become familiar with a rather small number of medications, learn to use them effectively when necessary, and recognize and manage problems associated with their toxicity.

The drugs are discussed under the headings that emphasize their major indications as defined by the predominant symptoms they control. These agents can be grouped under the following headings: antipsychotic, antidepressant, antimanic, antianxiety, and agents effective in the treatment of alcohol syndromes. Electroconvulsive therapy (ECT) and its rare emergency indications conclude the discussion.

MEDICATION THERAPY

Antipsychotic agents

Indications for antipsychotics. Feeling familiar with two or three antipsychotic agents allows their practical use. Because these medications have significant side effects, including the long-term side effect of tardive dyskinesia, the indications for using them are restricted. The following diagnostic categories are best treated with antipsychotic medications: schizophrenic disorders, schizoaffective disorders, bipolar affective disorders (mania or depression with psychotic features), depression, organic brain syndrome, severe anxiety, and certain specific nonpsychiatric conditions.

Psychiatric conditions

SCHIZOPHRENIC DISORDERS. When a schizophrenic disorder is diagnosed, initiation of antipsychotic medication is appropriate. It is rare in this day and age that a schizophrenic patient appears in the emergency department without ever having been diagnosed or treated previously. Therefore it is most important to clearly establish the drug history of the patient. It may be that restarting medication or increasing its present level is more effective than changing it. If a patient has been diagnosed as schizophrenic in the past and has been on maintenance therapy with antipsychotic medication for many months or years, the physician should look for signs and symptoms of tardive dyskinesia. This involves lip smacking, involuntary protrusion of the tongue, or a chewing motion of the month. Many times the patient who has a chronic psychiatric history is edentulous. The denture wearer may appear to have the same buccal-lingual movements as the patient with tardive dyskinesia. If the diagnosis of tardive dyskinesia is made, the medication does not have to be stopped or changed immediately, but the patient should be referred to a psychiatrist for further evaluation and treatment.

SCHIZOAFFECTIVE DISORDER. Patients with schizoaffective disorder have confused thinking, as do all schizophrenic individuals. The distinguishing features of this group are disordered thinking combined with inappropriate periods of depression or elation. These patients may be taking both antipsychotic and antidepressant medications. This dual treatment approach is only appropriate for relatively few patients, and the diagnosis of schizoaffective disorder is rarely if ever made in a one-visit consultation. Unless such a diagnosis has been made previously, it is more important to continue or adjust the dose of a single antipsychotic agent than to initiate or change an antidepressant medication.

BIPOLAR AFFECTIVE DISORDER (manic depressive illness). The patient who is developing a euphoric mood or is delusional, takative, or belligerent may have symptoms of mania. These symptoms may require the use of high doses of antipsychotic medication. Lithium is the therapeutic agent of choice for bipolar affective disorder, but after the initiation of therapy, the patient may not show clear-cut improvement for 4 or 5 days. It is more important, therefore, to control the patient's symptoms of mania, such as agitation, hallucinations, or combative behavior, with antipsychotic medication in the emergency department. Treatment with lithium should be started after admission. This can best be initiated in the controlled setting of a psychiatric inpatient unit. In an acute manic episode very high doses of lithium may be required. Such high doses require that the patient be monitored closely in the hospital.

DEPRESSION. Sometimes people with severe depression (including the manic depressive disorder) become delusional, paranoid, or combative. These people may need treatment with antipsychotic medication to control their behavior during the few hours they are in the emergency department. No harm is done by using this medication, and it should control the psychotic symptoms enough to allow treatment with the agents of choice—antidepressants.

ORGANIC BRAIN SYNDROMES. Acute delirium secondary to amphetamine, lysergic acid diethylamide (LSD), phencyclidine, and other hallucinogens responds to antipsychotic medication, although some authorities prefer treatment with antianxiety agents like diazepam (Valium) or withholding drug treatment altogether. Antipsychotic agents are effective in psychosis associated with other organic causes as well. Sometimes these medications can be quite justifiably given even though the underlying organic cause is not yet determined. The antipsychotic agent can bring disruptive symptoms under control and allow further evaluation to proceed. Dementia may also be treated in this way, helping to suppress hallucinations and delusions and to alleviate some of the confusion associated with this illness. This can be done while the evaluation of dementia is under way. Low doses of antipsychotic medication for patients with dementia may help them to remain functional longer than those not treated with antipsychotics.

SEVERE ANXIETY. In low doses antipsychotic medication may be useful in cases of massive anxiety. This is certainly not the usual treatment of choice but can be helpful for patients who are severely anxious, are in states of severe panic, and have histories that indicate that minor tranquilizers have been ineffective. When used for extreme anxiety, the dose of antipsychotics should be very low, and further evaluation of the patient for an organic cause of the anxiety should proceed.

Nonpsychiatric indications for the use of antipsychotic medication

GILLES DE LA TOURETTE SYNDROME. Gilles de la Tourette syndrome is manifested by both vocal and behavioral tics, cursing, gesturing, barking like a dog, echolalia, echopraxia, or sudden inappropriate movement. This often begins in late childhood or early adolescence but may appear later. It is an illness best treated with haloperidol (Haldol) in low to moderate dosages like 2 to 4 mg twice daily, with referral to an appropriate neurologist or psychiatrist for long-term follow-up care.

HUNTINGTON'S OR SYDENHAM'S CHOREA. Symptomatic relief can be obtained for patients with Huntington's or Sydenham's chorea by the use of low or moderate doses of antipsychotic medication.

NAUSEA AND VOMITING. Prochlorperazine (Compazine) is the most commonly used antipsychotic medication for nausea and vomiting. It is not uncommon to see a child come to the emergency department with symptoms related to the side effects of this medication. He may have extrapyramidal side effects or a movement disorder (such as chewing the tongue), extraocular crisis, paraspinal muscle spasm, facial spasm (producing what may look like an inability to swallow), or "lock jawism." Intravenous or intramuscular diphenhydramine (Benadryl) in a 25 to 50 mg dose should relieve these alarming symptoms rapidly.

INTRACTABLE HICCUPS. Low to moderate doses of chlorpromazine (Thorazine) have been found to be useful in the treatment of intractable hiccups.

ACUTE INTERMITTENT PORPHYRIA. The use of antipsychotic medication in acute intermittent porphyria can sometimes help modify secondary symptoms.

TETANUS. Chlorpromazine and barbiturates have been found to be useful in the management of severe tetany and painful muscle spasms associated with tetanus.

HYPERPYREXIA. Treatment with antipsychotics can sometimes be useful in severe hyperpyrexia. The cooling effect is from the secondary results of chlorpromazine on the temperature-regulating capacity of the hypothalamus. The drugs also inhibit shivering when a lowering of the body temperature to below normal is desired.

History and general considerations. In 1952 Delay and Deniker reported the remarkable effect of the phenothiazine agent chlorpromazine in the treatment of psychosis.[1] The introduction of this agent into clinical psychiatry virtually revolutionized psychiatric therapy and ushered in our present concepts of modern psychopharmacology. The basic structure of the phenothiazines is presented in Fig. 21-1. Substitutions at positions R_1 and R_2 create the various specific phenothiazines used in current clinical practice. The addition of a single chloride atom at position R_2, for instance, changes the drug from the highly sedating, weakly antipsychotic agent promazine (Sparine) to the markedly antipsychotic agent chlorpromazine. The phenothiazines are grouped into subclassifications on the basis of their side chain at position R_1 as shown in the following box.

CHEMICAL CLASSES OF ANTIPSYCHOTIC AGENTS

Phenothiazines*	Nonphenothiazines
Aliphatic	Butyrophenones
Chlorpromazine (Thorazine)	Haloperidol (Haldol)
Piperidines	Thioxanthenes
Thioridazine (Mellaril)	Thiothixene (Navane)
Piperazines	Dihydroindolones
Fluphenazine (Prolixin)	Molindone (Moban)
Prochlorperazine (Compazine)	Dibenzoxazepines
	Loxapine (Loxitane)

*Grouped by side chain at position R_1 on Fig. 21-1.

Since the 1950s, five other major chemical classes of antipsychotic drugs have been introduced. They are the following: thioxanthenes, butyrophenones, dihydroindolones, dibenzoxazepines, and diphenylbutylpiperidines. These classes and representative agents are also listed in the boxed material on p. 286.

Detailed and specific effects of antipsychotic drugs on the central nervous system (CNS) that diminish psychosis are unknown to a large extent. Most of the evidence accumulated to date suggests that their ability to antagonize the actions of dopamine as a neurotransmitter in the basal ganglia and limbic positions of the forebrain[2] produces their antipsychotic effect.[3-5]

Phenothiazines also affect the chemoreceptor trigger zone (CTZ) of the medulla, making many of these agents like prochlorperazine effective in the treatment of nausea or emesis.

Potency. One of the most important considerations for selecting a particular antipsychotic agent is its milligram for milligram effectiveness in antagonizing dopamine and treating psychosis. The most potent antipsychotics are haloperidol (Fig. 21-2) and fluphenazine; among the least potent are chlorpromazine and thioridazine. In general, the more potent antipyschotics produce less sedation and fewer anticholinergic side effects. In contrast to these desirable clinical attributes, the higher potency antipsychotics typically produce more prominent extrapyramidal side effects like acute dystonia. The relationship of these effects to antipsychotic potency is shown in Fig. 21-3. Equivalent doses of major antipsychotic drugs are listed in the following box.

ESTIMATED EQUIVALENT DOSES OF REPRESENTATIVE ANTIPSYCHOTIC DRUGS

Haloperidol	2 mg
Fluphenazine	2 mg
Thiothixene	5 mg
Loxapine	15 mg
Molindone	25 mg
Thioridazine	100 mg
Chlorpromazine	100 mg

Adapted from Mason, AS, and Granacher, RP. *Clinical handbook of antipsychotic drug therapy*. New York: Brunner/Mazel, Inc., 1980, Table 3, p. 33.

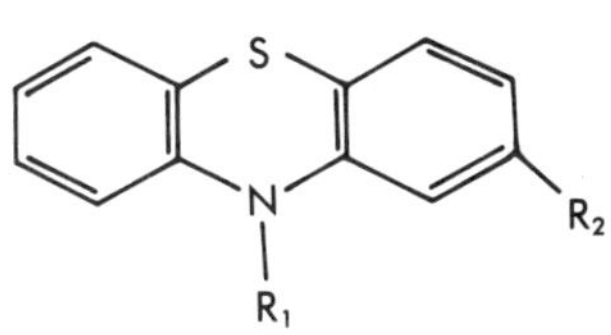

FIG. 21-1. Basic phenothiazine molecular structure showing side chain positions at R_1 and R_2.

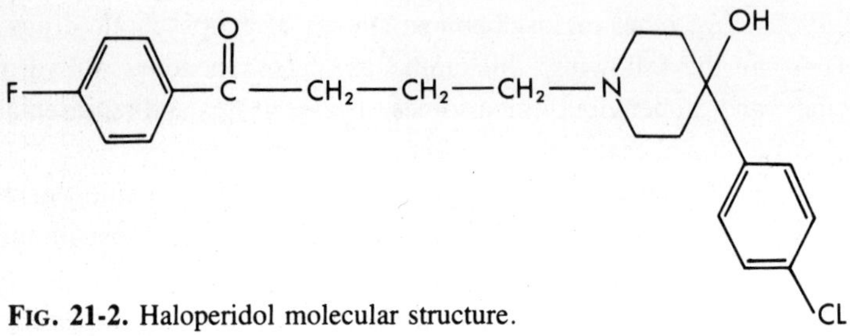

FIG. 21-2. Haloperidol molecular structure.

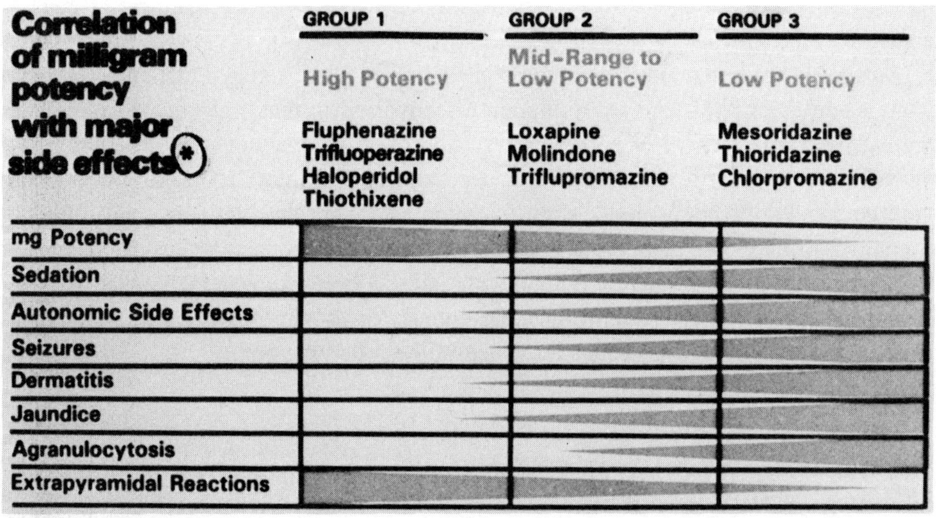

FIG. 21-3. Relative potency of antipsychotic agents in relation to side effects. (Adapted from Zavodnick, S. Comparison of neuroleptics. In Ayd, FJ (Ed.), *Haloperidol update: 1958-1980*. Baltimore: Ayd Medical Communications, 1980, Ch. 2.)

Side effects and overdoses. In general, the antipsychotic agents are relatively safe and have a high therapeutic index. Some side effects like dystonia are almost predictable and occur within hours or days after administration of the drugs. Others like tardive dyskinesia are unpredictable, may occur after several years of drug therapy, and seem unrelated to the specific agent used. In emergency psychiatry the most important side effects are those that affect the neurological and cardiovascular systems.

Neurological side effects. The neurological side effects of antipsychotic medications and their emergency treatment are listed in Table 21-1.

ACUTE DYSTONIA. Acute dystonia is probably the most common side effect of antipsychotic agents encountered in the emergency department. This dramatic side effect is sudden in onset, is more likely to occur in younger patients, and is often painful and disturbing to the person. The effect usually involves intense and sustained contractions

TABLE 21-1. Neurological side effects of antipsychotic drugs

Side effect	*Clinical features*	*Emergency treatment*
Acute dystonia	Muscular spasm of the neck, facial muscles, and back; patient has appearance of wry neck, protruding tongue, or trismus; more common in younger patients	Diphenhydramine 25 to 50 mg intramuscularly or intravenously or benztropine (Cogentin) 1 to 2 mg intramuscularly
Akathisia	Motor restlessness; inner compulsion to move, incessant movement, pacing or rocking; "ants in pants" sensation	Same as for acute dystonia (above)
Parkinsonism	Shuffling gait, mask-like face, "pill-rolling" tremor, muscular rigidity, bradykinesia	Antiparkinsonian agents (after consultation)
Tardive dyskinesia	Usually tics and involuntary movements of face, lips, or tongue; perioral tremor, "rabbit syndrome," regular tremor of lips and/or facial area; can be choreoathetosis or dystonia	No consistently effective treatment

of the muscles of the face, tongue, neck, or back. The patient may appear to have a "wry neck" or be unable to withdraw the tongue.

The effect may involve the eyes. The patient may experience an involuntary rolling of the eyes upward under the eyelids and may be unable to see during such an oculogyric crisis. A patient may also develop torticollis of the neck, protrusion of the tongue, or actual chewing of the tongue. He may develop a "locked jaw" (trismus) or laryngospasm. The dystonic movements disappear during sleep and decrease with voluntary control. They also seem to become more prominent with emotional stress. These symptoms occur almost invariably within the first few days after taking the medication.

Sometimes a patient develops an acute dystonic reaction after taking a "street drug." A particularly notorious example occurs when the patient takes 10 mg of haloperidol (a blue tablet) and thinks he is taking 10 mg of diazepam (also a blue tablet). When the acute dystonic reaction occurs the following day, the patient may be reluctant to relate the ingestion of any drugs. The history is then obtained only with repeated encouragement and explanation and by talking to the patient's relatives or friends in the waiting area.

The emergency management of the acute dystonic reaction usually involves the parenteral injection of 25 to 50 mg of diphenhydramine or 1 to 2 mg of benztropine. The intravenous injection of 50 mg of diphenhydramine is particularly rapid and effective. It causes a dramatic reduction of muscular spasm and the patient's abrupt return to normal muscular tone and posture.

AKATHISIA. Akathisia is motor restlessness. The patient usually complains of constantly needing to walk or move about and having an extremely tense or anxious feeling. He can become frantic and feel that he almost needs to run despite his feelings of exhaustion. He is usually up in the examining room pacing, wringing his hands, and looking anxious. The patient with akathisia may telephone his private physician so incessantly that he is sent to the emergency department for evaluation and treatment.

CASE EXAMPLE 1

A 52-year-old woman with a psychiatric history and previous record of a benign breast lesion called her surgeon ''at least 20 times'' one Saturday afternoon to complain that she was passing blood and ''all sorts of rotten things'' from her bowels. The surgeon finally referred her to the emergency department.

A history revealed that the patient was taking phenothiazines prescribed by one physician for her ''nerve problem.'' She also had received ''a shot'' of two medications the day before from another physician (the injections were later determined to be fluphenazine and benztropine).

On admission the patient paced back and forth in the examining cubicle; she pulled back the curtain continually to ask questions of the emergency staff. The examination, including proctoscopy, revealed no blood, mucus, or unusual material or lesions in the rectum. The patient literally ''could not sit still'' and said she felt like she ''had ants in her pants.''

Her diagnosis was akathisia and schizophrenia. The patient was given 50 mg of diphenhydramine intravenously. It quieted her quickly, and the symptoms of restlessness subsided.

The middle-aged patient taking antipsychotics seems at particular risk for akathisia. In this patient akathisia typically develops between the first and tenth week of treatment. The danger of this side effect is that many physicians react to it as they would to increased anxiety and treat it with higher doses of antipsychotic medication or minor tranquilizers. Antipsychotics make the syndrome worse, and antianxiety agents have little effect. The antipsychotic agent should be reduced or discontinued, and the reaction may be treated with diphenhydramine or benztropine.

PSEUDOPARKINSON'S SYNDROME. Parkinsonian-like features occur in pseudoparkinsonian syndrome, which is a common side effect of antipsychotic agents. Such a patient exhibits a masklike immobile face, shuffling gait, and a ''pill-rolling'' tremor of the hands. The patient sometimes shows mental dullness, cogwheel rigidity, and psychomotor retardation. These side effects are common in the elderly patient and usually occur between the first and fourth week of treatment.

The reaction is best treated by the patient's own psychiatrist who can monitor and adjust the doses of both the antipsychotic and antiparkinsonian drugs. In the emergency department either benztropine or diphenhydramine may provide temporary treatment.

TARDIVE DYSKINESIA. One serious complication of antipsychotics that does not appear to be related to any particular level of potency is tardive dyskinesia. It occurs abruptly after several years of treatment but has been reported as quickly as 3 months. Tardive dyskinesia manifests by continuous involuntary movements mainly of the face, lips, and tongue but may involve the trunk or extremities. Symptoms are made worse with stress, fatigue, or intentional movement and recede during sleep.

The incidence of tardive dyskinesia among the older chronic psychotic population is approximately 20%. The condition is usually reversible if diagnosed early. There is presently no unified opinion as to the etiology, but some hypothesize that it is caused by dopaminergic hypersensitivity and decreasing cholinergic activity. If possible, the antipsychotic medication should be gradually discontinued. The side effect is best managed by a psychiatrist experienced in these effects.

Cardiovascular side effects. The most prominent cardiovascular side effect of phenothiazine antipsychotic agents is orthostatic hypotension. The patient may pass out when trying to stand up after the acute psychosis has been treated with a large dose of intramuscular chlorpromazine. The treatment of such a reaction includes elevation of the legs and administration of intravenous fluid. Pressors with predominant beta stimulation effects like epinephrine and isoproterenol are contraindicated in the management of these reactions because it is felt that the hypotension is the result of alpha blockade. Beta stimulation further lowers blood pressure by dilating beta-responsive vasculature in skeletal muscle. The severe hypotension may result in cardiac arrest.

In general, phenothiazines are felt to have a negative intropic effect on the myocardium, and cardiomyopathy has been reported. The antipsychotic agents should be used with some caution for the patient with myocardial infarction, congestive heart failure, or a history of serious heart disease. Chlorpromazine has been shown to cause electrocardiogram (ECG) changes in some patients. These changes include lengthening of the QT interval, widening and notching of the T wave, and high doses flattening and even inverting the T wave.

Other side effects. Other side effects reported for antipsychotics include dry mouth, dysphagia, gynecomastia, amenorrhea, blurred vision, sexual dysfunction, occasional weight gain, and urticaria or other forms of skin eruptions. Chlorpromazine has been associated with cholestatic jaundice and dermal photosensitivity.

Overdose. Phenothiazines have a wide therapeutic margin. When a patient takes only phenothiazines in an overdose, there is rarely a fatal outcome. When other classes of medication like tricyclics or barbiturates are taken as well, the likelihood of lethality is increased considerably. The basic management for antipsychotic overdose includes protection of the airway and gastric emptying. Special problems encountered with antipsychotics, however, include disturbing extrapyramidal signs, seizures, hypotension, and respiratory depression.

Overdosing with high-potency antipsychotics like haloperidol may first show severe extrapyramidal signs, such as opisthotonus, oculogyric crisis, and muscle rigidity. Diphenhydramine can be given in an intravenous bolus dose of 50 to 100 mg delivered by slow push over 5 minutes.

Seizures may be treated by phenobarbital or phenytoin (Dilantin) as needed. Hypotension can be managed with intravenous fluid challenge, the antishock garment, or, if absolutely necessary, an alpha adrenergic agent like norepinephrine (Levophed). Beta agonists like epinephrine or isoproterenol are strictly contraindicated because they open vascular beds responsive to beta stimulation, reduce peripheral resistance, and thus further decrease the blood pressure.

Dosage routes, absorption, metabolism, and excretion. Many of the antipsychotic agents have an erratic and unpredictable absorption rate when given orally. Ingested food, antacids, and agents that decrease gut motility increase the breakdown of antipsychotics and limit their absorption. By contrast, intramuscular absorption is rapid and far more predictable than oral administration. The deltoid muscle is the preferred site for injection for high-potency antipsychotics when a rapid onset of action is required. The blood flow in that region is about two to three times greater than through a comparable area of gluteal muscle. When given by injection in the deltoid, a high-potency antipsychotic agent like haloperidol is absorbed in 20 to 30 minutes. For the purposes of rapid tranquilization in the emergency department, therefore, the intramuscular route of administration is preferred. Haloperidol has not yet been approved by the Food and Drug Administration for intravenous use.

Most antipsychotics are metabolized in the liver by the formation of sulfoxides or glucuronides or by hydroxylation. Those agents or diseases that impair hepatic function can decrease the metabolism of antipsychotics and cause higher levels of the drug in the blood. Agents that increase hepatic microsomal activity cause an increased metabolism of the antipsychotic agents and, thus, decrease their level in the blood.

Most of the antipsychotic drugs are highly protein bound and soluble in lipids. This accounts for their long half-life and the virtual impossibility of removing these agents by dialysis. For similar reasons plasma levels are difficult to measure and may lead to inaccuracies.

Interaction with other drugs. Antipsychotic agents may alter the effects on metabolism of other medications. Table 21-2 lists various drug interactions related to antipsychotic treatment. Some of these effects may be important in the emergency management of patients taking antipsychotic agents.

TABLE 21-2. Drugs that may interact with antipsychotic medication

Drug	*Possible interaction*
Alcohol	Increased sedation and CNS depression
Amphetamines	May potentiate stimulant effects of amphetamine at low antipsychotic levels
Antianxiety agents	Potentiates sedative effects
Antacids	May inhibit absorption of antipsychotics
Anticholinergics	Benztropine may decrease level of antipsychotic in blood; hydroxyzine (Vistaril) may decrease the effectiveness of antipsychotics
Antidepressants	Tricyclic hepatic metabolism may be inhibited by antipsychotics
Antihistamines	Combination of orphenadrine and chlorpromazine causes severe hypoglycemia
Barbiturates	Increased metabolism of antipsychotic drugs
Narcotics	Increased sedation and CNS depression
Phenytoin	Slower metabolism of phenytoin
Propranolol	Increased hypertension

Adapted from Mason, AS, and Granacher, RP. *Clinical handbook of antipsychotic drug therapy*. New York: Brunner/Mazel, Inc., 1980, pp. 242-243.

Effects on laboratory tests. Antipsychotics may cause metabolic effects or contribute substances to the body that alter certain laboratory tests. Phenothiazines, for instance, seem to elevate serum cholesterol and glucose levels. The urine of a patient taking these drugs turns pink or brown when left standing for a period of time. The agents may alter various other laboratory tests, according to the methods used in individual clinical laboratories.

Rapid treatment of psychosis. As discussed in detail in previous chapters, acute psychosis is a clinical condition characterized by a defect in the patient's information processing and is accompanied by symptoms and signs that may include anxiety, agitation, bizarre thoughts, behavioral abnormalities, loose associations, abnormal affect, delusions, or hallucinations. The causes of psychosis include organic mental disorders usually associated with a medical condition or intoxication that produces the disordered thinking, and functional or idiopathic mental illnesses like schizophrenia in which the defect is unknown. The most common functional mental illnesses that can produce psychosis are affective disorders (mania and depression) and schizophrenia.

The importance of distinguishing organic from functional psychosis in the emergency department has been stressed; the underlying medical condition causing the psychosis can be managed, and thus the cause of the psychosis is treated. The symptomatic treatment of the psychosis, however, can be the same for both major groups. The treatment modes for psychoses may be of two types. The traditional method involves administering rather small initial oral doses of an antipsychotic medication and then increasing the dosage daily until a remission occurs. The alternative method is the "rapid method"[6] that provides intramuscular dosages of high-potency antipsychotics every 30 or 60 minutes until a satisfactory clinical response occurs, or the symptoms persist despite rather massive dosages of antipsychotics. Because psychosis is a painful condition that involves high risk for the patient, the rapid method is preferred for emergency intervention.

Rapid technique. Before administering the first dose of haloperidol, the clinician should identify major target symptoms of the patient's psychosis. These symptoms are clearly evident and probably cause the patient and staff a great deal of trouble. Examples of target symptoms include agitation, hyperactivity, manifest delusions, anxiety, bizarre speech, or hallucinations. As the treatment progresses, the clinician notes the improvement or remission of the target symptoms as a sign that the antipsychotic therapy is effective. This strategy for rapid treatment of psychosis is outlined in Fig. 21-4.

The adult patient is initially given 5 to 10 mg of haloperidol by intramuscular injection. A high-potency antipsychotic like haloperidol produces a maximum reduction in psychotic symptoms with minimal side effects like sedation, hypotension, or anticholinergic effect. The patient is observed and then reevaluated in 30 to 60 minutes. If the target symptoms identified initially have not diminished significantly, the patient receives a second intramuscular injection of 5 mg of haloperidol. The process is repeated until the major target symptoms subside or until a total dose of 40 to 50 mg of haloperidol has been given.

Marked improvement or remission of target symptoms that indicate a clinical re-

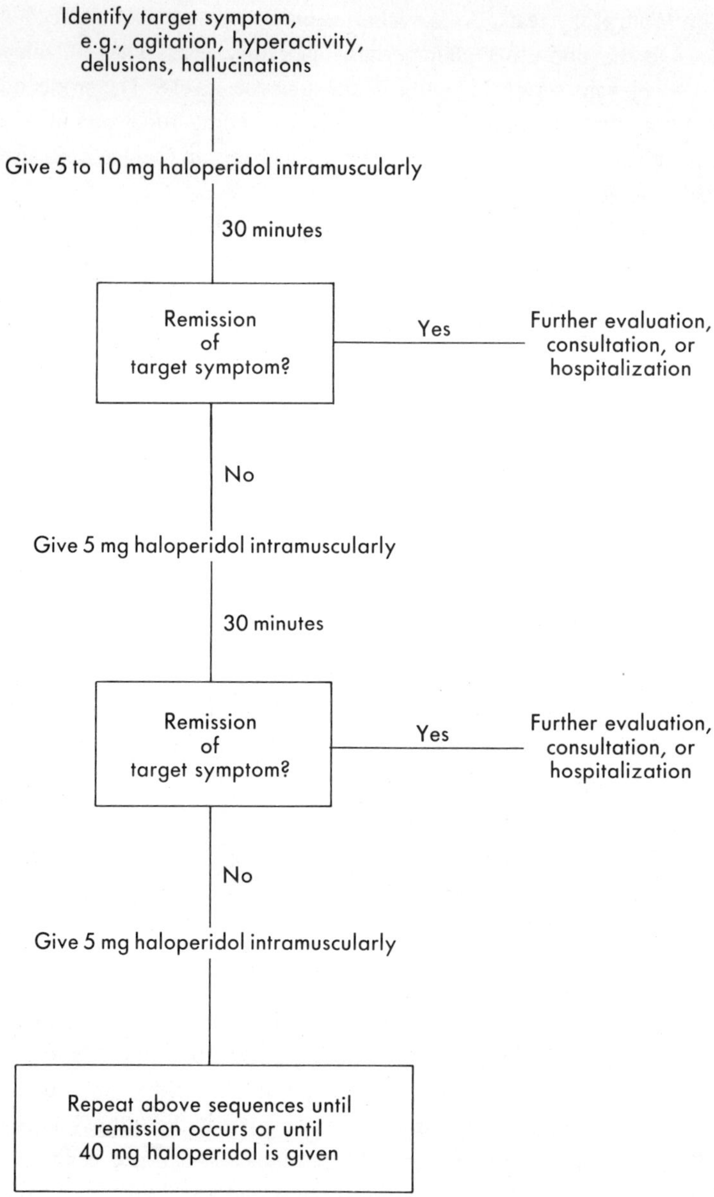

FIG. 21-4. Schematic of rapid tranquilization techniques.

sponse include diminished agitation, anxiety, hyperactivity, hallucinations, delusions, or confusion. With improvement the patient's thought content should be less bizarre, and the content of his speech should be more understandable.

Side effects. Acute dystonia is the most common side effect of the rapid technique of treatment. Various other pseudoparkinsonian signs like cogwheel rigidity or akinesia may develop. These effects can be prevented to some degree by the prophylactic use of intramuscular or oral benztropine given with the initial dose of haloperidol or treated when the dystonia develops with 50 mg of intravenous or intramuscular diphenhydramine.

Consultation, hospitalization, and maintenance of remission. One of the major disadvantages of rapid tranquilization in emergency practice involves the anticipated psychiatric consultation and admission. A consulting psychiatrist, unaware of the way the patient appeared earlier, could evaluate the medicated patient, minimize the seriousness of the condition, and send him home after a brief assessment. This scenario is particularly likely when the patient is transported some distance to a public mental health facility or a state hospital. For budgetary reasons and other considerations, the psychiatric staff at such public facilities generally tries to limit the number of patients admitted. When seeing a relatively asymptomatic patient transferred for admission, the receiving psychiatrist may discharge him on arrival.

These problems are minimized when the emergency physician works out a procedure in advance with consulting psychiatric colleagues. For instance, the psychiatrist could be called and informed of the major features of the psychosis after the emergency physician's initial assessment of the patient. Both physicians can then agree on a plan for rapid treatment of the symptoms and for subsequent hospitalization.

Once admitted, the patient's remission is generally maintained by giving an oral dose 12 hours after the last dose of intramuscular medication. In the first few days of treatment the daily dose of oral medication usually equals the total intramuscular dose required in the first few hours of treatment.

CASE EXAMPLE 2

A 34-year-old man was brought to the emergency department because he was "acting crazy." The patient had a vague psychiatric history and claimed he had "seen shrinks in the past—in Vietnam." He said he knew he "wasn't thinking right" because he had the feeling that other people were "after him." He "just wanted to load up his gun and start shooting."

There was no history suggesting any ongoing medical disorder. The patient and his friend denied recent drug use, and a physical examination was essentially unremarkable. The patient kept pacing anxiously around the room. A 10 mg dose of haloperidol was given by intramuscular injection. The patient slept for a short time (about 30 minutes). He awoke and claimed he still felt agitated; he appeared restless. Another 5 mg dose of haloperidol was given, and the patient slept for several hours and awoke with a clear sensorium and no obvious signs of mental disorder. He appeared somewhat embarrassed about his behavior and requested help with his nerves. The patient was seen in the emergency department by the consulting psychiatrist who arranged further treatment and an office appointment.

The ultimate success of treatment depends on the patient's compliance with his antipsychotic regimen on an outpatient basis and a satisfactory relationship with his psychiatrist or mental health worker.

Rapid antipsychotic treatment in organic mental disorders. Rapid antipsychotic treatment is indicated in certain organic mental disorders as well as functional ailments when the objectives of rapid treatment are only the symptoms and signs of psychosis. Haloperidol is generally contraindicated in psychosis caused by anticholinergic toxicity but has been successful in severe psychosis caused by phencyclidine or other hallucinogens. Mild psychosis associated with these drugs may be managed by withholding medication and maintaining close observation of the patient.

Antidepressants

Antidepressant drugs are the treatment of choice for major depression. Tricyclics, tetracyclics, and other antidepressant agents in adequate doses generally become effective after 3 to 4 weeks of therapy and act through a mechanism that is not well understood. When antidepressant agents are ineffective in relieving severe depression, electroconvulsive therapy (ECT) may be the only alternative.

Tricyclics. The three-ring structure of the tricyclic antidepressants illustrated in Fig. 21-5 is remarkably similar to that of phenothiazine and involves the following: an ethylene group in the middle ring of imipramine replaces the sulfur atom of the phenothiazine. Though similar in two-dimensional drawings, the molecules have different three-dimensional configurations and stereochemical properties.

Though the tricyclic agents were first synthesized in the late nineteenth century, the antidepressant effects were not recognized until the late 1950s. Since then, they have become the agents of choice for major depression. The mechanism of action for the tricyclics is not completely understood. The dominant hypothesis is that depression is perhaps caused by deficiency of certain neurotransmitters (serotonin and norepinephrine) in particular regions of the brain. Any treatment that increases the amount or effectiveness of these neurotransmitters, therefore, should relieve depression. Methods to increase the number of active transmitters include inhibition of enzymes that break down the neurotransmitters (monoamine oxidase [MAO] inhibitors) or prevention of their reuptake after their release by the presynaptic neural membrane. Tricyclics inhibit this reuptake and, therefore, leave more available neurotransmitter within the synapse.

According to the theory, the increased neurotransmitter activity within the brain improves the patient's mood and reduces the severity of the depression. The theory's shortcomings are that some antidepressants do not potentiate the effects of biogenic amines, and other reuptake inhibitors of norepinephrine (like cocaine) cause euphoria and stimulation but do not relieve other predominant vegetative symptoms of depression

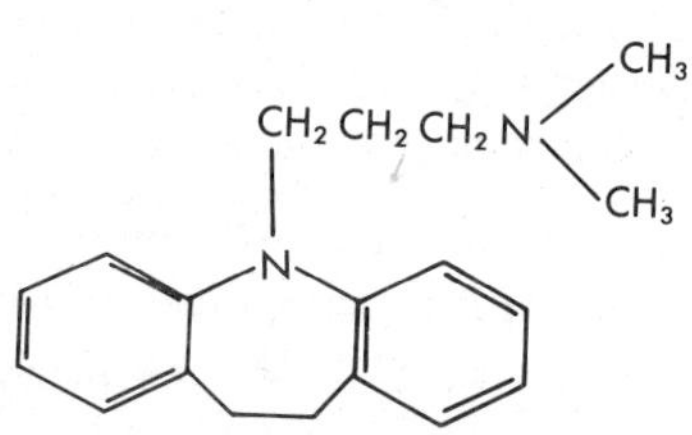

FIG. 21-5. Molecular structure of a representative tricyclic agent, imipramine.

like insomnia or decreased appetite. Another puzzling aspect of tricyclic therapy is that the drugs do not produce their peak anti-depressive effect until they have been taken in adequate doses for 2 to 4 weeks. Since the therapeutic effects are delayed and the side effects are unpleasant, the patient should be under the care of someone who can encourage him to take adequate doses of medication and bear with the therapeutic regimen.

Uses of tricyclic antidepressants in emergency medicine. Most authorities do not recommend initiating the patient's tricyclic treatment program in the emergency department. They cite the following three major reasons: the side effects discourage the patient rapidly, and he discontinues the medication and does not keep his follow-up appointment with the psychiatrist; the medication does not take full effect for 2 to 4 weeks; and the depressed patient may opt to overdose with his tricyclic medication and become severely poisoned.

In contrast to the view against beginning this medication immediately is the justification that the emergency physician should be able to make the diagnosis of major depression according to the DSM-III criteria. These criteria are clear cut and unambiguous. If the patient is able to cooperate in the interview, the physician should be able to elicit responses that determine whether or not the patient has had dysphoric mood (sadness) and four of the specific symptoms of depression for at least 2 weeks. When a treatment program for the patient is agreed to in advance by the emergency physician and the consulting psychiatrist, treatment can justifiably begin as soon as possible.

Up to a 3-day supply of tricyclics can be prescribed, and the patient must be able to see a psychiatrist within that period. When the patient is seen in a follow-up appointment, the psychiatrist can tell what side effects the patient is experiencing at the time of examination. One other justification for beginning treatment in the emergency department is that tricyclics have some immediate therapeutic value, including a sedating effect that may benefit the patient quickly. The sedative effect of agents like amitriptyline, for instance, should be of immediate help to the patient whose insomnia is a prominent or disturbing part of the disorder.

DOSE AND ADMINISTRATION. Four tricyclics in common use are amitriptyline (Elavil), imipramine (Tofranil), doxepin (Sinequan), and desipramine (Norpramin). The initial dose of the drugs ranges from 50 to 75 mg taken at bedtime. The dose is typically increased by 25 mg every 2 to 3 days until a 150 mg dose is reached. The medication is usually taken as a single dose 2 hours before bedtime. Adjustments upward or downward can be based on adequacy of the antidepressant response and the severity of side effects. Most treatment failures occur because the patient takes too small a dose or discontinues treatment too early.

The patient typically takes oral doses of antidepressants, but intramuscular preparations are available for the unusual patient who is so severely depressed that he refuses to take oral medication. An oral dose of tricyclics is usually absorbed within 2 to 8 hours. These lipophilic drugs are widely distributed throughout the body. They are strongly bound to plasma proteins and are metabolized in the hepatic microsomal system.

SERUM LEVELS. Because the drugs are highly bound to plasma proteins and some of their metabolites are clinically active, it is often difficult to interpret and use plasma concentration for adjustment of therapy or assessment of overdose. When both imipramine and its demethylated metabolite are measured, therapeutic effects are usually seen at concentrations between 100 and 200 ng/ml.

SIDE EFFECTS

Anticholinergic side effects. Anticholinergic side effects are commonly experienced in patients taking tricyclics. These effects include dry mouth, metallic taste, blurred vision, constipation, tachycardia, and urinary retention. Narrow angle glaucoma may be precipitated by these agents, especially in the susceptible elderly patient. The complaint of eye pain in a patient taking tricyclics must be evaluated thoroughly. The various tricyclics differ in the strength of their anticholinergic effects (Table 21-3).

Sedation. The degree of sedation caused by the agents generally parallels the magnitude of the anticholinergic effect. Sedation is a desirable early therapeutic effect when insomnia is a major component of the depression.

Cardiotoxicity. Tricyclic antidepressants produce a variety of cardiovascular changes in depressed patients.[7] The significant cardiotoxicity of these agents, when taken in large quantities, is a primary factor in the potential lethality of an overdose.

Rather benign ECG changes that are commonly seen in depressed patients taking therapeutic doses of tricyclics include prolongation of the QT interval and inversion or flattening of the T wave. A variety of arrhythmias and blocks has been reported and includes atrial fibrillation, supraventricular tachycardia, and bundle branch block. The tricyclics tend to reduce myocardial contractility and blunt cardiovascular reflexes that maintain blood pressure when some patients rise to the standing position. The result in some patients is orthostatic hypotension. Cardiovascular effects of tricyclic agents that are well tolerated in young patients may be dangerous in elderly patients or in those with preexisting cardiac disease, such as valvular heart disease, cardiomyopathy, and coronary artery disease. Patients who are over 45 years of age usually should have an ECG recorded before initiating therapy.

Miscellaneous. Jaundice has been reported as a side effect of imipramine. Improved appetite and weight gain are part of the drug's therapeutic effect in depressed patients. The tricyclics may elevate test results of hepatic function like alkaline phosphatase, serum glutamic-oxaloacetic transaminase (SGOT), serum glutamic-pyruvic transaminase (SGPT), and bilirubin.

TABLE 21-3. Tricyclic antidepressants, their dose ranges, and anticholinergic effects

Agent	*Dose range (mg)*	*Anticholinergic effect*
Amitriptyline	75 to 300	++++
Imipramine	75 to 300	+++
Doxepin	75 to 300	++
Desipramine	75 to 300	+

DRUG INTERACTION. Various drug interactions with tricyclics are listed in Table 21-4. Certain drugs potentiate the effects of tricyclics by interfering with their plasma binding, thus making more free drugs available. Such effects are caused by aspirin, phenytoin, and phenothiazines. Other drugs increase the effects of tricyclics by interfering with their hepatic metabolism. These drugs include methylphenidate (Ritalin) and oral contraceptives.

Barbiturates stimulate the hepatic microsomes to metabolize tricyclic agents more rapidly then normal, thus decreasing their effectiveness. Tricyclics potentiate the sedative effects of barbiturates and other hypnotics. The combination of tricyclics with MAO inhibitors can cause a severe toxic reaction characterized by fever, convulsions, and coma; this combination of agents is best avoided.

OVERDOSE. The tricyclics have a rather narrow therapeutic margin. Full clinical antidepressant effects may require a dose of 300 mg per day. Yet serious toxicity can be seen with ingestion of 1000 mg, and death has been reported following ingestion of 2000 mg. Thus a 4- to 7-day supply of medication may constitute a lethal dose when too much is taken. As a general rule, the psychiatrist should not dispense more than a week's supply at a time to a severely depressed patient.

The severe toxic effects of tricyclic overdose are cardiac dysrhythmias, seizures, and coma. Typical cardiac dysrhythmias include sinus tachycardia, premature ventricular contraction, and ventricular tachycardia. The severity of the intoxication can be inferred from the width of the QRS complex. A QRS duration of greater than 100 milliseconds reflects dangerous plasma levels and severe cardiotoxicity.

The early management of tricyclic overdose includes the basic and often stated principles of airway maintenance, intravenous fluids, gastric emptying, and cardiac monitoring. Activated charcoal and a cathartic can be given to reduce absorption of any drug remaining in the gastrointestinal tract. Physostigmine, given in a slow intravenous bolus of 1 to 3 mg, may suppress seizures and arrhythmia and may lighten the coma.

TABLE 21-4. Interaction of various drugs with tricyclic agents

Drug	*Effect*
Alcohol	Possible increased effects of alcohol
Antiarrhythmics, quinidine-like	Arrhythmias, ectopy, negative inotropic effect, conduction defects
Digitalis	Increased heart block and ectopy
Anticholinergic agents	Additive effects
Anticoagulants	May require increased anticoagulant dose
Anticonvulsants	Increase in seizure frequency
Antihypertensives—clonidine, methyldopa, hydralazine	Diminished antihypertensive effect, postural hypotension
Antipsychotics	Increased cardiotoxicity, CNS depression, hypotension, anticholinergic effect, possible sudden death

Sodium bicarbonate is given in sufficient dosage to elevate the pH to 7.50 and to maintain a pH of at least 7.45. An initial bolus of 1 to 2 mg/kg of sodium bicarbonate should be followed by a constant bicarbonate infusion that contains 50 mEq of sodium bicarbonate and 750 ml of 5% dextrose in water. Lidocaine and phenytoin are antiarrhythmics of choice when alkalization is ineffective. Propranolol and cardiac pacing are indicated when these other methods fail.[8]

External heating or cooling measures are required for disorders of thermoregulation associated with overdose. Since the tricyclics have such a wide distribution and long half-life, these patients need hospital admission and cardiac monitoring for a minimum of 24 hours beyond the last evidence of cardiac arrhythmias. Even asymptomatic patients with allegedly minimal ingestions should be observed and monitored in the emergency department before medical clearance and psychiatric evaluation.

Sometimes the patient with tricyclic toxicity has mild poisoning and moderate tachycardia caused by the tricyclic's anticholinergic effect. When not admitted, this patient should be monitored in the emergency department for 6 hours. If a subsequent ECG shows a resolution of the tachycardia, no other changes occur (e.g., widening of the QRS to greater than 0.10 seconds or frequent premature ventricular contractions), and the patient appears otherwise well (alert, awake, and oriented), he can be evaluated by the emergency physician or psychiatrist and cleared medically for psychiatric admission or discharge as indicated.

Tetracyclic drug. Antidepressant agents closely related to the tricyclics are the tetracyclic drugs formed by adding a fourth ring to the tricyclic structure. These tetracyclic or "quadracyclic" agents may produce a more rigid molecular arrangement that perhaps has more specificity and selectivity than tricyclic agents.[9] The most common tetracyclic in clinical use is maprotiline (Ludiomil). The indications for its use, side effects, and toxicity are similar to those for the tricyclics.

Other antidepressants. Nontricyclic antidepressants have been developed that should be safer for the patient who has severe clinical depression. One such agent is trazodone (Desyrel), a phenylpiperazine derivative of triazolopyridine. The drug has antidepressant activity but far less cardiotoxicity and a much wider therapeutic margin than the tricyclics. In rats, for instance, half the lethal dose is greater than 500 mg/kg. The dose range for antidepressant effects in humans is similar to that of the tricyclics. The treatment for overdose of this agent includes gastric lavage and forced diuresis, induced by furosemide and saline solution.

Lithium

Lithium is most accurately described as an antimanic drug. Its clinical effectiveness in the treatment of manic patients was first described by John Cade, an Australian psychiatrist in the late 1940s. Despite this early recognition of its clinical effectiveness, lithium was not widely accepted as treatment for mania in the United States until the 1970s. In the 1940s some patients used lithium salt as a sodium substitute with disasterous consequences. One of the reasons for its slow acceptance as an antimanic agent was its demonstrated danger for patients who used lithium salt as a substitute for sodium chloride in salt-restricted diets.

Lithium belongs to the alkali metal group, and because of several side effects associated with other preparations, the carbonate salt, Li_2CO_3, is the preparation used clinically in the United States. Lithium is rapidly absorbed from the gastrointestinal tract. Peak serum levels occur in 30 minutes, and a plateau concentration is reached in 12 to 24 hours. However, because the ion crosses cell boundaries slowly, clinical antimanic effects may not be seen for 6 to 7 days. The exact mechanism of its effect is unclear, but it is thought to be active at neuronal synapses in the brain to decrease norepinephrine and to increase serotonin.

Lithium is most appropriately used in the treatment and prophylaxis of bipolar affective disorder (manic depressive syndrome). Since lithium therapy may last a lifetime, a treatment program is usually initiated in the hospital, where the patient can be thoroughly evaluated and serum lithium levels can be measured frequently. Antipsychotic agents are far more effective for the treatment of acute manic episode in the emergency department or in the early stages of hospitalization.

Lithium is used primarily for the treatment and prevention of mania. Other clinical uses of lithium include the treatment of unipolar depression (which has no manic episodes), some types of schizoaffective disorder, and temporal lobe epilepsy. Other uses of lithium are being investigated.

Dose and administration. Lithium is rapidly absorbed from the stomach and is cleared unchanged by the kidney. Both sodium and lithium pass through the glomerulus, and 80% of each is reabsorbed in the proximal tubule. Lithium competes with sodium for reabsorption. As more sodium is delivered to the proximal tubule, less lithium is reabsorbed and relatively more lithium is excreted in the urine. Thus as the dietary intake of sodium increases, the reabsorption of lithium decreases (lithium excretion in the urine increases). When sodium depletion is present, less sodium is delivered to the tubule, and lithium reabsorption increases. This increased absorption may cause lithium toxicity. Adequate renal function is necessary for the proper clearance of lithium, and the dose must be carefully adjusted, according to the patient's renal status.

The standard lithium capsule contains 300 mg of lithium carbonate. The average patient requires a daily dose of 900 to 1200 mg. In acute manic states a loading dose of 1500 to 1800 mg per day can be given to establish adequate serum levels. Lower doses are given to elderly patients because of their decreased renal clearance. Lithium is best taken three or four times per day to avoid toxic serum levels that may peak after a single large dose.

The thyroid concentrates lithium to levels many times greater than the plasma level. Some problems that are seen by emergency department physicians may, therefore, include thyroid disease with detectable goiter as a side effect. Before initiating lithium therapy, it is advisable to obtain certain laboratory tests, including a complete blood count (CBC) with differential, serum electrolyte concentrations, renal function tests, ECG, and thyroid function tests. Since there is a 4% incidence of goiter in patients taking lithium, a manual thyroid examination should be documented. The optimum serum levels should be between 0.8 and 1.2 mEq/liter, although the requirements may be much higher in an acute manic state. In the emergency department serum blood levels may be an important aid in management.

Initially, lithium levels are obtained after 5 days of oral loading or as soon as signs of toxicity develop. The serum should be collected 12 hours after the last dose of lithium. During a stabilization period of 1 to 3 weeks, lithium levels are measured every 3 to 4 days. During the following 6-month maintenance phase, levels can be measured every 2 to 4 weeks and finally every 3 months for the duration of therapy.

The only absolute contraindication to lithium use is severe renal impairment. Other relative contraindications are myocardial infarction, extrapyramidal syndrome (parkinsonism), cerebral or cerebellar damage, dementia, hypothyroidism, pregnancy, or breast-feeding. If absolutely necessary, lithium can be continued during pregnancy, but its use during the first trimester provides the highest risk to the fetus. After birth, the infant should be given formula because breast milk contains high levels of lithium.

Side effects and toxicity. Side effects and toxicity frequently correspond to serum levels. However, it is not unusual for patients to experience uncomfortable side effects even in the "therapeutic zone." Side effects most often reported are gastrointestinal distress, dry mouth, fine hand tremors, mild polyuria, increased thirst, pretibial edema, and hand edema. These symptoms usually subside in 1 to 2 weeks. If they remain, they may often diminish after the dose of lithium is decreased. Hand tremors can be treated with 15 to 60 mg per day of propranolol.

Once the serum lithium level is in excess of 1.5 mEq/liter, more serious complications take place. These toxic effects may be additive and push levels to even more dangerous heights. For instance, polyuria may dehydrate the patient, causing increased toxicity. Gastrointestinal effects are common at levels of 1.5 mEq/liter and beyond. Vomiting and diarrhea may exacerbate toxicity by hemoconcentration and increased lithium reabsorption secondary to sodium loss. Some of these effects and their associations with the serum level are listed in the following box.[10]

Neurological effects seem to be dose related. Initially, there may be "drugged" feelings, coarse tremors, ataxia, muscle weakness, confusion, blackouts, increased deep tendon reflexes, fasciculations, blurred vision, and scotomas. As levels rise, there is increasing confusion, seizures, myoclonus, choreoathetosis, incontinence, and eventually coma.

Cardiovascular effects are rare below levels of 4.0 mEq/liter. Cardiovascular effects usually are benign flattening or inversion of T waves. With extreme toxicity there may be hypotension and cardiovascular collapse.

Renal effects include a mild polydipsia or polyuria that develops in the therapeutic range. At higher levels diabetes insipidus may develop. Lithium must be discontinued or decreased to reverse this effect.

Endocrine effects may be noted. A physical finding sometimes noted in a patient taking lithium is a diffuse, nontender goiter in a euthyroid patient. Apparently lithium

SIGNS AND SYMPTOMS OF DOSE-RELATED LITHIUM INTOXICATION

Initial response to therapy*

Fine tremor of hands
Dry mouth
Mildly increased thirst
Mild polyuria
Transient mild nausea

Blood level mEq/liter†

1.5 Nausea
Vomiting
Diarrhea
2.0 Polyuria
Blurred vision
Muscular weakness
Drowsiness
Dizziness
Vertigo
Increasing confusion
Slurred speech
Transient scotomas
Blackouts
Fasciculations
Increased deep tendon reflexes
2.5 Myoclonic twitches
Myoclonic movements
Choreoathetoid movements
Urinary and fecal incontinence
Increasing restlessness, followed by stupor, followed by coma
3.0 Epileptiform seizure
Cardiac arrhythmias
4.0 Hypotension
Peripheral vascular collapse

From Hall, RCW, Perl, M, and Pfefferbaum, B. Lithium therapy and toxicity. *American Family Physician,* April 1979, *19*(4), 135.
*Not toxic signs.
†May occur in different order or at lower serum levels in susceptible individuals.

decreases production of thyroid goiter hormone. The decreased levels of T_3 and T_4 cause increased thyroid-stimulating hormone (TSH) secretion. Goiter usually disappears with thyroid supplementation or discontinuation of lithium. Lithium may cause a mild leukocytosis.

Laboratory tests. Abnormalities of certain laboratory tests may be early indicators

TABLE 21-5. Lithium's effect on certain laboratory tests

	Increase	*Decrease*
Serum	Creatinine	Cortisol
	Fasting blood sugar	Creatine clearance
	Magnesium	Potassium
	TSH	T_4, T_3 uptake
	White blood cells (WBC)	Uric acid
Urine	Glucose	
	Protein	
	Vanillylmandelic acid (VMA)	

of lithium's toxic effect. Renal function tests must be performed often to ensure adequate ability to excrete lithium. Some effects of lithium on laboratory tests are listed in Table 21-5.

Drug interaction. When given in combination with antipsychotic agents, lithium can increase the incidence and severity of extrapyramidal effects, such as acute dystonia and hyperglycemia.

Diuretics like thiazides or furosemide promote the excretion of sodium and result in the retention of lithium and its potential toxicity. Neuromuscular blockade induced by agents like succinylcholine or pancuronium is prolonged in patients taking lithium. Aminophylline seems to increase the excretion of lithium.

Overdose and intoxication. Lithium intoxication can be acute as a result of overdose or rapid salt loss or it can be chronic with effects developing over months or years. Chronic intoxication may cause serious renal injury that results in reduced creatinine clearance or nephrogenic diabetes insipidus. Polyuria may be the first clue to chronic lithium toxicity. The large volumes of urine characteristically have a constant specific gravity (1.010). Sodium depletion may result in increased lithium reabsorption. When a patient with chronic lithium intoxication is identified, hospitalization is necessary to thoroughly evaluate his renal status.

Acute toxicity can result from overdose or from salt loss. Vigorous exercise in a warm climate, for instance, may cause excessive sweating. In such a condition the loss of body sodium may be significant enough to precipitate lithium toxicity. Acute overdose results in the following signs and symptoms: neurological changes include muscular twitching, hyperactive reflexes, confusion, seizures, and coma; cardiac changes include conduction disturbances, ventricular tachyarrhythmias, and congestive heart failure.

Treatment. The initial treatment of acute lithium intoxication is rapid infusion of normal saline solution. The goal is to induce a lithium diuresis and prevent hypotension. Three to 6 liters of saline solution given intravenously over the first several hours may be required to induce a satisfactory diuresis. Mannitol may be added to the infusion to promote osmotic diuresis. Gastric lavage and routine blood studies, including a lithium level, magnesium level, and serum osmolality, should be performed. Although alkaline diuresis may be attempted, the results of hemodialysis are extremely effective in this setting. The relatively small lithium cation has a small molecular weight, no protein binding, and high water solubility. It passes easily into the dialysate. In acute, life-threatening lithium overdose, hemodialysis is definitely the treatment of choice when available.

Antianxiety drugs

Episodic anxiety is a common human experience. The "fight or flight" reaction sometimes associated with anxiety prepares us for dangerous situations and, in proper doses, motivates us for our daily tasks. In excessive measures anxiety becomes a troublesome and sometimes disabling symptom associated with psychiatric illnesses like generalized anxiety disorder, panic disorder, and certain phobias. The term *anxiety* is rather ubiquitous and causes many of the problems involved in defining anxiety and the indications for required treatment. As a rule, when there is such an excess of anxiety that it interferes with the individual's ability to function or causes severe psychic distress, the patient requires further evaluation and treatment.

A patient may present a host of psychological and physiological symptoms associated with their anxiety. Psychological symptoms include apprehension, dread, feeling of impending doom, fear, worry, fright, jumpiness, panic, restlessness, or a sense of being threatened or scared without reason. Physiological symptoms and signs include nausea, palpitations, abdominal cramps, breathlessness, weakness, chest pain, tachycardia, faintness, syncope, headache, dry mouth, diaphoresis, anorexia, urinary frequency, choking, pallor, and diarrhea.

These symptoms are seen in any number of combinations and must be differentiated from organic illnesses. A significant number of patients, initially diagnosed as having an anxiety disorder, are later found to have dysrhythmias, anemia, stimulant abuse (caffeinism or others), hyperthyroidism, pheochromocytoma, hypoglycemia, pulmonary embolism, electrolyte imbalance, or mitral valve prolapse. The majority of these conditions are treated by correcting the underlying abnormality, though antianxiety drugs may be employed in conjunction with medical therapy.

The benzodiazepines are currently the antianxiety agents of choice. They are clinically effective, do not cause drug addiction when used properly, and have a high margin of safety even when taken in overdose. In emergency medicine certain antihistamines like hydroxyzine are widely used and quite effective in certain settings. Barbiturates and meprobamate, by contrast, carry the potential for drug addiction and can be highly lethal when taken in overdose. Because acceptable alternative drugs are available, the barbiturates are no longer drugs of choice for anxiety. Various antianxiety agents and information regarding them are listed in Table 21-6.

Benzodiazepines in general and diazepam in particular have been among the most frequently prescribed medications in the United States. Their use or abuse has been the subject of multiple studies, congressional outcry, and media attention. Physicians vary

TABLE 21-6. Various antianxiety agents, their half-lives, rapidity of effects, and usual daily doses

	Equivalent dose (mg)	*Half life*	*Rapidity of effect*	*Usual daily dose (mg)*
Long-acting (metabolites)				
Chlordiazepoxide (Librium)	10.0	12 to 24	+3	15 to 150
Diazepam (Valium)	5.0	20 to 100	+5	4 to 40
Chlorazeptate (Tranxene)	7.5	30 to 200	+4	15 to 60
Prazepam (Centrax)	10.0	30 to 200	+1	20 to 60
Short-acting (no metabolites)				
Oxazepam (Serax)	15.0	8 to 15	+2	30 to 120
Lorazepam (Ativan)	1.0	12	+3	2 to 6

in their attitudes toward these drugs so widely that their approach falls within broad limits defined by "pharmacologic Calvinism" on the one hand and "psychotropic hedonism" on the other.[11] Although the individual physician's attitude determines prescribing habits, there are certain rational uses for antianxiety agents.

The indications for the benzodiazepines are fairly restrictive, but because of the wide therapeutic margin and confusion over the types of anxiety, these agents are inappropriately given to many patients. One of the indications for antianxiety agents is short-term, situation-induced anxiety. Patients who have difficulties on their jobs, have been fired, or are having severe acute marital problems face extreme anxiety-producing situations. They may benefit by a short course of an antianxiety agent like diazepam or chlordiazepoxide, especially when combined with some form of brief psychotherapy.

Episodes of brief situational anxiety, occurring in otherwise healthy persons, can be legitimately treated with benzodiazepines. A similar justification is often made for patients who experience anticipatory anxiety before encountering a phobic stimulus. The patient who has a morbid fear of crowds, for instance, may experience considerable relief by taking an antianxiety agent before plunging into a crowded party or department store. The medication is best used, however, when the patient is also undergoing some form of brief psychotherapy and panic and generalized anxiety disorders are not present.

In the past, psychological theories were proposed to explain panic attacks, but current theory now favors the medical illness model.[12] These panic attacks are best treated by antidepressants like imipramine and some form of counseling. In cases in which a phobia initiates a full-blown panic attack, the treatment of panic disorder with imipramine is more appropriate than the use of antianxiety agents.

Antianxiety agents can be used as preoperative medication. They tend to allay anticipatory anxiety and facilitate the induction of anesthesia. Similarly, they are commonly used in procedures to facilitate muscular relaxation during endoscopy or in the reduction of fractures and dislocations.

The benzodiazepines are also useful for seizures and alcohol withdrawal delirium, which are well known to emergency physicians. Diazepam is the most frequently used drug for acute seizure control, but oxazepam is actually a more effective anticonvulsant.

The mechanism of action for benzodiazepines is largely unknown. Many researchers now feel that there is binding of these drugs to specific synaptic receptors in the brain, primarily in the limbic system (septum, amygdala, hippocampus), the cortex, and the reticular activating system. The potency of the various benzodiazepines seems to be related to the affinity they have for these receptors. Binding to the receptors causes a gamma aminobutyric acid (GABA) agonist effect that in turn reduces the activity of serotonin. Electroencephalograms (EEGs) performed after initiating treatment have demonstrated slow waves, fast beta waves, and generalized low voltage.

Dosage and administration. The benzodiazepines are the preferred antianxiety agents for clinical use. The agents commonly used are generally equivalent in their efficacy against anxiety but vary in other pharmacological criteria. Their major differences relate to the following three factors: their rapidity of absorption, the presence of active metabolites, and the duration of their activity. Those drugs that have short half-lives and no active metabolites (oxazepam and lorazepam) are probably safer for elderly patients and for those with hepatic disease.

The long-acting benzodiazepines have long half-lives (up to 100 to 200 hours) and at least one active metabolite. These drugs are generally more appropriate for use in younger patients without liver disease. Diazepam is the most frequently used long-acting benzodiazepine because of the rapid onset of symptomatic relief. This property has been attributed to its higher lipid solubility compared to the other agents. The usual dosage is 2 to 5 mg orally given twice or three times a day in cases of moderate anxiety. The long half-life of many of the benzodiazepines can be an advantage that allows decreased frequency of administration. The gradual diminution in effect that may occur over days decreases the possibility of rebound symptoms. One evening dose of medication allows the sedative side effect to improve sleeping patterns and produces a residual antianxiety effect the following morning.

The benzodiazepines may be given orally, intramuscularly, or intravenously. Because of their excellent absorption in the gastrointestinal tract, the oral route is satisfactory if the patient complies with therapy. In some cases a high gastric pH or decrease in gastric acid can decrease absorption of benzodiazepines. Antacids, cimetidine, or achlorhydria can cause such a condition. Cimetidine may also interfere with the metabolism and subsequent elimination of chlordiazepoxide. In some cases intravenous administration of benzodiazepine may damage blood vessels. Animal experiments have shown endothelial damage to vessels. In humans the concern is thrombophlebitis. The risk of thrombophlebitis can be reduced by ensuring that patients have no thrombotic risk factors like oral contraceptive use, recent surgery, or inability to walk and by decreasing the number of injections. Undiluted diazepam is injected at a rate of 0.5 ml per minute into a freely running intravenous solution to avoid hypotension. Risk is also decreased by injection into a larger vein of the arm, rather than the arteries or veins of the hands. Intramuscular injection is an option that does not provide as reliable a dose delivery as the other two routes because of unpredictable absorption rates.

Adverse effects. Most patients who begin taking benzodiazepines report some sedation and drowsiness. Reflexes and mental alertness are decreased. After a period of time, patients generally become physically tolerant to the sedation experienced initially. In some cases patients experience more disturbing effects like hypotension, dizziness, allergic reactions, abdominal pain, tremor, ataxia, liver damage, or blood dyscrasia. In the early stages of therapy when sedation and decreased mental acuity are prominent side effects, the patient must be cautioned not to operate heavy machinery or drive a car.

Tolerance to the anxiety effects of the benzodiazepines may occur. In such cases the patient experiences continuing anxiety in spite of the medication and may begin increasing the dosage without the physician's knowledge. In some cases this may result in psychological dependence, physical dependence, or habituation. Physical dependence may be encountered in the patient who takes huge amounts of medication (10 to 20 times the regular dose) over several months. When the patient reports the first symptoms of tolerance to the antianxiety effects of these medications, the drugs should be stopped, and an alternative treatment mode must be sought. Troublesome, persistent side effects like continued sedation, hypotension, or allergic reactions are also reasons to discontinue the drug and search for alternative treatments.

Withdrawal, when it occurs, is experienced after a lag period of 3 to 5 days in cases of the long-acting benzodiazepines. Tachycardia, tremor, nausea, diaphoresis, depression, and seizures are common symptoms. Rebound insomnia is the most common symptom, however, and is most severe with the short-acting antianxiety agents. The treatment for withdrawal symptoms involves reinstitution of the drug, followed by more gradual tapering of the benzodiazepine or in some cases the temporary prescription of a barbiturate.

Teratogenicity has not been conclusively shown with the benzodiazepines. Some research has noted an association with development of cleft lip and palate in newborns. However, like all drugs, antianxiety agents in pregnancy are avoided when possible.

Relatively few laboratory tests are adversely affected by antianxiety medications. There may be increases in serum alkaline phosphatase, SGOT, SGPT, or serum and urine bilirubin levels.

Drug interactions. Most dangerous situations and fatalities noted with diazepam have been with the use of more than one drug. Alcohol is the primary drug found in lethal combination with diazepam. Barbiturates and narcotics are also combined with benzodiazepines in lethal overdoses (Table 21-7).

Overdose. Benzodiazepines are used rather frequently in accidental or intentional overdoses. They are available to many patients and when taken alone, without other drugs or alcohol, rarely cause death. When taken with alcohol or other drugs, however, they can cause serious cardiac and respiratory depression. The treatment of overdose includes the standard measures to prevent absorption, hasten elimination, and support the patient until the effects of the drugs subside.

A patient with a history of suicide attempts, severe depressions, or use of many

TABLE 21-7. Interaction of antianxiety medications with other drugs

Drug	*Effect*
Alcohol	Increased CNS depression
Antihistamines	Increased CNS depression
Neuroleptics	Increased CNS depression
Tricyclic antidepressants	Increased CNS depression
Barbiturates	Increased CNS depression, hypotension
Phenytoin	Increased CNS depression, increased toxicity

drugs should probably not be given antianxiety agents. If the drugs are prescribed, the quantity should be small, and the patient should be followed carefully.

Useful agents in alcohol syndromes

Chlordiazepoxide. Chlordiazepoxide is the traditional agent of choice for the treatment of alcohol withdrawal syndrome and alcohol withdrawal delirium. Relatively large doses of chlordiazepoxide are needed to control the symptoms. In the average size person, a 50 to 100 mg dosage of chlordiazepoxide is given every hour until the patient is quiet. Thereafter, a 50 mg dosage is given every 6 hours. Since absorption from the muscle may be erratic, the oral route of administration is preferred. For intravenous therapy slightly lower dosages may be preferred initially.

Diazepam. Diazepam is an appropriate agent to quiet a patient in the early stages of withdrawal. A small intravenous dose of 5 mg may be given initially to evaluate the extent of its effect on the patient. If the initial dose is ineffective, a second dose can be given.

Haloperidol. If chlordiazepoxide does not quiet the delirious patient with alcohol withdrawal, 10 to 20 mg of haloperidol four times daily may be effective.

Thiamine. Alcoholics may be thiamine deficient. Fifty mg of thiamine intravenously or 50 to 100 mg intramuscularly can be given initially with 50 mg given intramuscularly each day until the syndrome subsides. Thiamine treats and prevents the Wernicke syndrome of ataxia, ophthalmoplegia, and memory loss associated with thiamine deficiency in the alcoholic.

ECT

In the late 1930s ECT was the treatment of choice for severe depression. The introduction of effective antidepressant drugs into clinical practice (MAO inhibitors and tricyclics) gave ECT a secondary role in the treatment of depression. The indication for ECT is generally the patient's failure to improve on full doses of antidepressant medication.

The emergency indications for ECT are few indeed. One indication for emergency ECT could be a patient who is so severely depressed that he cannot be stopped from trying to hurt himself even in the hospital setting. Another emergency indication, perhaps, is the patient who is so severely depressed that he does not eat, drink, or swallow medication. When a rapid alleviation of such depression is necessary, therefore, ECT may provide the most effective therapeutic answer.

SUMMARY

The effectiveness of psychoactive medication has radically altered psychiatric practice and brought the discipline into the medical model. The search for the underlying biomolecular pathology in the functional or idiopathic illness continues, however, and pharmacotherapy of psychiatric illness can only become more specific and effective. In emergency psychiatry the proper use of psychoactive medication and effective management of toxicity have made the treatment of the psychiatric patient vastly more satisfying for both the practitioner and the patient.

REFERENCES

1. Delay, J, and Deniker, P. Trente-huit cas de psychoses traitées par la cure prolongée et continué de 4560 RP. Le Congress des Al. et Neurol. de Langue Francais. Ir *Compte rendu du Congres,* Paris, 1952, Masson et Cie.
2. Baldessarini, RJ. Drugs and the treatment of psychiatric disorders. In Gilman, AG, Goodman, LS, and Gilman, A (Eds.), *The pharmacologic basis of therapeutics*. New York: Macmillan Publishing Co., Inc., 1980.
3. Barchas, JD, et al. (Eds.). *Psychopharmacology: from theory to practice*. New York: Oxford University Press, 1977.
4. Baldessarini, RJ. *Chemotherapy in psychiatry*. Cambridge, Mass.: Harvard University Press, 1977.
5. Herrington, RN, and Lader, MH. *Drug treatment in psychiatry—psychotropic drugs* (Part 5). In Van Praag, HM, et al. (Eds.), *Handbook of biological psychiatry,* New York: Marcel Dekker, Inc., 1981.
6. Anderson, WH, and Kuehnle, JC. Current concepts in psychiatry: diagnosis and early management of acute psychosis. *New England Journal of Medicine,* Nov. 1981, *305*(19), 1128-1130.
7. Risch, SC, Groom, GP, and Janowsky, DS. The effects of psychotropic drugs on the cardiovascular system. *Journal of Clinical Psychiatry,* 1982, *43*(5), 16-31.
8. Vance, M, and Kunkel, D. The pharmacology and toxicology of tricyclic antidepressants. In Rund, DA, and Wolcott, BW (Eds.), *Emergency medicine annual,* New York: Appleton-Century-Crofts, 1983.
9. Pinder, R, Brogden, R, and Speight, T. Maprotiline: a review of its pharmacological properties and therapeutic efficacy in mental depressive states. *Drugs,* 1977, *12,* 321-352.
10. Hall, RC, Perl, M, and Pfefferbaum, B. Lithium therapy and toxicity. *American Family Physician,* April 1979. *19*(4), 135.
11. Rosenbaum, JF. Current concepts in psychiatry: the drug treatment of anxiety. *New England Journal of Medicine,* Feb. 1982, *306*(7), 401-403.
12. Sheehan, DV. Current concepts in psychiatry: panic attacks and phobias. *New England Journal of Medicine,* July 1982, *307*(3), 156-158.

APPENDIX I

DSM-III CLASSIFICATION

axes I and II categories and codes

All official DSM-III codes and terms are included in ICD-9-CM. However, in order to differentiate those DSM-III categories that use the same ICD-9-CM codes, unofficial non-ICD-9-CM codes are provided in parentheses for use when greater specificity is necessary.

The long dashes indicte the need for a fifth-digit subtype or other qualifying term.

DISORDERS USUALLY FIRST EVIDENT IN INFANCY, CHILDHOOD OR ADOLESCENCE

Mental retardation

(Code in fifth digit: 1 = with other behavioral symptoms [requiring attention or treatment and that are not part of another disorder], 0 = without other behavioral symptoms.)

317.0(x) Mild mental retardation, ______

318.0(x) Moderate mental retardation, ______

318.1(x) Severe mental retardation, ______

318.2(x) Profound mental retardation, ______

319.0(x) Unspecified mental retardation, ______

Attention deficit disorder

314.01 with hyperactivity
314.00 without hyperactivity
314.80 residual type

Conduct disorder

312.00 undersocialized, aggressive
312.10 undersocialized, nonaggressive
312.23 socialized, aggressive
312.21 socialized nonaggressive
312.90 atypical

Anxiety disorders of childhood or adolescence

309.21 Separation anxiety disorder
313.21 Avoidant disorder of childhood or adolescence
313.00 Overanxious disorder

Other disorders of infancy, childhood or adolescence

313.89 Reactive attachment disorder of infancy
313.22 Schizoid disorder of childhood or adolescence
313.23 Elective mutism
313.81 Oppositional disorder
313.82 Identify disorder

From American Psychiatric Association. *Diagnostic and statistical manual of mental disorders* (3rd ed.). Washington, D.C.: The Association, 1980.

Eating disorders
307.10 Anorexia nervosa
307.51 Bulimia
307.52 Pica
307.53 Rumination disorder of infancy
307.50 Atypical eating disorder

Stereotyped movement disorders
307.21 Transient tic disorder
307.22 Chronic motor tic disorder
307.23 Tourette's disorder
307.20 Atypical tic disorder
307.30 Atypical stereotyped movement disorder

Other disorders with physical manifestations
307.00 Stuttering
307.60 Functional enuresis
307.70 Functional encopresis
307.46 Sleepwalking disorder
307.46 Sleep terror disorder (307.49)

Pervasive developmental disorders
Code in fifth digit: 0 = full syndrome present, 1 = residual- state.
299.0x Infantile autism, ______
299.9x Childhood onset pervasive developmental disorder, ______
299.8x Atypical, ______

Specific developmental disorders
Note: These are coded on Axis II.
315.00 Developmental reading disorder
315.10 Devlopmental arithmetic disorder
315.31 Developmental language disorder
315.39 Developmental articulation disorder
315.50 Mixed specific developmental disorder
315.90 Atypical specific developmental disorder

ORGANIC MENTAL DISORDERS
Section 1. Organic mental disorders whose etiology or pathophysiological process is listed below (taken from the mental disorders section of ICD-9-CM).

Dementias arising in the senium and presenium
Primary degenerative dementia, senile onset,
290.30 with delirium
290.20 with delusions
290.21 with depression
290.00 uncomplicated
Code in fifth digit:
1 = with delirium, 2 = with delusions, 3 = with depression, 0 = uncomplicated.
290.1x Primary degenerative dementia, presenile onset, ______
290.4x Multi-infarct dementia, ______

Substance-induced
Alcohol
303.00 intoxication
291.40 idiosyncratic intoxication
291.80 withdrawal
291.00 withdrawal delirium
291.30 hallucinosis
291.10 amnestic disorder
Code severity of dementia in fifth digit: 1 = mild, 2 = moderate, 3 = severe, 0 = unspecified.
291.2x Dementia associated with alcoholism, ______

Barbiturate or similarly acting sedative or hypnotic
305.40 intoxication (327.00)
292.00 withdrawal (327.01)
292.00 withdrawal delirium (327.02)
292.83 amnestic disorder (327.04)

Opioid
305.50 intoxication (327.10)
292.00 withdrawal (327.11)

Cocaine
305.60 intoxication (327.20)

Amphetamine or similarly acting sympathomimetic
305.70 intoxication (327.30)
292.81 delirium (327.32)
292.11 delusional disorder (327.35)
292.00 withdrawal (327.31)

Phencyclidine (PCP) or similarly acting arylcyclohexylamine
305.90 intoxication (327.40)
292.81 delirium (327.42)
292.90 mixed organic mental disorder (327.49)

Hallucinogen
305.30 hallucinosis (327.56)
292.11 delusional disorder (327.55)
292.84 affective disorder (327.57)

Cannabis
305.20 intoxication (327.60)
292.11 delusional disorder (327.65)

Tobacco
292.00 withdrawal (327.71)

Caffeine
305.90 intoxication (327.80)

Other or unspecified substance
305.90 intoxication (327.90)
292.00 withdrawal (327.91)
292.81 delirium (327.92)
292.82 dementia (327.93)
292.83 amnestic disorder (327.94)
292.11 delusional disorder (327.95)
292.12 hallucinosis (327.96)
292.84 affective disorder (327.97)
292.89 personality disorder (327.98)
292.90 atypical or mixed organic mental disorder (327.99)

Section 2. Organic brain syndromes whose etiology or pathophysiological process is either noted as an additional diagnosis from outside the mental disorders section of ICD-9-CM or is unknown.

293.00 Delirium
294.10 Dementia
294.00 Amnestic syndrome
293.81 Organic delusional syndrome
293.82 Organic hallucinosis
293.83 Organic affective syndrome
310.10 Organic personality syndrome
294.80 Atypical or mixed organic brain syndrome

SUBSTANCE USE DISORDERS

Code in fifth digit: 1 = continuous, 2 = episodic, 3 = in remission, 0 = unspecified.

305.0x Alcohol abuse, ______
303.9x Alcohol dependence (Alcoholism), ______
305.4x Barbiturate or similarly acting sedative or hypnotic abuse,
304.1x Barbiturate or similarly acting sedative or hypnotic dependence, ______
305.5x Opioid abuse, ______
304.0x Opioid dependence, ______
305.6x Cocaine abuse, ______
305.7x Amphetamine or similarly acting sympathomimetic abuse, ______
304.4x Amphetamine or similarly acting sympathomimetic dependence, ______
305.9x Phencyclidine (PCP) or similarly acting arylcyclohexylamine abuse, ______ (328.4x)
305.3x Hallucinogen abuse, ______
305.2x Cannabis abuse, ______
304.3x Cannabis dependence, ______
305.1x Tobacco dependence, ______
305.9x Other, mixed or unspecified substance abuse, ______

304.6x Other specified substance dependence, ______
304.9x Unspecified substance dependence, ______
304.7x Dependence on combination of opioid and other nonalcoholic substance, ______
304.8x Dependence on combination of substances, excluding opioids and alcohol, ______

SCHIZOPHRENIC DISORDERS

Code in fifth digit: 1 = subchronic, 2 = chronic, 3 = subchronic with acute exacerbation, 4 = chronic with acute exacerbation, 5 = in remission, 0 = unspecified.

Schizophrenia,
295.1x disorganized, ______
295.2x catatonic, ______
295.3x paranoid, ______
295.9x undifferentiated, ______
295.6x residual, ______

PARANOID DISORDERS

297.10 Paranoia
297.30 Shared paranoid disorder
298.30 Acute paranoid disorder
297.90 Atypical paranoid disorder

PSYCHOTIC DISORDERS NOT ELSEWHERE CLASSIFIED

295.40 Schizophreniform disorder
298.80 Brief reactive psychosis
295.70 Schizoaffective disorder
298.90 Atypical psychosis

NEUROTIC DISORDERS: These are included in Affective, Anxiety, Somatoform, Dissociative, and Psychosexual Disorders. In order to facilitate the identification of the categories that in DSM-II were grouped together in the class of Neuroses, the DSM-II terms are included separately in parentheses after the corresponding categories. These DSM-II terms are included in ICD-9-CM and therefore are acceptable as alternatives to the recommended DSM-III terms that precede them.

AFFECTIVE DISORDERS

Major affective disorders

Code major depressive episode in fifth digit: 6 = in remission, 4 = with psychotic features (the unofficial non-ICD-9-CM fifth digit 7 may be used instead to indicate that the psychotic features are mood-incongruent), 3 = with melancholia, 2 = without melancholia, 0 = unspecified.

Code manic or mixed episode in fifth digit: 6 = in remission, 4 = with psychotic features (the unofficial non-ICD-9-CM fifth digit 7 may be used instead to indicate that the psychotic features are mood-incongruent), 2 = without psychotic features, 0 = unspecified.

Bipolar disorder,
296.6x mixed, ______
296.4x manic, ______
296.5x depressed, ______

Major depression,
296.2x single episode, ______
296.3x recurrent, ______

Other specific affective disorders

301.13 Cyclothymic disorder
300.40 Dysthymic disorder (or Depressive neurosis)

Atypical affective disorders

296.70 Atypical bipolar disorder
296.82 Atypical depression

ANXIETY DISORDERS

Phobic disorders (or Phobic neuroses)
300.21 Agoraphobia with panic attacks
300.22 Agoraphobia without panic attacks

300.23 Social phobia
300.29 Simple phobia

Anxiety states (for Anxiety neuroses)
300.01 Panic disorder
300.02 Generalized anxiety disorder
300.30 Obsessive compulsive disorder (or Obsessive compulsive neurosis)

Post-traumatic stress disorder
308.30 acute
309.81 chronic or delayed
300.00 Atypical anxiety disorder

SOMATOFORM DISORDERS
300.81 Somatization disorder
300.11 Conversion disorder (or Hysterical neurosis, conversion type)
307.80 Psychogenic pain disorder
300.70 Hypochondriasis (or Hypochondriacal neurosis)
300.70 Atypical somatoform disorder (300.71)

DISSOCIATIVE DISORDERS (OR HYSTERICAL NEUROSES, DISSOCIATIVE TYPE)
300.12 Psychogenic amnesia
300.13 Psychogenic fugue
300.14 Multiple personality
300.60 Depersonalization disorder (or Depersonalization neurosis)
300.15 Atypical dissociative disorder

PSYCHOSEXUAL DISORDERS
Gender identify disorders

Indicate sexual history in the fifth digit of Transsexualism code: 1 = asexual, 2 = homosexual, 3 = heterosexual, 0 = unspecified.

302.5x Transsexualism, ______
302.60 Gender identity disorder of childhood
302.85 Atypical gender identity disorder

Paraphilias

302.81 Fetishism
302.30 Transvestism
302.10 Zoophilia
302.20 Pedophilia
302.40 Exhibitionism
302.82 Voyeurism
302.83 Sexual masochism
302.84 Sexual sadism
302.90 Atypical paraphilia

Psychosexual dysfunctions

302.71 Inhibited sexual desire
302.72 Inhibited sexual excitement
302.73 Inhibited female orgasm
302.74 Inhibited male orgasm
302.75 Premature ejaculation
302.76 Functional dyspareunia
306.51 Functional vaginismus
302.70 Atypical psychosexual dysfunction

Other psychosexual disorders

302.00 Ego-dystonic homosexuality
302.89 Psychosexual disorder not elsewhere classified

FACTITIOUS DISORDERS
300.16 Factitious disorder with psychological symptoms
301.51 Chronic factitious disorder with physical symptoms
300.19 Atypical factitious disorder with physical symptoms

DISORDERS OF IMPULSE CONTROL NOT ELSEWHERE CLASSIFIED
312.31 Pathological gambling
312.32 Kleptomania
312.33 Pyromania
312.34 Intermittent explosive disorder
312.35 Isolated explosive disorder
319.39 Atypical impulse control disorder

ADJUSTMENT DISORDER

309.00	with depressed mood
309.24	with anxious mood
309.28	with mixed emotional features
309.30	with disturbance of conduct
309.40	with mixed disturbance of emotions and conduct
309.23	with work (or academic) inhibition
309.83	with withdrawal
309.90	with atypical features

PSYCHOLOGICAL FACTORS AFFECTING PHYSICAL CONDITION

Specify physical condition on Axis III.

316.00	Psychological factors affecting physical condition

PERSONALITY DISORDERS
Note: These are coded on Axis II.

301.00	Paranoid
301.20	Schizoid
301.22	Schizotypal
301.50	Histrionic
301.81	Narcissistic
301.70	Antisocial
301.83	Borderline
301.82	Avoidant
301.60	Dependent
301.40	Compulsive
301.84	Passive-Aggressive
301.89	Atypical, mixed or other personality disorder

V CODES FOR CONDITIONS NOT ATTRIBUTABLE TO A MENTAL DISORDER THAT ARE A FOCUS OF ATTENTION OR TREATMENT

V65.20	Malingering
V62.89	Borderline intellectual functioning (V62.88)
V71.01	Adult antisocial behavior
V71.02	Childhood or adolescent antisocial behavior
V62.30	Academic problem
V62.20	Occupational problem
V62.82	Uncomplicated bereavement
V15.81	Noncompliance with medical treatment
V62.89	Phase of life problem or other life circumstance problem
V61.10	Marital problem
V61.20	Parent-child problem
V61.80	Other specified family circumstances
V62.81	Other interpersonal problems

ADDITIONAL CODES

300.90	Unspecified mental disorder (nonpsychotic)
V71.09	No diagnosis or condition on Axis I
799.90	Diagnosis or condition deferred on Axis I

V71.09	No diagnosis on Axis II
799.90	Diagnosis deferred on Axis II

INDEX

T